Essays on the
Rise and Decline of
Bedside Medicine

Essays on the Rise and Decline of Bedside Medicine

by
Mark D. Altschule, M.D.
With a Foreword by Stewart G. Wolf, Jr., M.D.

Published by Totts Gap Medical Ressearch
Laboratories Inc.

Distributed by Lea & Febiger
Philadelphia-London
1989

Totts Gap Medical Research Laboratories Inc.
RD#1
Box 1120G
Bangor, PA 18013

Foreword

MOST WRITERS ON THE HISTORY OF MEDICINE trace a sequence of conceptual or practical advances in biomedical science, building their narrative around the lives and works of the discoverers who, by inference, are credited with having advanced the care and cure of patients. Altschule inaugurates a new way of looking at the history of medicine. He offers a synthesis of the writings and behavior of influential physicians that reaches over 400 years. He traces a remarkable fluctuation of interest among physicians in what they can learn about medicine from their patients. From time to time in history and here and there in the western world, physicians have been attentive to the patients' message; at other times the message has faded as medical practitioners and teachers have become preoccupied with scientific and technological matters tangential to the care of their patients.

Altschule writes as a serious scholar with a sense of humor and a feeling for the absurd. His style is informal, almost jaunty, and his insight is penetrating. The book is peppered with entertaining and sometimes riveting asides, including accounts of Copernicus and Galileo as medical students in Padua, and the revelations that John Locke anticipated Freud by teaching that anxiety (inquietude), or the need to avoid it is a main motivating force in human behavior.

Altschule begins his account in 1552 with DuMonte's teaching of medicine at the bedside in the hospital of San Francisco in Padua. DuMonte attracted students from all over Europe, as did Bottoni and Oddi, his successors, who continued his educational practices. Later, however, their successors abandoned the bedside of the patient in favor of text books and lectures. Fortunately bedside teaching had so impressed one of DuMonte's students, a Dutch physician, Johann Von Heurne, that he and his son transferred the practice of bedside teaching back home to Leiden. Again such patient-centered clinical teaching achieved great popularity among the young, who came to Leiden from far and wide.

A Scottish physician, Thomas Browne, who studied both in Padua and Leiden was also impressed by the value of including the patient in the educational process. He brought DuMonte's methods to Edinburgh where, in the 18th century, bedside teaching gained that city a position of world wide prominence in the education of young physicians. Nevertheless, as had occurred in Padua and Leiden, later generations of clinical teachers minimized the importance of bedside teaching, so again the practice floundered. By this time, however, seeds had been planted in France and in Canada that brought on another flowering and, by the end of the 19th century, bedside teaching was again in full bloom. It was especially so in the United States where, in Baltimore, William Osler enshrined it and wrote about it in his *Principles and Practice of Medicine*, the most widely read medical textbook of the 20th century.

The counterpoint to bedside teaching was played by those who believed that knowledge of the care of the sick would emerge exclusively from the growth of the sciences. The strength of this contention also varied from era to era. It was popular in 19th century Germany, but had been preached earlier in France and was later proclaimed in America under the influence of William H. Welch, Abraham Flexner and others whose strong influence on the shaping of the John Hopkins Medical School may have been responsible for Osler's departure for England in 1912. Altschule quotes a letter to Hopkins' president Remsen in 1911 in which Osler had "warned against the appointment of medical faculties on the basis of their laboratory research reputations instead of on their interest in students and patients."

Altschule searches through four centuries of medical history for the balanced physician, one with a strong commitment to science, who also possesses the skill and sophistication to listen, to observe, and to interpret the clinical evidence with the help of, but not in subordination to the laboratory.

When competent physician-scientists emerged from time to time in Europe and America, great days dawned for medicine. Altschule cites the influence of Thomas Browne's disciples, Thomas Sydenham and John Locke, whose work in the 18th century was followed by a major spurt in the quality of medical practice. At the same time there were important advances in physics and chemistry that led to the emergence of experimental physiology, as promoted by ALbrecht Von Haller in Bern, Switzerland. Haller was a cultivated bibliophile who served as librarian for the city of Bern. He practiced medicine with a rich educational background that included study in Basel, Tubingen, Paris, London and in Leiden under Boerhaave, a pupil of Von Heurne.

The trouble started when a rivalry broke out among the extremists, the physicians, on the one hand who emphasized exclusively observation and tradition, and who considered the sciences to be only accessory to medicine; and on the other hand the experimental scientists, who believed that an understanding of chemistry and molecules would explain disease and cure the patient. The struggle was seen vividly in France at mid 19th century at a time when the seemingly endless and clearly fruitless conflicts between various versions of vitalism and mechanism were winding down.

Many of the German medical leaders, Virchow, Cohnheim and others were attempting to reduce clinical medicine to the principles and laws of inanimate science, physics, chemistry and mathematics, their assumption being "that all patients with a given set of measurements are alike," whereas, as Altschule points out, any experienced physician knows that no two patients with the same disease are ever alike. "Most of all" as Altschule contends, "the reliance on numbers on a chart permits, or even worse, encourages physicians to absent themselves from the personal care of their patients."

Altschule identifies a few men with the wisdom and vision to see through the smoke of conflicting advocacies. Among them, John Shaw Billings, who, says Altschule, "emphasized the importance of making observations as they occur in nature, a process today scornfully called bird watching by ultrascientific biologists." In an incisive, perceptive and engaging style, he offers persuasive evidence that in the practice of medicine, science and technology can support, but must not supplant the dialogue between patient and physician.

The heyday of the scientist-physician in America which was followed by a period of extraordinary progress in clinical medicine began, according to Altschule, when Francis Peabody of the Harvard Medical School established the Thorndike Laboratory at the Boston City Hospital. Having declined the chairmanship of medicine at Hopkins and Yale, Peabody remained in Boston to be succeeded at the Thorndike by such distinguished scientist-physicians as Minot, Castle and Finland. Altschule also singles out George Pickering who in 1978, near the end of his distinguished career, emphasized the lack of replicability of clinical, in contrast to scientific data, adding "understanding such variabilities is the art of medicine." As Altschule puts it: "learning the patient's message is the basic quality of good medical practice." He identifies and quotes other late lamented physician-scientists who had the balanced vision and had heard the patient's message, among them Columbia University Nobel laureate, Dickinson Richards.

Altschule, himself, is such a physician-scientist. Not surprisingly, he was born into a cultivated and cosmopolitan family that emigrated from the Ukraine to England and the U.S. early in this century. His relatives were pharmacists, physicians, artists and educators. Mark himself received a beginning education in the humanities at home before his formal schooling began. His college years were spent in the highly competitive environment of the College of the city of New York. He studied medicine at Harvard, graduating cum laude in 1932.

As Altschule suggests early in his book, periods of decline of clinical medicine may be related more to prevailing educational practices than to the rapid growth of science. Half a century ago American medical education was dominated by professors who were called diagnosticians. They were held in high esteem, not because of their ability to attach a name to their patient's illness, but because of their perspicacity, depth and breadth of education and experience and their interest in people that enabled them to know and to understand their patients thoroughly. Diagnosis, as derived from the Greek, does not mean to name but to know thoroughly. Many of the best of these professors were also scientists in their own right.

During World War II some of the best and brightest candidates to ultimately succeed such broadly educated teachers had been recruited midway through their residency training for duty alternate to military service through the Berry Plan, which assigned them to work for two or more years in an intramural laboratory of the NIH. Their efforts were focused on a sharply restricted problem, such as the purification of a single enzyme, and their clinical experience was restricted to caring for a few selected patients in a narrow subspecialty of medicine.

Many of those talented young men, whose clinical education had been truncated, but intensified in a very restricted area, eventually joined the clinical faculties of medical schools, often serving as division heads, or even department chairmen. When those doctors were called upon to make teaching rounds on the general medical services, however, their limited clinical experience seemed to accentuate an already prevalent tendency among young physicians to "cover themselves" by asking for the consultations of specialists or for a battery of tests and procedures. Responsibility for the care of individual patients was thus diffused. It still is today. Physicians are practicing the medicine of the "lateral pass," while neglecting the rich mine of clinical information available in a skillfully conducted dialogue with the patient. The shortened time in the presence of the patient provides them little opportunity for encouraging, or for building a patient's confidence, let alone helping him understand what he suffers from, what is being done about it and what his prospects for the future may be. The alienation that ensues may have destructive consequences for patient and physician alike.

The pages that follow put these present-day developments in vivid historical perspective. Dr. Altschule has dug up new and intriguing information on some of the characters in the fascinating medical drama. He has the ability to see beyond intellectual fads and popular ways of thinking. His work, his ideas, and his words have always had a provocative and stimulating freshness as well as candor and lack of cant. He is known to some as an iconoclast, which indeed he is, when icons are symbols of the tyranny of tradition. Altschule's work, however, identifies him more as a builder of intellectual bridges and a champion of the patient. He does not deprecate the important and useful contributions of the laboratory to clinical medicine, but he contends that uncritical use of the laboratory in medicine has impaired clinical practice by attenuating the doctor-patient relationship. Thus, he does not advocate less scientific thinking in modern medical practice, but deplores the displacement of clinical perspicacity and dialogue with the patient by the technological tools provided by science which, unlike the stethoscope, sphygmomanmeter, ophthalmoscope, endoscope, and even microscope, are not used by the practitioner, but are operated by technicians who may barely glimpse the patient and scarcely speak to him or her.   Such aids, when appropriate, may be of great value; but their selection and interpretation and the synthesis of the data that emerges must be the responsibility of the physician caring for the patient.

The decline of clinical medicine is thus not the fault of science or even of too much science. The fault lies in the forfeiture to technology of the most important element in medical practice, a thorough understanding of the patient. In Altschule's words, ..."medical practice that derogates, or interferes with doctor-patient relations, is medicine deformed."

STEWART G. WOLF, JR., M.D.

Acknowledgements

For having read this book in manuscript and for their valuable criticisms and suggestions, I thank Richard J. Wolfe, Garland Librarian and Elin L. Wolfe, Archivist at the Boston Medical Library. In addition to her editorial assistance, Mrs. Wolfe generously discharged the responsibility of identifying and verifying the references with great skill. Many thanks are also extended to Professor Saul Benison of the University of Cincinnati.

Publication of the book was delayed for some months because of a lack of financial support for publication. Its appearance, therefore, is due to the generosity of Dr. Norman Zamcheck, Director of Cancer Research, Mallory Institute of Pathology and Associate Clinical Professor of Medicine at Harvard and Dr. John P. McGovern, Professor and Chairman of the Department of the History of Medicine at the University of Texas Graduate School of Biomedical Sciences at Houston, who volunteered to cover the entire cost of publication. I am especially grateful to Dr. Stewart J. Wolf, Jr., Director of Totts Gap Institute, Bangor, Pennsylvania, who not only wrote the Foreword to introduce the book, but who found an appropriate publisher, helped mobilize the funds and performed many other services leading to publication.

Dr. Ronald F. Kotrc, former director of the Francis Clark Wood Institute for the History of Medicine at the College of Physicians of Philadelphia and founding editor of Centrum, Inc. in the same city, edited the manuscript of this book and prepared the plates for publication by Lea & Febiger. My special thanks are extended to Dr. Kotrc and to Kenneth Bussy, editor of Lea & Febiger.

Mark D. Altschule

CONTENTS

Part II

AUSTRIAN AND GERMAN INFLUENCES IN NINETEENTH-CENTURY MEDICINE

Introduction

THIS BOOK DOES NOT PURPORT to be a traditional history of medicine. Rather, its main burden is in accord with some of Garrison's words in the Preface to the fourth edition of his monumental *An Introduction to the History of Medicine* (1929). He wrote (on page 7), "The greater physicians of the past, reasoning from what seems to us very faulty premises, somehow got their patients well, otherwise they would have had no clientele or following. The thing is to ascertain, if possible, just how they did it."

How, then, may we ascertain how they did it? Obviously, by studying the history of *medical practice*. As Muller's *The Uses of the Past* (1952) discusses in its second chapter, the usefulness of history in solving problems of this sort is paramount, for the past is contained in the present, and the future is implicit in it. Although it is appropriate that Garrison, the historian, should have raised the question, anyone could have done so. Only history, however, can answer it. Regrettably, the answer to Garrison's crucial question is not to be found in the works of the great medical historians of this century. The histories available today comprise either lists of the broad, all-encompassing theories to which some medical historians devote their attention, or else lists of the scientific discoveries that other medical historians believe created by themselves a new medicine or some main branch of it.

The making up of lists of concepts that marched along the road of history, pushing the ones before them off the road, can produce only historical accounts that, although popular, are misleading. Garrison, at another place in the Preface to the fourth edition of his book, wrote, "Anyone who studies secular history will find that the wisest heads and shrewdest wits of important periods were perfectly aware of the salient lines of medical doctrine current at that time. In poetry, drama, and novels, or what [Victorian poet Algernon] Swinburne called 'creative and imaginative literature,' we often get, in fact, the very best sidelights on the medicine of the period." This idea, the truth of which is proved easily, is not valid for the history of medical practice because it implies that much or most of that history should be the history of concepts. According to this notion, medicine's history should be what physicians who mainly practiced medicine and physicians who mainly taught medicine thought about disease, or perhaps only thought that they thought about disease. A history of medicine so conceived is, however, a history mainly of error, dogma, and superstition. Although histories of this sort are useful (they would not have been written otherwise), practitioners like me usually find them irrelevant, often boring, at times embarrassing, and most important of all, not descriptive of what doctors do when they practice medicine. Furthermore, when the study of concepts of the past, erroneous or otherwise, is pursued, scholars are encouraged to seek explanations for the rise (and fall) of these concepts. We must remember that any explanations of the origins of specific human thoughts are in danger of being delusions, at least to some degree. Even when the delusional component is minor, an unprovable speculative component remains paramount.

Nevertheless, events occurring outside medicine, most of them accidental, do affect the thinking and concept formation of doctors. In fact, that is a main argument of this work. However, those occurrences will not be explained as the results of the operation of a Platonic collective intelligence (conscious or unconscious), but as the inevitable changes produced within one segment of society by changes in any other. This thesis should require no defense, although we must recognize that the processes it describes may be erroneous. Many medical historians, including Garrison, equate discoveries in biological sciences with advances in medicine. The view that the early development of modern medicine is best represented by a list of discoveries in biological science (since most were made by physicians) makes the history of medicine resemble a great clock with its arms moving in sudden jerks, each jerk creating a new time. The invalidity of this view becomes apparent when, owing to the 19th-century proliferation of medical professorships, the discoveries that made the men famous became smaller and smaller, and were expressed in histories in such terms as, "He was the first in Germany to suture the patella," or, "He made many studies in metabolism."

As Wightman has pointed out in *The Emergence of Scientific Medicine* (1971), "It is easy to write, and much easier to read the still too common history in which a succession of 'fathers' of this, that, and the other appear; the reader is kept in a state of heightened excitement as one dramatic 'breakthrough' follows another." But, this is journalism, not history. I will attempt to demonstrate that "common history" is both cause and consequence of today's inaccurate ideas about medicine, and is probably a cause of medicine's confused present and dubious future.

One thing became clear early in the studies that I made for this book. The discoveries in science, whether true or false, had, as a rule, no immediate effect on clinical practice, although they might have influenced, for better or worse, medical education. Harvey's work on the circulation had no effect on medical practice: it led to the cure of no more sick people and encouraged no more sick people to go to physicians. Harvey had an excellent practice not because of his discoveries, but because he was a fine physician. In fact, one of the two 17th-century English physicians who created medicine, Sydenham (the other was Locke), went to the extreme of disparaging the role of the sciences. However valid Sydenham's views may have been in the 1600s, they were clearly less valid 100 years later and became even less so, at an accelerating rate, thereafter. There is little doubt that the reverse is true: The advancement of general knowledge and the development of specific sciences are both affected by scientific discoveries made by physicians and others who have worked in medicine-related sciences. In the past, scientific discoveries often influenced more what some physicians said about their profession than what they did in practicing it. We are, however, more interested here in what physicians in practice do than in what some physicians think physicians do. By this criterion, balancing the good against the harm it did after it was finally accepted by physicians, Harvey's discovery of the closed circulation may be regarded as less important to practitioners than Theobald Smith's less famous two discoveries: (1) that an arthropod may spread an infectious disease (Texas tick fever), thereby foreshadowing the ultimate prevention of malaria, and (2) that the injection of killed microorganisms may, like that of live ones, confer immunity. (Pasteur already had shown that artificially weakened, but still alive, microorganisms could do that.) However, it is futile to try to rank scientific discoveries on any absolute scale pertaining to their value both as science and as an influence on medical practice, and no such attempt will be made here.

Although I recognize the role of the "accessory" (French), "collateral" (English), or so-called "basic" sciences in influencing medical practice for better or for worse, I do not believe they are the substance of medicine. Moreover, treating the history of medicine as if it were the same as the history of biological sciences is certain to create confusion. Where does one place non-physicians whose discoveries have impinged on, or at least been usable in reference to, medical problems? Such figures as Hales, Lavoissier, Metchniksoff, Roentgen, and Mendel come to mind. What about the anonymous Peruvian Indians who told the Jesuits about the tree bark that cured fevers, the ancients who told us about the pain-killer opium, the village wise woman who told Withering about the foxglove? Were they medical scientists? And how do we handle the physicians who gave up medicine to become basic physicists, pure and simple - de Fourcroy, Poisseiulle, Bernouille, and von Helmholtz - for example, or for that matter, physicians who became novelists - Smollet, Goldsmith, Chekov, Maugham? Are all of their contributions to be regarded as medical because these men, at one time in their lives, professed medicine?

The known data are arranged in order, making some more, others less, prominent than other writers have done in the past or omitting them entirely. No data are created, and few dug up from obscurity. The data used were selected only because of their clinical bearing, and though not new, their arrangement and the varying importance given them here affords the present work a semblance of a new history. Hopefully, this does not give the appearance of creating a new history for the sole purpose of explaining, justifying, or discrediting some current situation. (A revised history is always an important weapon used by reformers or revisionists who want to induce acceptance of their unorthodox views. I refer here to the biased process of selection used by these persons and not to the deliberate lying of propagandists.) In this book the facts, insofar as they can be ascertained, speak for themselves. They describe what happened: how the attitudes that determined medical practice arose and changed. There is bias, however. It concerns what I, together with a considerable number of well-known physicians, conceive the nature of medicine to be.

These comments properly raise the question about what it is we are discussing. How is the medicine that we are considering defined? In my opinion, the best definition, and in any case the one I will use throughout, is that presented by Lawrence J. Henderson at Harvard around 1930. It should be noted that Henderson, although a graduate of the Harvard Medical School, never practiced medicine, but instead became probably the greatest physiologist our country has produced. Nevertheless, he perceptively described medicine as a sociological process, the interaction between a physician and a patient. In medicine practiced this way, we must understand that neither of these two persons functions alone: The physician has physician consultants, laboratory specialists of various grades, nurses, office personnel; the patient has family, friends, perhaps lovers, associates in work, neighbors.

The physician uses information of all types - chemical, physical, biological, psychological, economic, and above all clinical. In fact, he uses information of any type whatsoever which he may find helpful. At different times in the interaction with the patient, the physician may use solely or mainly one type of knowledge to the partial or complete exclusion of the others. Nevertheless, the entire clinical process is an interaction. Although the patient may not be present physically at all times, he is present usually and always involved. Also, the various peripheral components of this small social system participate in the doctor-patient interaction in various degrees at different times - on occasion, not at all.

The fact that medicine is defined here as what happens to and around sick people is not original as a basis of a historical account. It is worthy of note that one historian, Harris Coulter, has written a history (1975, 1977) from the viewpoint of an empiricist, although he is not a practitioner and, in fact, not a physician. Coulter's conclusion was that histories of medical theories are misleading because they pretend - falsely - to show how our understanding of disease steadily has been approaching perfection through science. This view was dealt with harshly (by Brieger [1978], a historian, of course), but we intend to maintain a similar one here.

There have been many definitions of disease in modern times (Rothschuh, 1975). Hufeland called it a quantitative deviation from the normal in structure or function; this was a slight change from Boerhaave's concept of a disturbance in internal equilibrium, which likewise was taken over by Virchow. There is a host of philosophical definitions of disease in the literature from Plato's time to the present, for philosophers, and physicians who like to dabble in philosophy have expressed a variety of ideas about the nature of medicine, mostly in German. (William James, more than a century ago, pointed out that the German language encourages philosophizing.) The most recent French contribution in this area has no evident usefulness. Foucault's *Origins of the Clinic* (1973) has an attractive title that is completely misleading, for it tells us nothing about clinical medicine. The text is a dreamy account of the author's free associations, with old words used solipsistically and ideas always expressed with confused vagueness and, at best, simple imprecision. We are not concerned here with any of these ideas about disease, but rather what happens between a patient (a person who believes himself to be sick or who believes that he might become sick) and a doctor (a person who has been trained by schooling and by experience to deal with such persons). Poynter's collection of essays on the social implications of medicine (1973) makes it plain that today physicians and certain non-physicians can attain positions of great power and authority in medicine without ever having seen a patient up close, except by accident. One may encounter this fact with amusement, wonder, or scorn; I regard it as unworthy of praise.

Medicine-related science has good press today. Clinical medicine, on the other hand, needs to be explained and described and even justified. This work attempts to carry that out by means of a developmental approach that automatically will omit some material that today has come to contaminate thinking about clinical medicine.

The current practice of exaggerating the importance of laboratory research, both past and recent, is misleading. It ignores what practicing physicians have been talking and writing about for centuries, recording their clinical observations in hundreds of reports, printed or in manuscript diaries. Hundreds of other such reports were never recorded, but were given orally before physicians' clinical clubs, societies for medical improvement, and other professional associations. These practitioners took very seriously the accumulation and sharing of clinical experience, recognizing that it was not only the basis but the very content of their practice. Hundreds of these reports of individual patients by individual practitioners are available in historical collections but are rarely referred to and even more rarely given any importance except as curiosities. Some of them are curiosities. For example, *Cases and Observations of the Medical Society of New Haven County in the State of Connecticut* was printed by J. Meigs in 1788 when the Society was four years old. It includes Dr. Ebenezer Beardsley's paper, given on April 5, 1786, "Case of an Enteritis." This clinical report contained the complaint that the medical professors had advanced medical knowledge very little, and that the Society of medical practitioners would have to do it:

> That article in our constitution, which obliges every member of the society, to exhibit a history of all the remarkable cases which occur in his practice, must, if duly observed, conduce in the highest degree to promote the design and end of our institution. If we are faithful, accurate and persevering in our observations, we shall soon be furnished with a number of facts and histories, which at some future period, may be very interesting and beneficial to the public, and do

> honor to the society. It is much to be re-
> gretted that hitherto, the faculty, in this
> country, have contributed so little to the
> general stock of medical knowledge. Our
> predecessors would have rendered an impor-
> tant piece of service to us, and to future
> generations, if they had made and transmitted
> down, faithful histories of the diseases which
> prevailed in their times.

We recognize, however, that this complaint might apply
only to New Haven.

The guiding principle of this book, that medicine is
the interaction between two persons, imposes an obligation
to describe the participants in this special transaction.
Whereas we know a great deal about the physicians involved - as illustrated by the considerable amount of biographical material here presented - we know almost nothing specific about the ordinary people who were the
patients. Perhaps we can surmise something about these
persons by knowing about the physicians who contributed
most to the development of clinical medicine.

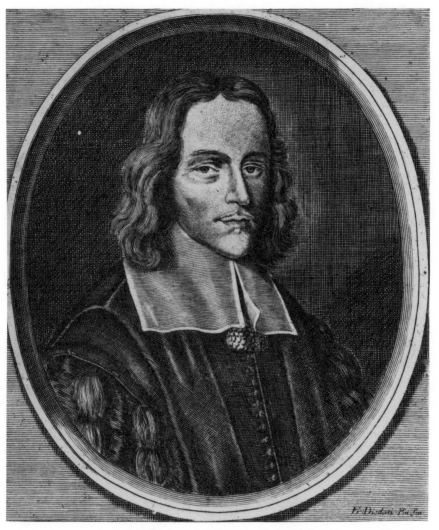

Thomas Willis, 1621-1675

CHAPTER 1: Medicine in Seventeenth-Century England

THE STATE OF ENGLISH MEDICINE in the 17th century naturally re-
flected in large measure events of the 16th, and so we
must consider the latter.   In this connection the name of
Linacre stands first (Copeman, 1960; O'Malley, 1965; Maddison *et al.*, 1977).   Linacre received the M.D. degree both
at Padua and Oxford.   His studies in Italy from 1487 to
1499 encouraged his appreciation of the Renaissance hu-
manism and the development of his scholarly aptitudes.
Physician to Kings Henry VII and Henry VIII, his influence
extended well beyond their tenures.   He became a main
force in the transmission of Renaissance learning, both in
medicine and in other fields, in 16th-century England.   He
is today remembered for his role in the founding of the
College of Physicians in 1518, and the endowment of the
Linacre Lectures at Oxford and Cambridge.   Linacre's own
contributions included a Latin grammar and, in medicine,
accurate translations of Galen's work that he either produced or stimulated others to make.   Thomas Elyot, a layman probably trained in medicine by Linacre, wrote *The
Castle of Health*, the most popular work of the period
(Lehmberg, 1960) among those who could read, but who
probably did not follow its arbitrary recommendations.
    Another of the classical humanists of the times was
John Caius (O'Malley, 1965).   Fifty years younger than
Linacre, Caius also had taken his degree in Padua and then
followed in his footsteps as the restorer of the accuracy
of Galenic translations available in England.   He wrote
The Disease Called the Sweate (1552), a work that was

the first original description of a disease written in England and in English. (Today we are not certain what disease it actually was.) It is clear that both Linacre and Caius did nothing to liberate medicine from the dead hand of Galen; in fact, by providing greatly improved translations of his works to replace the corrupt and garbled ones then available, they strengthened the hold of Galenism by giving it a new authority.

William Gilbert was an early physician who, although a highly regarded medical practitioner in his lifetime, is remembered only for his book *De Magnete*. Born in 1540 in Colchester of a middle-class family, he had his early education locally, after which he entered Cambridge University, where he took his two arts degrees and then, in 1569, his M.D. degree. Four years later he started his practice in London and quickly became recognized as a fine physician. He became fellow, censor, treasurer, and finally, in 1600, President of the College of Physicians. His large practice included Queen Elizabeth I, who despite recurrent ill health, survived to an advanced age, finally dying of an illness characterized by swollen neck glands. He also was appointed physician to James I on his accession, but died soon afterward. Gilbert had an engrossing hobby, mineralogy, and he accumulated a fine collection of specimens. His treatise on the lodestone, published in 1600, was the first modern physics treatise published in England. It quickly gained widespread recognition, was praised by Galileo, Bacon, and many others, and was republished on the Continent. The work was both a review of the literature and an account of Gilbert's own experiments. His studies led him to conclude that the earth was a huge magnet. On a practical level, he suggested that small magnets be used to determine latitude, and he invented several navigational instruments. He also wrote on a number of meterologic topics. Gilbert differs from those physicians of the 18th and 19th centuries who gave up medicine entirely to become famous physicists. However, we have no records of his clinical practice, for his papers were destroyed when London burned in 1666. He remains an example, like Copernicus, of a physician considered to be an excellent medical practitioner by his contemporaries, but remembered today only for one of his scientific hobbies.

During the 16th century Oxford became the leader of experimental medical studies in the Western World, and in the 17th century Boyle, Lower, Willis, Wren, Petty, Locke, Hooke, and Mayow all worked or taught there. Sydenham was also a member of this group for a time, taking his M.B. degree there in 1648. He also was given his M.D. degree by Cambridge in 1678. In the following centuries, Oxford retreated into its former mediocrity (Dewhurst, 1970). The regius professorships and Linacre lectureships established at both Oxford and Cambridge retarded rather than helped English medicine in the early 17th century, for the lectures still were based on Galen and Hippocrates. Until 1623 anatomy was not taught at all (Allen, 1946), and thereafter, for a half-century or more, very sparingly and irregularly. As Debus' *Medicine in Seventeenth-Century England* states, the Regius Professors of Medicine at Oxford were not regarded highly: One was called "a little insect," while another was referred to as "the very lolpoop of the University."

This did not change for the next century, although the 17th was one of enormous change in England. It saw the rise of Protestantism and growth of Parliament's power in the first half. The decapitation of Charles I was followed by Cromwell's Commonwealth, the restoration under Charles II, the repressive trends under James II, and the full development of the constitutional monarchy under William and Mary. During much of the century the people were divided into two main groups: the Tories, who were Royalists, generally Anglican and conservative; and the Whigs, who were Parliamentarians, Protestant, and liberal or, in some cases, rabidly radical except in religion, in which they were often brutally repressive (as in Ireland). The more radical of them espoused causes and used language remarkably like that of many young Americans of the 1960s. The radicals' influence diminished when Cromwell bested them in pitched battles, but the revolutionary change in thinking and lifestyles persisted.

Medicine was divided, with most of the leaders of medical sciences remaining Royalists, whereas the man who was to create modern clinical medicine, Sydenham, was a

Parliamentary trooper.   Together with Locke, today regarded as a philosopher rather than as a physician, Sydenham led medicine into an era of empirical observation. The Tories listed among them the great names of 17th-century English medicine - Harvey, Willis, Lower, and Mayow, for example.   They were conservative, but not reactionary, and actively participated in the destruction of the moribund prevailing Galenism by pursuing the newly popular experimental and observational sciences.   Their findings made them famous and contributed ultimately to advances in medical knowledge, albeit with little or no effect on that part of medical practice concerned with diagnosis and treatment.   Also among the Tories were the Regius Professors at Oxford and Cambridge, who, for the most part, continued to be a succession of nonentities whose conceptions of medicine were largely those of Galen.

The Whigs included an unknown number of country doctors as well as a great medical reformer, Sydenham, who strongly espoused the Puritan view of things - utilitarian as well as utopian, and against privilege.   He took the utilitarian view that observation of sick people, not dead people or live experimental animals, must be the essence of medicine.

Seventeenth-century England was not only a period of political revolution and counterrevolution, but was also one of revolution in both medicine and science, changing them forever.   Webster's *The Great Instauration* (1975) has given us - with remarkable breadth combined with meticulous detail - an account of the changes that occurred at midcentury.   The political triumph of Puritanism perhaps has overshadowed the revolution in medicine - in sciences both pure and applied - in education, and in social theory; but all of those were lasting, unlike the political revolution.   The change was especially marked and lasting in medicine.

The state of English medicine in the early 17th century is difficult to describe in simple terms, for it was both unchanged and changing.   On the one hand, Galenism, the prevailing dogma for 15 centuries, although badly shaken, still persisted.   At its peak, as Temkin's *Galenism* (1973) makes clear, it was not only a general philosophy, but a specific body of information (much of it false) of interpretive conjecture (most of it nonsense) and of therapeutic procedure (most of it without value). The fact that only the wealthy could afford medical care probably is the reason that mankind in Europe survived during those centuries. Although Galenism came under attack first from the peculiar chemical theorizing of Paracelsus and then, in the 16th century, from the expansion of anatomical study beginning before Vesalius and accelerating after him, the teaching at medical schools of anything but Galenism was forbidden until the end of that century. Galenic teaching still continued throughout the 17th century, and the practice of Galenic medicine was widespread throughout the 18th century. Even Sydenham used Galenic concepts to explain disease. Galenism cannot be derogated merely because the doctors it produced were unable to treat many diseases adequately, since today many better educated doctors cannot treat many diseases. Nor can it be said that its concepts were totally erroneous, since many modern ones are at least largely so. The chief complaint about Galenism was that it prevented clear thinking: It considered all diseases to be manifestations of humors that had been thinned, thickened, curdled, agglutinated, dispersed, or translocated, the difficulty being that the humors did not exist. Likewise, the other principles, spirits, souls, or fragments thereof which caused the appearance of illness by being altered, suppressed, or moved to the wrong places, were likewise imaginary. There is no indication that there was any widespread skepticism regarding the existence of those factors; after all, had not Plato said that if anything has a name it must exist? When finally Paracelsus raged across Europe in the 16th century denouncing the errors of Galenism, he replaced them with his own absurdities, unacceptable to most English physicians. Galen's anatomical dogmas were destroyed by Vesalius and his followers, but the rest of his system persisted in the English universities (Allen, 1946; Rook, 1969a; Brown, 1977). Thus, Glisson, Regius Professor of Medicine at Cambridge for 40 years (1636-1676) made excellent studies of the liver, but still accepted the physiological elements of Galen's dogma (Brown, 1977). However, new and even more peculiar dogmas were arriving from abroad: Descartes' writings on man as machine were welcomed when introduced into England by Ent, a Belgian refugee who had been educated at Cambridge and, like many leading physicians of the time, earned the M.D. degree at Padua. The introduction of Cartesian concepts was most opportune. Although structure could be described only in terms of what one saw, function at the time could be described only in terms of what one imagined. Descartes provided material for that process, as did others such as Borelli, a pupil of Galileo and an associate of Malpighi. Thus was founded the iatromathematical (or iatrophysical) school of medicine, whose hold on the academically minded English physician was exemplified in the work of Keill.

Trained at Cambridge and Leyden, Keill became the author of the most popular English anatomy text of the late 17th century. In 1698 he also translated the chemistry text written by Lemery of Paris. Later, in his writings on physiology, he entered into calculations of the muscular work of the heart and other organs using the iatrophysical method. Despite his preoccupation with unfounded iatrophysical imaginings, he apparently was a good physician (Valadez and O'Malley, 1971). Evidently, the dogmas of iatrophysics had little effect on clinical practice.' The same is true of the dogma known as iatrochemistry, which came into being in the 17th century owing largely to the writings of von Helmont, an ex-Capuchin monk-turned-physician. Having made some valuable, if primitive and partly misinterpreted, chemical observations, he proceeded to create an imaginary system of human physiology based on the then-known erroneous chemistry. His general approach was to study patients by the primitive chemical means then accepted. To his credit, he refused to use metaphors taken from inorganic chemistry to explain life processes, as many later iatrochemists did (Niebyl, 1973). In his works published in 1662, he not only attacked the concept that disease was merely a disturbance of the humors, but also substituted the concept that diseases were each an entity, with some external factor responsible for their spread. Pagel's book, *The Religious and Philosophical Aspects of von Helmont's Science and Medicine* (1944), makes it clear that he had no great following. Whatever ideas he had were stated so vaguely and so enveloped in mystical and poetic language as to be barely intelligible, or worse. For example, he held that the *ens*, or cause of disease, appeared to be not a living thing but a self-existent force or principle, whatever that was; however, his idea that there were specific diseases became accepted in a variety of ways as the years progressed. His concept of an *archeus*, the vital principle in each person or each organ, was referred to by some 17th-century English physicians, although it was accepted by few. He did, however, establish the concept of a *gas* (a misspelling of chaos) and made the valid physiological observations that digestion was affected by gastric acid.

Although men like de le Boe and Boerhaave of Leyden, and Willis of London, were iatrochemists who explained things in terms of the primitive and generally erroneous chemistry of the times, there was nothing to indicate that these men were other than outstanding clinicians. In fact, Willis was not only a Leyden-type iatrochemist; he was also a Cartesian iatrophysicist, but remained an outstanding clinician. (In those days dogma did not spoil good clinicians.)

The English medicine of the 17th century (as well as that of the 16th) was influenced also by the views of Paracelsus. He was hailed by some, such as Bostocke in his *Difference Between the Ancient Phisicke and the Latter Phisicke* (1585), for his overthrow of the superstitious "heathenish" physic of Galen, which was stated to be based upon the heathenish philosophy of Aristotle. Bostocke particularly was angry at Aristotle because he would not accept anything that could not be demonstrated. As Pagel has shown in his *Paracelsus* (1938), that writer's system was designed to explain all creation - the macrocosm and the microcosm - and, only secondarily, medicine. The English Paracelsans, for the most part, accepted a role for chemistry, which was to help medicine fulfill *its* role, that of searching out the secrets of nature. To them, bodily functions were chemical functions, and diseases were chemical malfunctions that only chemical medicine could heal, a view not unlike one that is prevalent today. On the Continent, unlike in England, the broader claims of Paracelsan theory usually were favored, although some Englishmen went just as far as any German enthusiast. When John Donne compared Copernicus and Paracelsus, for example, he thought the latter was the greater. Debus' *English Paracelsans* (1965) is an excellent source, as is his later paper (1972). Another work, *Science, Medicine and Society in the Renaissance* (1972), edited by Debus, goes into the various aspects of Paracelsan ideas and other contemporary matters. For the most part, the English Paracelsans limited their activities to the use of chemical remedies in preference to, or in addition to, the botanical remedies of Galen. After all, Bacon had said that the future of medicine was in using chemistry to develop new remedies: Medicine's growth would be enhanced by chemical analogies of the most primitive sort, which would explain the workings of the body, as was done by such iatrochemists as Willis.

The chaotic state of English medicine in the 18th century has been presented clearly by Trail (1965). Most practitioners adhered to the content and tenets of Galenic medicine - with its indifference to exact diagnosis and its advocating of irrational polypharmacy - as manifested by the official *Pharmacopoeia* of the College of Physicians. The published works on treatment said little of value and, as Sydenham later showed, the rich, who could afford medical care, often were worse off than the poor, not that all physicians were satisfied with the published material. Lack of communication, local prejudice, and a general spirit of revolt against authority all combined to interfere with the development of good medical practice. The contradictions among recommendations by the official bodies that were supposed to regulate medicine all added to the confusion, as did the persistent belief in astrology. A beneficient confusion also was introduced when, as the result of the Reformation, dissenters were forbidden to enter Oxford or Cambridge: A great number of academies were created for them and were so organized, with laboratories and botanical gardens, as to introduce a new element into medical education.

The situation in English medicine is summarized in the papers that make up the books, *Medicine in Seventeenth-Century England*, edited by Debus (1974), and *Oxford Medicine*, edited by Dewhurst (1970), as well as such separate papers as those of Doll (1973). Davis' *Circulation Physiology and Medical Chemistry in England* (1973) and the articles by Brown (1970, 1977), Moravia (1978), French (1972), and Anning (1957) describe the theories that were considered at the time to be important to an understanding of the bodily functions in health and disease. Those theories, which only after a struggle had replaced the superstitions of the Galenic system, were pitiful attempts to use the fragmentary and often inaccurate data of physics and chemistry then available and were, in fact, nothing but superstitions themselves. Regrettably, that material makes up a large part of the medical writings of the 17th century. Men who probably were fine physicians left a record of mainly nonsense in writings that tell us nothing about the practice of medicine in the 17th century. This superstitious material is important because it reminds us that physicians of all eras who are required or constrained to teach also are constrained to explain. Since no explanation of basic processes can be based on anything approaching complete information, all such explanations must be superstitions to a greater or lesser degree. Whatever such explanations may provide in teaching the immature, they advance knowledge only when the testing of these explanations uncovers new information that controverts them. Although Paracelsan and Helmontian superstitions had little discernible effects on the practice of medicine, they have held the attention of medical historians; thus, we know little about medical practice in those eras.

Lester King has produced an interesting variant on the practice of analyzing the ideas found in medical writings of the 17th century. He has analyzed these ideas in terms of today's formulations of philosophic thought. His views have been expanded in his books, *The Medical World of the Eighteenth Century* (1958), *The Growth of Medical Thought* (1963), and *The Road to Medical Enlightenment* (1970), as well as in articles (1963, 1965). This material is an account of what 17th-century physicians *said* they thought, but not necessarily what they actually thought. King's analyses are highly important for the history of ideas, but they tell us little about the practice of medicine, and so do not bear upon this work.

During the 16th and throughout most of the 17th century, Padua was the university at which English physicians and medical students supplemented their inadequate Oxford and Cambridge educations (O'Malley, 1970). At the time, Padua was controlled by Venice which, after its conquest of Padua, wisely maintained it as its state university. Padua was a center of extraordinary tolerance, as opposed to Rome, which was repressive. Foreigners, including Vesalius, the Belgian, held some of the principal chairs at Padua. Due to a peculiarity of University rules, many Protestants from all over northern Europe received their Padua degrees from the German Count Palatine, while the Catholics received their degrees from the Bishop of Padua. One interesting requirement in that era of traditionalism was the fact that professors were forbidden to give the same lecture in consecutive years. The faculty was remarkable: Bagellardi, the author of the first printed pediatric text; Fracastoro, the father of epidemiology; Vesalius, the great anatomist; Ramazzini, the pioneer reporter of occupational disease; and later, the great pathologist Morgagni, one of the founders of modern medicine. Another fundamental aspect of modern medicine had its inception in Padua - long before Leyden, which is given the credit - when da Monte, otherwise obscure today, taught the students at the bedside in the hospital of San Franciscus. Da Monte (also known as Montanus) died in 1552 and was succeeded at Padua by his pupils Bottoni and Oddi, who continued his practice of bedside teaching. (They also taught pathological anatomy.) Bedside medical teaching was carried from Padua to Leyden by van Heurne (or Heurnius), who with his son Otto, established the practice in that city. The fact that da Monte was an extraordinary clinical teacher is mentioned briefly, if at all, it today's authoritative writings. The exception is Wightman's *The Emergence of Scientific Medicine.* The elite of English medicine - physicians to kings and other notables, founders and members of the Royal College of Physicians, and leading teachers and practitioners - were more likely to have had Paduan training than any other variety, until the rise of Leyden at the end of the 17th century.

In his *The Development of Medicine as a Profession* (1966), Bullough gave an account of ancient and medieval medical teaching; however, since our interest is in bedside teaching, only one passage will be quoted: "Marcus Valerius

Martial wrote, 'I was ailing: But you at once attended me, Symmachus, with a train of a hundred apprentices °or students§. A hundred hands frosted by the North Wind have pawed me: I had no fever before, Symmachus; now I have.'" There is no indication that bedside teaching was practiced at the undergraduate level before the 16th century.

Among the medical alumni of Padua was Copernicus, who first entered the University of Cracow in 1491 and studied philosophy, mathematics, painting, and drawing. Five years later he went to Bologna and then to Padua, where he studied medicine, among other subjects. He took a doctorate in canon law in 1503 at Ferrara, since the degrees were less expensive there than at Padua. After his return to Poland in 1505, he served as a canon, practiced medicine and, when time permitted, pursued studies in astronomy. He was secretary and physician to his uncle, the Bishop of Warmia. While at Padua he had studied under the surgeon de la Torre, for whom da Vinci had made his famous anatomical drawings. (De la Torre died young, and if he had ever had a plan to publish an anatomical atlas - some decades before Vesalius - he died without doing so.)

One of Copernicus' fellow students was Fracastoro, the famous physician-poet of the Renaissance and the founder of epidemiology. Copernicus had a number of famous men as patients and was evidently much in demand as a physician and as a consultant to other physicians. Today he is remembered as a great astronomer, author of the treatise on the revolution of the earth, finished in 1520, circulated in manuscript, and finally published in 1543, shortly before his death. During much of his adult life his main activity was the practice of medicine (Bruce-Chwatt and Bruce-Chwatt, 1973).

It is interesting to note in passing that Galileo, a man whose work Copernicus greatly influenced, also studied medicine. However, he chose not to become a physician. His father was a famous musician, and he had young Galileo educated in music, literature, and the pictorial arts before sending him to Pisa to study medicine. (At that time music and mathematics were considered to be closely related.) Young Galileo preferred mathematics to medicine and left his medical studies when he was 21 years of age, in 1585.   His professional life was in mathematics and the sciences, including the latter's technology.   Today Galileo's background in the humanities and in medicine rarely is mentioned.

Another Pole who studied at Padua was Struthius, important because of his measurements of arterial blood pressure made over 400 years ago.   Born in Poznan in 1510 of the wealthy Strus family, he later Latinized his name to the form by which he is now known.   He studied at the University of Cracow from 1527 to 1531, earning two degrees in arts.   In 1532 Struthius went to Padua for his medical training and in 1535 was granted the degree of Doctor of Medicine and Philosophy, whereupon he immediately was made Professor of Theoretical Medicine there, much as Vesalius immediately was made Professor of Anatomy and Surgery after receiving his doctor's degree in 1537.   Returning to Poznan in 1545, he soon became Poland's leading medical practitioner, his patients including such persons as Isabella, daughter of King Sigismund I of Poland and wife of King Zapolya of Hungary.   He was called to treat Sultan Sulaiman II in Constantinople, but declined to go to Madrid to treat King Philip II of Spain. He preferred to remain in Poland, where he became Physician to King Sigismund II, Burgomaster of Poznan. Struthius' treatise, *Sphygmicae Artis* (1555) was a study of the pulse, but in it is found a discussion of how to estimate the arterial pressure by placing weights upon a pulsating artery until the pulsations are abolished (Schott, 1977).   Thus is discovered that the basis of today's method of measuring blood pressure, the method of occlusion, was known four centuries ago, the physiologic concept having been worked out by a perceptive clinician.

To many historians of medicine, the 17th century in England was the century of Harvey, with Willis and his associate Lower a little "below" him, and then perhaps Glisson and a scattering of others who are familiar to most of us only because their names are memorialized in some disease or some part of the body.   Harvey is in a different category, usually represented as one of the greatest medical scientists of all time and the pioneer in the introduction of modern science into medicine.   Yet his influence during the 17th century was far from universal, since many of his contemporaries or successors either ignored or actually rejected his ideas about blood circulation. (It should be noted that these ideas were not completely new; the general concept is to be found in the writings of Cesalpino and Bruno °Pagel, 1950§.) It is ironic that the acceptance of Harvey's thesis by some - Browne, the physician-turned-philosopher, and Fludd, the Rosicrucian mystic (Huntley, 1951) - was due to the appeal of the idea of the then-praised Circle of Perfection. This is not the same as saying, as Pagel did (1950, 1968), that Harvey himself chose that idea because of *his* reverence for this Circle. It has been said that Harvey favored Aristotelian philosophy (Pagel, 1976), but that had no evident bearing on his medical practice. Stevenson (1976) has provided an excellent discussion, with the inevitable ambiguous question about whether Harvey was the great medical scientist that worshipping historians suggest. Such information, however, is irrelevant to this study, which is concerned with how he practiced medicine and what particulars allowed him to be considered an outstanding physician (Keel, 1965; Keynes, 1966). There is no way to gauge that in detail, although it must be assumed that he did not use his knowledge of circulation in practice, for there was no way in which he could have done so. Willis tried to apply Harvey's discovery, but he did so in his research and not in clinical practice.

Willis was another of the great Oxford group who gave that university scientific prominence in the 17th century. Although a physician, he did not teach medicine, but rather was Professor of Natural Philosophy. (A fine biography has been done by Wisler °1968§.) Much attention has been devoted to Willis' studies on the brain and nerves, as discussed in Feindel's edition of his *Cerebri Anatome* (1965), Keele's review of that subject (1967), and the articles by Meyer and Hierons (1965a,b). Willis' anatomical studies were received enthusiastically on the Continent, but less so in England. His nonsensical chemical theorizing based on the fragmentary chemistry of the time (iatrochemistry) alienated many English authorities but, if anything, appealed to the Germans. His reputed discovery of the circle of Willis clearly had been made by others before him, beginning with Fallopius a century earlier (Meyer and Herois, 1962). His reputed first use of the term "pineal organ" was preceded by Crooke's use of the term a half-century before him.

Willis was evidently a great physician. He was Court Physician under Charles II, and his *London Practice* showed him to be a perceptive clinical observer. His reports on disease states were based on clinical history and inspection alone: He described the sweet taste of diabetic urine and the clinical pictures of diseases as diverse as myasthenia gravis and puerperal sepsis, and "redescribed" hysteria, melancholia, and the mental deterioration of what is now called schizophrenia. Willis should be ranked, therefore, high among clinical observers who never ceased to learn from patients, rather than being given the ambiguous standing he has earned as a medical scientist. That ambiguous standing was the result of the brilliance of his anatomical studies being tarnished by the fallacious reasoning of his iatrochemistry.

Consideration of Willis' place in the history of medicine requires mention of Wren. Known as the man who rebuilt St. Paul's Cathedral after the great fire of London, he was also Willis' friend, dissecting assistant, and illustrator (Bennett, 1876). He was for some years President of the Royal Society, the inventor of intravenous drug administration (in dogs), Professor of Anatomy, microscopist, designer of telescopes and other instruments, maker of anatomical models, (an) inventor of transparent beehives, surgical pioneer (in dogs), architect, nutritionist, veterans' friend and, in short, "one of the most accomplished and illustrious characters in history" (Gibbon, 1970).

Lower was another of the famous Oxford physicians of the 17th century. Entering Oxford in 1649, he soon became an assistant to Willis and worked for and with him until his death in 1675. In 1666 Willis took up the practice of medicine in London, and in 1667, two years after he received his M.D. degree, Lower followed him there. On Willis' death, Lower succeeded him as Court Physician, and he was recognized as London's greatest practitioner. He lost his Court position after the death of Charles II in 1685, but continued to practice less remuneratively until January of 1691. We know a great deal about Lower's work on fevers, blood transfusion, and especially the heart. His anatomical studies of the heart and his researches on the reasons for the change in the blood's color as it traverses the lungs have given him lasting fame. Almost nothing is known about the way he practiced medicine.

Mayow is a man whose status as a physician is difficult to define. Although he prepared himself at Oxford for a career in the clergy, he also attended the medical lectures there and may have studied with Willis, Oxford's Professor of Natural Philosophy at the time. Despite his not having an M.D. degree, Mayow practiced medicine, but only during the season at Bath. He wrote two medical works, one on the chemical constitution of the supposed healing waters at Bath and the other on rickets, but neither was outstanding. It is probable that he did not consider himself primarily a physician. Today he is recognized as a pioneering physiologist because of his writings on the mechanics of breathing and more particularly on the physiology of respiration. He showed that the effects on air of combustion and respiration were similar and postulated that air contained a substance that he called "nitroaerial spirits," which was required in both processes. He held that the air gave up this material to the blood in the lungs and that the blood delivered it to the tissues. A century later his ideas were revived by Laviossier, and the discovery of oxygen by Priestley gave them a firm basis. Mayow died young, only nine years after his graduation from Oxford, "having a little before been married, not altogether to his content." His early death makes it difficult to assign him a place in the history of clinical medicine. Some physicians of the past, like some today, have worked mainly in physiologic science during their "salad days," later making it an appendage to the more interesting pursuit of clinical practice, to the enhancement of both. There is no way of knowing whether Mayow's career would have followed this course, and even if it had, historians probably would have ignored his clinical pursuits, much as they did those of Gilbert.

Neuberger (1944) has given us an interesting account of British-German relations in medicine in the 17th century. Whereas the flow of knowledge in surgery was mainly from Germany to England, and the writing of

Paracelsus still had some adherents in England, the movement of physiological knowledge (as in the works of Harvey and Willis) was the reverse. Although the philosophy
of Bacon only had limited acceptance in Germany, one of
its offshoots - the clinical viewpoints of Sydenham - came
to give much of German medicine its character, and the
influence of those viewpoints grew for 100 years.

On the whole, it is difficult to gain an accurate
idea of medical practice in early 17th-century England.
The records are poor, and although some recipe and account books are available, there is little case material.
Two available compilations of case material are interesting
to compare: One was produced by John Hall, a physician of
good education and high reputation, as well as Shakespeare's son-in-law; the other is that of John Symcott, a
country physician of obscure education and humble status.
As Harriet Joseph (1964) and Virginia Jones (1977) pointed
out, Hall kept excellent case records; he had studied at
Cambridge and, apparently also abroad, probably at Padua.
Symcott, although he also studied medicine at Cambridge,
evidently could not afford the practical training available
only in Europe; nevertheless, he became highly competent.
As discussed by Poynter and Bishop in *A Seventeenth-Century Doctor and His Patients* (1951), he had a number of
prominent patients, including Parliamentarians and members
of the Cromwell family. As far as can be ascertained
from the case material, the diagnoses were based (albeit in
terms of the humoral theory) on what the patients revealed in his history as well as what inspection revealed:
Examination determined the patient's general appearance,
the external features of the body, respiration, character of
the pulse, state of the tongue, location of pain, if any,
signs of fever, the appearance of the excreta, and signs of
muscular paralysis. Shed or withdrawn blood was examined
grossly, and tumors, liver, and spleen were evaluated by
palpation. In short, in addition to the history, the clinical
evaluation depended on inspection and palpation, with some
superficial and probably misguided attention to the blood
and excreta. Some physicians evidently still used astrology
as a main basic science of medicine. Later on, possibly
under the influence of Sydenham's ideas either as such or

brought back by Leyden students, the case material became fuller.

The 17th-century practitioner of medicine about whom most is known is Sir Thomas Browne. Born early in the century, he entered the study of medicine in 1623 at a time when formal medical education in England was so decadent that Sydenham was constrained to remark, "One had as good send a man to Oxford to learn shoemaking as practicing physic" (Dewhurst, 1962). Bad as that situation was, it was worsened by the fact that no attendance at all at any institutions of learning was required for the M.D. degree, although the King could bestow it and, more amazingly, the Archbishop of Canterbury also. Those who could afford it traveled to the Continent to be educated in medicine, and Browne was one of those. He went first to Montpellier, one of the three earliest university medical schools founded in Europe. (The other two were at Paris and Bologna.) Montpellier's main attraction at that time was its fame and the tolerant spirit that permitted Protestant students to function there; the former was not justified, since Montpellier's teaching of anatomy was inferior, and its teaching of therapeutics merely had replaced Galenic superstitions with Paracelsan dogma. Patin, at Paris, remarked that one could learn more in three months observing a practitioner's methods than in four years at Montpellier. Browne did not register for a degree and stayed probably for only one year.

Browne apparently went to Padua in 1632. At that time many students from all over Europe (especially Germany, which had been ruined by the Thirty-Years' War) came to experience what was the best teaching in the world in anatomy and surgery. The extent to which Browne might have benefitted from the general atmosphere or from the specific courses is not known, for he left Padua probably late in 1632 and registered in Leyden at the end of 1633. Leyden was in the process of capturing from Venice its trade and prosperity and, by supplanting Venice's famous university situated in Padua, its intellectual leadership. A few weeks after registering, Browne received the M.D. degree after defending his thesis. He returned to England in 1634 and started his practice in Norwich. Little is known about what he did in that ca-

pacity.   Keynes, his earlier biographer, has speculated the
following:

> The medicine of his day consisted in the
> grave and untroubled administration of tactful
> words and a limited number of drugs for as
> many disorders, and was undisturbed by the
> scurry of new theories and experiments which
> at the present day makes the profession at
> once so attractive and so distracting.   It is
> accumulation of possibilities that paves the
> way for uncertainty, and their knowledge was
> so limited that there was little scope for an
> obscure   diagnosis....There   is   no   indication
> that, any more than his contemporaries, did
> he perceive the fallacies of such a practice
> as phlebotomy, which had been a panacea
> since the days of Galen fifteen centuries be-
> fore.   Every   age   has   its   cure-alls;   after
> blood-letting came purging drafts, and after
> purges has come the assertion that we eat
> too much.

To what extent did untroubled, reassuring word and
manner counteract the adverse effects of excessive bleeding and purging?   We shall never know.   How often were
the bleeding, purging, blistering, and so forth, so severe as
to be harmful?   We may suspect but, again, we shall never
know.

What little historical material is available on the
doctor-patient relationship of that era is never more than
a bare recital of medications given and bleedings and
clysters performed.   Discussion of the prominent theories
and the well-known men of 17th-century English medicine
throws very little light on the subject of our interest, the
doctor-patient   relationship   as   expressed   in   clinical
medicine.   The great English physicians discussed here, at
least those considered to be great today, were products of
Padua, either as such or in spirit.   Yet those men are
known mainly for their scientific discoveries and not at all
for their clinical expertness.   Was a higher value placed
on the former than the latter then, as is common now?

Padua today is not famous for its da Monte, but for its Vesalius, the Belgian; for Vesalius' successor, Fabricius of Aquapendente; for Galileo, then the mathematician; for Sanctorius, the physiologist; for Ramazzini, the industrial physician; for the great botanist, Vesling, the Westphalian. The spectacular discoveries of those men, and the equally spectacular discoveries of English physicians trained by them or inculcated with their spirit appeal to the modern view that holds, not that science has an important role in everyday life, including medical practice, but that science has the *most important* role in these activities. A similar view might have been current then, for the famous Englishmen exerted themselves greatly in the pursuit of scientific discoveries; nevertheless, we have their patients' approval, implied or stated, of their clinical activities. It must be concluded that those great medical scientists took clinical medicine seriously, but, except for Willis' *London Practice*, there is no way in which to judge that. Clinical medicine, although obviously being both practiced and taught, did not become the most important aspect of medicine until two other Englishmen, Sydenham and Locke, made it so in the same century.

In this connection it is important to note that the renaissance of English medicine led by Harvey, Willis, and Lower, although probably encouraged by the popularity of Baconian philosophy, derived its origin and its impetus from the happenings in northern Italy, which had reached a high point long before Bacon made his ideas known. On the other hand, another component of the 17th-century renaissance of English medicine was clearly the child of the Revolution and was fathered by Baconian philosophy. This second component was the great clinical renaissance, initiated by Sydenham, abetted by Locke, and based on empirical observation and the collection of clinical data.

It has been shown that 17th-century English medicine developed despite the persistence of the ancient twin forces of dogma and ignorance. Although the ignorance was lifting, old dogmas were being replaced by new ones. The old prevailing dogma, the Galenic, denied the existence of specific diseases, although different symptoms might occur at different times. Physicians, although still thinking in Galenic terms of humors and principles, began to describe specific individual diseases not merely as names but as groups of distinctive manifestations.   Thus in 17th-century England, Glisson described infantile rickets and Willis described a half-dozen diseases.   But this tendency was neither new or limited to England.   For example, an unknown German physician gave an accurate description of hemophilia before that, and other definitive descriptions were made even earlier, as will be noted elsewhere.   Nevertheless the pace at which clinical descriptions were written clearly was accelerating.   It is possible that several factors might be responsible: the spread of printing, which made it easy for physicians to record and disseminate their views; and, the spread of anatomical writings, which often included mention of pathological anatomy and the associated symptoms.   Thus, Vesalius, in the second edition of his *Fabrica*, included observations of the pathological findings in a number of disease states.   (It must not be forgotten that Vesalius was a busy practitioner whose main income was earned by treating patients.)   The post-mortem examination often became part of the case study, and physicians felt impelled to report their clinical observations together with the post-mortem findings.   When Bonet of Geneva collected in 1579 the clinicopathological reports previously made by many physicians, he encouraged further reports and also set a pattern that Morgagni followed so brilliantly 200 years later.

Whatever the factors that led to the increasing number of reports accurately describing individual diseases, there is no doubt that from the middle of the 17th century onward the responsibility for this development lay mainly with Sydenham and his followers.   However, it must be recognized that Sydenham was a man who entered the scene at the right time - that of the midcentury revolutions: one a revolution that led to political oscillations, and the other, much more important for this discussion, to new patterns of seeking and handling information.   It is possible, but not likely, that this second revolution might have developed in England without the writings of the philosopher Bacon and, on the Continent, without the writings and travel of the physician and philosopher Locke.   Nevertheless, the then-popular empirical philosophies justified what happened in medicine.   One point must be clarified: Although for more than a century Locke has been represented as a great philosopher (which he was) and an occasional, almost dilettantish physician, he was actually an excellent clinician. The evidence is that he was an active physician, limited in his activities by ill health, and more cerebral than most. It is probable that his thinking as a physician helped him to become a great philosopher.

Little is known about Sydenhams's early life, although his family was prosperous and prominent in county affairs: parliamentary and anti-Royalist in politics, participating in military actions against the King's armies. Four brothers served in the Parliamentary Army, and their mother was killed in a Royalist raid. Regarding Sydenham himself, the details of his early life were long obscured, so much so that his biography (written by Samuel Johnson) erroneously has him fighting on the Royalist side (McHenry, 1969). Later biographers, however, diligently have worked out many of the details, culminating in Dewhurst's *Dr. Thomas Sydenham* (1962, 1966), a detailed study of the sources.

Sydenham entered Oxford in 1643, but left after a few months to go to war. Returning a few years later, he stayed one year and received the Bachelor of Medicine degree in 1648 and also was granted a fellowship, apparently with no duties. Although in contact with the virtuoso scientists and physicians then active in Oxford, he did not join them. Recalled to military duty, he was commissioned a captain in the cavalry and, after being wounded, retired. He received a pension in 1655, married, and started a medical practice in London. It is evident that he had little formal training, but he must have been an outstanding physician, because he was hightly successful. His success continued despite the adverse social circumstances imposed by the Restoration.

Attempts have been made to analyze the way Sydenham carried on his studies and his practice. A recent discussion by Bates (1977) makes the attempt in accordance with today's formal philosophic concepts, but King (1970), himself no mean philosopher, wisely concluded that several philosophic systems are represented in Sydenham's writings: this suggests that Sydenham's views on medicine grew out of his practice, and not out of a phi-

losophy. Sydenham was described as outspoken, argumenta-
tive, often sarcastic, and sometimes abrasive in manner.
He is quoted as having advised against going to Oxford for
training as a physician, although he did approve going
there for training as a shoemaker. Another of his comments, this one in answer to a question by a student about
what to read to become a good doctor, was to read Don
Quixote. That unexplained comment has been sufficiently
puzzling to give rise to a variety of complicated, and dubious, interpretations (Edelstein, 1944). Another student,
Sloane (later Sir Hans Sloane, whose great collections
later established the British Museum) applied to Sydenham
for a clinical apprenticeship, carrying with him a letter
that described him as "a ripe scholar, a good botanist, and
a skilled anatomist." Sydenham read it and said, "This is
all very fine, but it won't do. Anatomy, botany - nonsense, sir. I know an old woman in Covent Garden who
understands botany better, and as for anatomy, any butcher
can dissect a joint just as well. No, young man, all this
is stuff: you must go to the bedside. It is there alone
you can learn disease" (Wolfe, 1961). Actually, although
he expressed himself similarly on other occasions, he was
not opposed to the experiments of the Oxford scientific
virtuosi and the other medical scientists - he merely considered them irrelevant to medicine. He did consider the
then-current iatrochemical theorizing nonsense, but he was
not above theorizing himself from time to time; the difference being that he did not insist on those theorizings, and
not only welcomed but invited criticisms of them (Keele,
1974). He was a close friend of some of the medical scientists - Boyle, Wren, and Locke, with whom he had a
special relationship. Whatever the others thought of him
as a person, they all respected his honesty, his devotion to
medicine, and his brilliant clinical performance. If if had
not been for this performance, all of his writings would
have been mere words.

One of Sydenham's highly interesting comments, one
that was to be ascribed to many others in succeeding centuries, was this: "A disease, however much its cause may
be adverse to the human body, is nothing more than an effort of Nature, who strives with might and main to restore
the health of the patient by the elimination of morbific

matter" (Keele, 1974). Except for the last clause, the comment is strikingly modern. He stated on several occasions that the proximate cause of infections was "morbific particles," today interpreted by some to mean microorganisms. His rejection of such popular causes as the wrath of God, the positions of the stars, and other mystical factors was noteworthy. It is probable that Sydenham took some ideas from his friend Boyle (Keele, 1974), since they both held that relying on humoral changes to explain infections was an error. However, Sydenham was not entirely sure that Boyle's germ theory was correct. (For a discussion of the "Germ Theory" of disease, see Chapter 13.)

Sydenham tried to describe diseases as he saw them, without any preconceived hypotheses. He believed the task of the physician was only to cure disease, not to explain it. Accordingly, he regarded animal experiments, post-mortem examinations, microscopical studies, and chemical analysis as unnecessary, a conclusion certainly justified in his time. As a follower of Baconian philosophy, he derogated preoccupation with speculations of the ancients, not merely because they were wrong, but rather because they stultified clinical thinking. He found harmful the then-common practice of adducing disease manifestations from *a priori* formulations, because it stimulated worthless disputation and cast contempt on those who tried to do their work in a plainer way. Hence, to many of his contemporaries, Sydenham's custom of ignoring established concepts and trying to develop his own by observation and by therapeutic experiment was not only unorthodox but heretical. In pursuing his practice, Sydenham kept detailed clinical notes and made them the basis of his *Methodus Curandi Febris* (1666) and his *Medical Observations* (1676). He also published short works on a variety of diseases such as rheumatism, gout, venereal disease, hysteria, dropsy, and what was probably typhoid fever. His treatments were as simple as possible, and he avoided the dreadful purging, emesis, blistering, and blood-letting that hastened so many prominent persons toward the grave, by then a welcome prospect. In treatment, Sydenham recommended rest or, when indicated, exercise, plus light diets and a few medications such as iron (as steel filings or a syrup made by boiling them in wine), preparations of opium, and Peruvian bark.   (The quinine content of the last was highly efficacious against the malaria endemic in England, but problems arose because some apothecaries substituted an inefficacious ordinary bark made bitter with herbs for the true bark.)

Sydenham expected a "harvest of abuse" because of his unorthodox views on treatment but, unlike many of the other medical writers of the time, he provided case material to substantiate his conclusions.   Moreover, his clinical descriptions of many specific diseases impressed physicians who otherwise might have opposed him.   He rescued them from being trapped in the morass of undifferentiated humoral concepts of disease and from being misled by the will-o'-the-wisp of imaginary chemical formulations of disease processes developed by the iatrochemists.   His clinical teaching attracted important converts.   Two of Sydenham's apprentices, Sloane and Goodall, later became Presidents of the College of Physicians.   Trail (1965) and Rook (1969) list the many prominent physicians who became his followers, including Millington, Willis' successor as Professor of Natural Philosophy at Oxford, and Brady, Regius Professor of Medicine at Cambridge.   Sydenham's influence at Cambridge seemed especially strong (Rook, 1969).

The growth of Sydenham's reputation in England and abroad cannot be understood without appreciating the relationship between him and Locke.   So closely did they work together at times that there is some controversy about the extent to which Locke may have been responsible for some of Sydenham's medical ideas (Romanell, 1958; Cowen, 1959).   There seems to be little doubt that Locke helped Sydenham to write.   It is highly likely that Locke's experience with the success of Sydenham's kind of medicine convinced Locke of the validity of empirical philosophies in general, as Dewhurst indicates in his *Oxford Medicine* (1970).   It is impossible to define those matters exactly from the contents of letters and other currently available documents.   Rather, this work will show how Locke's participation in Sydenham's career became a factor that made the other's reputation more widely known, especially on the Continent.

Locke was born near Bristol in 1632, eight years after Sydenham.   He gained his B.A. degree at Oxford in

1656, but a decade before that had begun to show interest in medicine, as evidenced by his notes on the works of Wharton, Glisson, and Willis.   Also, his papers were found to contain prescriptions and medical recommendations from Lower, Boyle, and others, as discussed by Dewhurst in *John Locke* (1963).   While at Oxford he was friendly with some of the Oxford scientific virtuosi and some of the students who were later to become well-known physicians.   Such was the case despite the fact that during that time he held lectureships at Oxford successively in Greek and Rhetoric, and from 1661 to 1664, the post of Censor in Moral Philosophy at Christ Church.   At about that time he wrote *Essay on Respiration*, in which he discussed the work of his friends and indicated that he assisted Lower in some experiments (Dewhurst, 1960).

After a brief period in Brandenburg as secretary to a diplomat, he returned to Oxford and devoted his time mainly to scientific pursuits, including assisting Boyle with experiments in botany and chemistry in 1665.   In that year he applied for a doctorate in medicine, but his application was rejected because he had not fulfilled the requirements. Nevertheless, he began to give a course in chemistry and entered into the practice of medicine in partnership with Dr. David Thomas.   It was during Thomas' absence that Locke met one of his patients, Lord Ashley (later the Earl of Shaftesbury), who invited him to move to London as physician to his family.   Once in London, Locke attached himself to Sydenham, whose early writings on fever had attracted his attention.   Locke was the pupil and Sydenham the master, but they became close friends and colleagues and planned to co-author a medical treatise.   That was never done, although fragments of it and other collaborative writings are extant (Dewhurst, 1957, 1958, 1959; Wolfe, 1969).   The story of how Locke's original attraction to Willis' group and its iatrochemical ideas was replaced by one in favor of Sydenham's approach is described in Dewhurst's *Oxford Medicine* (1970).

Shaftesbury became Lord Chancellor in 1672 and, because Locke was in ill health, was able to persuade him to spend his time more as a statesman than as a physician. During that period Locke suggested a treatment that opened him to sarcastic criticism by modern writers, both

medical and others.   This was the now-famous episode of
the "wound powder."   It will be recalled that in the *Iliad*,
Achilles healed Telephus by scraping rust off the spear
that had wounded him and putting it into the wound.   Centuries later Paracelsus recommended that wounds be
treated not by putting powders or salves on them, but by
putting the medications on the weapons that had produced
the wounds.   Locke had become learned in the history of
medicine even before he became a practitioner.   He recalled the Paracelsan recipe, probably not from its original
source, but from the writings of the English Paracelsans of
the 17th century.   When Locke recommended treating the
sword, the patient's pain quickly was allayed.   It is not
known whether the wound healed with unusual rapidity.

When Shaftesbury fell from favor in 1675, Locke returned to Oxford where, after a brief interval, he was
granted the degree of Bachelor of Medicine.   However, his
ill health (chronic bronchitis with asthma and probably
bronchiectasis) forced him to retire from active professional life.   He traveled primarily in southern France from
1675 to 1679, during which time he visited the medical
school at Montpellier.   In his travels he often praised
Sydenham's ideas to physicians and probably others.   At
any rate, he continued to be interested in medicine.   In
Paris he was called to see an English noblewoman who had
grown dissatisfied with the care given her by a French
physician.   Unable to diagnose the condition, Locke wrote
to physician friends in London, and his description became
the earliest account of trigeminal neuralgia.   Returning to
England he rejoined Shaftesbury, whose plots to secure a
Protestant successor to Charles II failed and forced him to
flee.   In 1683, Locke considered it wise to go to Protestant Holland, where he remained until the "Glorious Revolution" of 1688 brought William of Orange to the throne of
England.   During that period he continued to give medical
advice (Stannard, 1963), and when he returned to England,
although ailing, he continued his interest in medicine, according to letters written close to the end of his life in
1704 (Cowen, 1957; Dewhurst, 1962).   It is noteworthy
how little writing of medical importance Locke did in the
25 years after the death of Sydenham.   That was due to
many factors: Locke's growing preoccupation with his

philosophical writings, his frequent change of locus, his ill health, which made him curtail some of his interests, and his less well-known preoccupation with the data of social and preventive medicine, regrettably not put into a format that could be useful (Dewhurst, 1962).

The part played by Locke in the dissemination of Sydenham's type of medical practice cannot be stated, but it must have been great, for Sydenham quickly achieved fame in most continental countries.   The most striking acceptance of Sydenham's views occurred in Leyden, where bedside medicine already had been introduced from Padua. There, Pitcairne, a political refugee from Scotland, became Professor of the Practice of Physic in 1691 and the next year startled the university by declaring that medicine must be free from philosophical sectarianism.   Although ironically he became an iatromathematician on his return to Edinburgh a few years later, he had had Boerhaave as a student before he left.   Boerhaave considered Sydenham the equivalent of Aesculapius, and from Leyden the enthusiasm for Sydenham spread to Edinburgh and Vienna and gave their medicine its character for years (Poynter, 1973).   In Italy, Baglivi likewise accepted Sydenham's clinical views promptly but, like Pitcairne, he, too, became an iatromathematician.   The changeability of Pitcairne in Edinburgh, and Baglivi in Padua, is interesting as an example of how easily dogma may be accepted by teachers of medicine.

In France the situation differed from that in Leyden, since different forces were operative.   One was Sydenham's fame *per se*, especially as emphasized by Locke in his travels in that country.   Another was Sydenham's statement that "It is necessary that all diseases be reduced to definite and certain *species* and that with the same care that we see exhibited by botanists in their phytologies; since it happens, at present, that many diseases, although included in the same genus, mentioned with a common nomenclature, and resembling one another in several symptoms and notwithstanding, differ in their natures and require a different medical treatment" (Poynter, 1973). That statement encouraged interest in logical classification. In the early 1700s de Sauvages proposed a classification of disease based on Sydenham's views.   That was the first of the modern classifications and soon was followed by others. Even more important, however, was the great admiration later expressed by 18th-century French intellectuals for the Leyden medicine of Boerhaave, the disciple of Sydenham.   Such admiration of Leyden medicine activated a reform of French medicine before the French Revolution, and it was directed in many ways by trends derived from Sydenham's writings.   The whole intellectual atmosphere of prerevolutionary France was influenced strongly by philosophers who owed their inspiration to Locke, and those philosophies made Sydenham's medicine not only acceptable but also the *only* one acceptable.   In different ways, all of them significant, Locke's influence favored the dissemination of Sydenham's ideas.

Switzerland's Haller, a pupil of Boerhaave, also publicized Sydenham's ideas, and he continued to do so after moving to the German university at Gottingen when it was founded and endowed by George I of England.   Regarding the rest of Germany, although Sydenham's works had been translated into German in Leipzig and Frankfurt in 1717, his ideas were never really to take hold until finally, around 1848, they reappeared there in a wondrously changed form.   In this connection, it should be noted that Locke's philosophy was not popular in Germany: Some of his ideas were attacked and he was called, scathingly, some kind of Unitarian (Jolley, 1978).

The role of a popular English philosophy - the empirical - in favoring the acceptance of new clinical ideas has been discussed here in relation to Bacon and the Sydenham-Locke approach.   Later it will be shown how the popular 18th-century sensist philosophy of France and the Kantian and Hegelian philosophies of Germany affected the development of medicine differently in those two countries.

The important part played by Locke in helping Sydenham to formulate his views and disseminate them by no means exhausts the ways in which Locke influenced medicine.   His role in the development of psychiatry also is noteworthy.   Locke's analysis of thinking in terms of the association of ideas not only stimulated the creation of the Associationist School of Psychology by David Hurtley, M.D.; what is more important for medicine, it led to the concept, basic in modern clinical psychiatry, that a fundamental manifestation of psychosis is disordered association, manifested as flight of ideas and impaired abstract formation (Hoeldtke, 1967). Locke was evidently the first to point out that anxiety *(he used the ancient word "inquietude") or the need to avoid it is a main motivating force in human behavior, a concept that today is described as a discovery by Freud.

Two main schools developed in 17th-century English medicine. One group of men, Harvey, Willis, and their associates and disciples, continued and expanded the northern Italian enthusiasm for scientific observation and had clinical careers that did not use much, if any, of the newly discovered material. That approach - to accumulate data - clearly was consistent with the then-popular Baconian philosophy. However, it did not prevent those who practiced that approach from accepting dogmas, and in that sense it was contrary to the intent of Bacon's philosophy. Moreover, the impetus for that kind of observation came from Italy, where it had started years earlier, actually before Bacon was born. The other school that developed in English medicine was that of Sydenham and his followers, who accumulated the data of clinical observation, ignoring the medicine-related sciences. Such an accumulation of data definitely was in keeping with Baconian philosophy, but it was contrary to it in its refusal to acknowledge the data of science, and more particularly in its unwillingness to formulate generalizations in the area of its own interest, clinical observation. It appears, therefore, that although both trends of 17th-century medicine were consistent with Baconian concepts, they were not determined by them. At most, Baconian concepts could have been used to justify two divergent trends in the approach to medicine. It is not valid to give any philosophy the role of the *creator* of medical concepts and procedures.

It must not be concluded that English medicine turned its back on its universities as Sydenham's approach became popular. The virtuosi of Oxford, who did much for the sciences, including those related to medicine, had their day and were succeeded by men of different character and interests. Two Oxford alumni of the 17th century deserve comment because of the parts they played in the medical scene in England. One of them, Floyer, began his writing before the beginning of the 18th century, but his influence was most felt later, in the beginning and the middle of that century.   Born in Staffordshire, he entered Queen's College, Oxford, in 1664 at the age of 15.   He earned his medical degree there in 1680 and later settled in Litchfield to practice.   Aside from the fact that he had advised Samuel Johnson to go to be touched by Queen Anne for cervical tuberculosis, he is known today for two of his books.   His earliest works, written between 1687 and 1696, are of no great consequence, being in the Galenic spirit. However, his *Treatise on Asthma*, first published in 1698 and again repeatedly until the mid-18th century, is note-worthy for its mention of spasm of the bronchi as the cause of the symptoms of asthma.   He noted the roles of heredity, atmospheric pollution, and apparent allergy as causes of asthma.   His book also contained the first record of post-mortem findings in emphysema - in a broken-winded horse.   Floyer's other important work was *The Physician's Pulse Watch*.   (Convinced of the necessity of counting the pulse accurately, he invented a special type of watch and published his invention in 1707.)   However, that book contained much more than studies of the pulse, since he also described variations in the rate and charac-ter of respiration and discussed their significance.   Re-garding the pulse rate itself, he described the effects of diet, blisters, sleep, age, and pregnancy, among other fac-tors.   Floyer's work on the pulse rate was not only ne-glected but ridiculed, until late in the century when men such as Heberden recommended it.   In contrast, his obser-vations on respiratory disorders were appreciated widely (Neuberger, 1948).

Radcliffe, another Oxford alumnus, became notable in other ways.   He was the son of a man of strongly inde-pendent opinions, who vigorously expressed his republican principles at a time when they were not popular.   Also, he developed an independent personality.   He attended local schools and then entered University College, Oxford, at the age of 15 in 1655.   He gained honors in logic, but after obtaining the B.A. and M.A. degrees and a fellowship, he turned to medicine.   He earned the M.D. in 1675, and in 1682 earned the title of "grand compounder."   More witty than wise, he was no scholar, and relied on his quick mind more than on learning.   Since most of the learning then being expounded was wrong, that might have been an advantage.   He began his practice in Oxford and soon managed to offend not only the local physicians but the University authorities.   He moved to London, and there his practice grew remarkably through his taking over that of the recently deceased Lower.   His witty conversation seemed to have curative effects; either that, or his quick mind enabled him to learn clinical medicine rapidly.   At any rate, he practiced successfully among the rich and famous, becoming both himself.   He effected some remarkable cures of the King and members of the Court, as well as some remarkable predictions about the imminent demise of some of them.   Radcliffe was a member of Parliament and became a Governor of St. Bartholomew's Hospital. When his health began to fail early in the 18th century, he passed much of his practice on to Mead.   Among the bits of advice he gave Mead was never to be civil to a patient, advice that often is followed today.   Radcliffe never married, and upon his death Oxford University inherited his huge fortune, the money going to the support of various enterprises including the founding of the Radcliffe Infirmary.   He is an example of a man educated at a grossly inadequate school but able to learn enough medicine in a busy practice to become far from inadequate.   Apparently he realized the necessity of clinical experience, as evidenced by his founding a hospital as a way of helping his old school, dormant for a century or more, to enter the mainstream of medical education.

Thus, an interest in clinical observation was developing among English university-trained physicians, a process that was to indicate appreciation of the fact that whatever their origins and training, the physicians of England were to become leaders in clinical medicine.

The history of English medicine during the 17th century usually is presented as an account of two opposing schools of thought: the academic or theory-bound, and the practitioners' or patient-oriented.   That formal division, regrettably, submerges other trends too ill-defined to be called "schools of thought."   There seem to have been numbers of practitioners who, without much thought of what school of medicine they followed, practiced good medicine.

One such practitioner was Woodall (Power, 1912). Born around 1569, he was in the British Army fighting in France 20 years later.   Afterward he traveled widely in France, Germany, and Poland practicing surgery, which he must have learned as an apprentice in the army.   He returned to England in 1603 and soon thereafter was appointed Surgeon-General to the East India Company.   He must have had considerable knowledge and skill, for in 1616 he also was made Surgeon to St. Bartholomew's Hospital.   He published textbooks of surgery in 1617 and 1628, and those remained the standards for many years for surgeons in practice, both at sea and on land.   His familiarity with reports from ships returning from long voyages called his attention to the fact that the accidental inclusion of limes in the diet of a single East Indiaman had prevented scurvy in circumstances that would have caused the disease on other ships.   Woodall exemplifies the facts that a lack of formal education is not a necessary bar to excellence in medical practice within limits and that the good clinician is one who takes advantage of accidental circumstances to enlarge his knowledge.   However, a self-directed man like Woodall probably would have been an outstanding clinician no matter what his training, as long as a large part of it involved observations on patients, and as long as he continued to learn from them.   Most physicians, however, need a good deal of guidance in their early years and afterward.   Irregular physicians who succumb to - or create - superstitions for their medical practice can do dreadful harm.

Garrison's comment that the physicians of earlier eras must have been doing something correct is supported by English 17th-century experience.   When England's hospitals were opened in response to requirements of Poor Law, the mortality rates improved (Thomas, 1980).   Clearly, the English physicians of 300 years ago were not practicing 20th-century medicine and even could not imagine its large scientific content.   This raises a question about whether today's so-called "scientific" physicians are doing something different from what they think they are doing.   The aspects of medical care which are responsible for clinical improvement may be different in different cases and certainly are not related to current scientific theory.

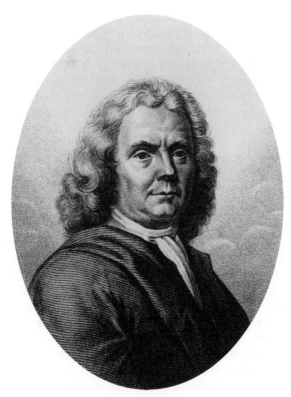

Hermann Boerhaave, 1668-1738

LEYDEN'S RISE TO PROMINENCE IN MEDICINE in the 17th and 18th centuries hardly could have been predicted. What most of us remember about the premodern Dutch nation is mainly the fierce conflict between the Dutch and the Spaniards, which began with Charles I of Spain, a Hapsburg, who was elected Holy Roman Emperor Charles V in 1519. A man suffering from deep and persistent melancholia, he had a poor start in life. His mother, known as Jeanne la Folle (or in Spanish, Juana la Loca) had a post-partum psychosis and was psychotic probably most of her life as a result. (Her portrait, hanging today in the Spanish Embassy in London, shows a young woman whose face and attitude suggest catatonia.) The Netherlands belonged to Spain, and the Netherlanders' Reformation activities were countered strongly by Charles and later by his son, Philip II. When Calvinism became entrenched in the Netherlands in the 1560s, the Spanish repression became increasingly severe. The Dutch War of Liberation began in 1572, with William of Orange elected Stadtholder, or Head of State. The war went on with increasing ferocity, until a peace, of sorts, was signed in 1579. The southern provinces of the Netherlands (now approximately Belgium) recognized Philip II, but the seven northern provinces did not; and, in 1581 they renounced their allegiance to Spain. England was in and out of the conflict in support of the Dutch (the Spanish Armada was destroyed in 1588). A truce was signed between Spain and the Netherlands in 1609 and, to everyone's amazement, it was kept.

Shut in by France and by the German states, the Dutch turned to the sea and, in a remarkably short time, established an empire in the East Indies and beyond. This gave them great wealth, since the overland routes from there to Europe had been closed by the Asian Moslem conquests. Moreover, the Dutch were the only ones allowed to trade in Japan. As a dividend, they brought back to Europe in 1682 the first specific knowledge of acupuncture. Dutch men of science, mathematicians, and painters of the 17th and 18th centuries were among the world's leaders. The University of Leyden was said to have been founded in 1578 by William the Silent, as a reward for the town's performance in resisting a siege. According to legend, William offered the town the choice of either remission of taxes for 10 years or the founding of a university; the town chose the latter. It is against that background that the sudden development of Leyden as a great medical center becomes understandable. Since the main concern of this work is bedside medicine, the discoveries of medical scientists, physicians, or others will not be presented in detail. The modern practice of so-called *sick-bed* teaching was started by da Monte in 16th-century Padua. It was continued for a time by his successors after his death, but was dropped owing to objections by church authorities. However, a Dutch student at Padua, van Heurne, carried the concept back to Leyden, where he taught anatomy, medicine, and surgery from 1581 to 1601. In 1630 van Heurne's son Otto, joining with Shrevelius, started bedside instruction twice weekly at Leyden, but this teaching seemed to have been extracurricular and unofficial until 1635, when two salaried professors began to carry it out under formal auspices. It is possible that the institution of bedside teaching at Montpellier in 1634 stimulated the authorities at Leyden to formalize the clinical instruction.

The first Professor of Medicine at Leyden was van Foreest (Forestus), who was appointed in 1575. He graduated at Bologna in 1543 and took additional study at Padua and Paris. Although author of a then-famous compilation of therapeutic opinion, he found medical practice more to his taste than teaching and, therefore, gave up his post. Another early professor was de Bondt (Bontius), a graduate of Padua appointed originally to the post of Professor of Physics and Mathematics at Leyden, but who later became Professor of Anatomy and Botany in 1581. Paaw, who had studied anatomy at Padua under Fabricius, Harvey's teacher, became Professor of Anatomy in 1597, leaving botany to de Bondt. A number of teachers of lesser note followed, and then, around the middle of the

17th century, the Leyden faculty of medicine began to achieve fame when de le Boë started teaching there. (He also was called Sylvius, not to be confused with the 16th-century French physician de Bois, likewise called Sylvius.) The career and works of de le Boë have not been studied extensively, but something about them is known (Gubser, 1966).

De le Boë was descended from wealthy Huguenots who had fled from Cambrai in France to Hanau in Germany. Following his early schooling in Germany, he studied medicine and philosophy at Sedan and, after some wanderings, studied medicine and botany at Leyden. While there, he wrote a pamphlet called *Various Medical Propositions* (1634) and in 1637 earned the M.D. degree at Basle with a thesis on the physiology of movement. He then became Professor of Anatomy at Leyden and quickly achieved a reputation as an outstanding teacher. (He described the aqueduct of Sylvius, the Sylvian fissure, and other structures.) It is difficult to evaluate his career: he has not been a popular subject for historians, being overshadowed by the phenomenal brilliance of his successor, Boerhaave. It is probable, moreover, that the attachment of his name to certain anatomical features has exaggerated the importance of anatomy in his career, although his contemporaries considered him to be the greatest teacher of that subject. He is perhaps best known today as the probable formal founder of the iatrochemical school. Although initially Professor of Anatomy at Leyden, he began to practice medicine at Amsterdam a few years after assuming that post, returning to Leyden after 14 years (in 1658) as Professor of Practical Medicine. He became Rector of the University in 1669.

When de le Boë took the Chair of Medical Practice at Leyden, he quickly became recognized as an enthusiastic bedside teacher. In his own words he stated the following (Grubser, 1966):

> Called some five years ago and more to the chair of medicine, I at length assumed it, and have endeavored with all my might to make sure that my auditors should profit as much as possible by my industry and labor and

go out as excellent physicians. To this end I pursued not only those things that it was truly necessary for them to investigate and find out, I went further in my way of teaching them, using especially a method not hitherto in use here nor perhaps elsewhere. I led them by the very hand into the practice of medicine, *i.e.*, I took them daily into the public hospital for the purpose of seeing the sick to whose complaints and other notable symptoms I directed attention, asking immediately afterwards what they had observed in the disorders of the patient; their views as to the causes and proper treatment and their reasons for the same. Whenever differences of opinion arose among them concerning these things, I, in a quiet way, pitted against each other those holding different opinions, in order that they might mutually satisfy themselves by as solid reasons as possible drawn from every source, finally giving my own judgment regarding the various views. With me they confirmed the happy results of the treatment, when God rewarded our labors by the return to health of the patients, or assisted in the examination of the cadavers when the patients finally paid the inevitable tribute to death.

His colleague, Schacht, described his method of instruction as follows:

When he came with his pupils to the patient and began to teach, he appeared completely in the dark as to the causes or the nature of the affection the patient was suffering from, and at first expressed no opinion upon the case; he then began by questions put to different members of his audience to fish out (*expiscabatur*) everything and finally united the facts discovered in this manner into a complete picture of the disease in such a way that the students received the impression that they had themselves made the diagnosis and not learnt it from him. (Baker, 1909)

De le Boë was thus the initiator of student participation in bedside teaching. An active experimenter in the field of chemistry, he created a system of medicine that blended data from simple chemical studies, such as fermentation and effervescence, with observations made by him and others on glandular secretions and nervous function. In particular, the findings of Harvey were given a central role in his thinking. In short, he was a great academician, uniting all available, seemingly relevant basic science, valid or invalid, in his explanations of the phenomena of disease, as well as the effects of drugs. For example, although he described tubercles in the lung and related them to consumption and the formation of cavities, he naturally knew nothing of the existence of the tubercle bacilli and chose to regard tubercles as having originated from the extravasation of blood. Owing to the fragmentary nature of chemical and physiologic data, he was forced to make such Galenic concepts as humors, spirits, and so forth, the bulk of his formulations. Nevertheless, he was remarkably convincing, and many physicians followed him. He did deny some of the old superstitions involving astrological concepts and, more particularly, the existence of witchcraft, and he rigorously rejected the mystical superstitions of Paracelsus and von Helmont.

De le Boë tried to explain all life, normal or diseased, in analogies based on what was observable in simple laboratory experiments (Lindeboom, 1972). In addition to fermentation and effervescence, he postulated that a basic process in all life was the interaction of acids and alkali. He believed that excessive acidity or alkalinity in the blood, as expressed in the humors, was the cause of dysfunction of the different organs bathed by it. He explained body heat as the result of the effervescent action of chyle on the blood. (This was different from the Galenic notion that the beating of the heart was responsible for heating the body, as proved, some believed, by the fact that the body cooled rapidly when the heart stopped beating. If that phenomenon were to be studied today by the use of modern statistical methods, the correlation co-efficient would be sensationally high, thereby proving, by today's reasoning, the truth of Galen's proposition and the falsity of de le Boë's.)

Despite all of this preoccupation with contemporary biological and chemical science and our conception of de le Boë as an early and leading iatrochemist, we must recognize the fact that he was a great clinical teacher at the bedside in his teaching ward. His real contribution to bedside teaching was to stimulate others to pursue it; hence, we are likely to forget his importance in keeping that kind of teaching alive after its introduction from Padua. Actually, it was not until the phenomenal advance in clinical medicine produced by Sydenham, his contemporary, that bedside teaching became highly important in medical history. The roles of de le Boë in Leyden and earlier of da Monte in Padua in the development of such teaching have been developed more in retrospect than in the then-contemporary accounts.

The facility with which men like de le Boë accepted iatromathematical and iatrochemical superstitions may surprise some of todays's physicians (who willingly accept today's superstitions). As for iatromathematics, we must remember the admiration given the work of Descartes, the Paris high-school dropout who became famous, then living in the Netherlands. When Descartes dreamed his dream of explaining all of biology and medicine in terms of physics and the mathematics that accompanied it, he stimulated a revolution in medical thinking. Many leaders of academic medicine became iatromechanists or iatromathematicians. In 1696 Baglivi wrote, "Since doctors have begun to examine the structure and action of the living body on the basis of geometrical and mechanical principles, they have not only discovered innumerable phenomena unknown to preceding centuries, but have also realized as far as its natural actions are concerned, the human body is nothing more than a complex system of mechanical and chemical movements that obey mathematical laws." In short, according to Baglivi, the body was a machine; however, the introduction of the then-current mathematics into biology and medicine served only to confuse medicine (Moravia,

1978).   That mathematical notion became established in academic medicine, despite Descartes' own view expressed earlier that it was far too difficult to explain a human being in that way, because the gap between the laws that governed the earth and the planets was too far removed from humans to permit an understanding of human nature. In 1707 Guglielmini, a Bolognese physician, wrote words that should have had an even more sobering effect on the iatromechanists.   He wrote about how in his youth Aristotelian concepts comprised all of medicine, but shortly afterward "physiologists proclaimed the necessity for closer contact with the physicists while repudiating the Aristotelian doctrines and introducing into the medical field the systems of Descartes and Gassendi, systems which have been distorted to a point at which they can no longer tell upon what physiological foundations a doctor bases his personal theories or establishes his therapy."   Despite those disclaimers, iatromechanism, iatrophysics, and iatrochemistry (it was difficult to separate them) became established as the mode used to explain clinical phenomena in basic terms.   The teachers, who were under great pressure to explain things, found those systems to be what they needed.

Striking evidence of the influence of the iatrochemical and iatromathematical schools is afforded by Jacob Bruno's revision of a famous medical dictionary by Castelli.   The dictionary was first published in Messina in 1598 and was a listing of all the known medical terms and their meanings, based on references in the available literature.   Bruno, Professor of Medicine at the University of Altdorf, revised that work in 1682 and again in 1687, much of his revision consisting of the addition of the content of the chemistry and physics of the time.

The death of de le Boë in 1672 created a situation that can be regarded with amusement in retrospect, but which should teach a serious lesson to boards responsible for academic appointments.   Craanen, de le Boë's successor, born in Cologne in 1620, was called to Nijmegen in 1661 to teach philosophy, geometry, and medicine.   Nijmegen was not an outstanding clinical center.   In 1670 he was appointed Professor of Logic and Metaphysics at Leyden after having made a reputation for himself as an expounder and explicator of Cartesian doctrines. He was not popular with either the students or the other men on the faculty of the University and had a reputation for abrasiveness and ill temper notable even in Leyden. In 1673 he was removed from his post in philosophy but was given de le Boë's old chair in Medicine. He preferred no bedside teaching and confined himself to explaining everything in terms of Cartesian principles. In 1683 he refused absolutely to conduct bedside teaching and in 1684 chose to teach geometry instead. Two years later he went to Brandenberg to become Physician to the Elector there. Before he left, he persuaded a small group of Dutch physicians to become iatromechanists, that is, medical Cartesians. Their certainty with regard to everything stultified for a time any strong tendency to enquiry and the progress that might have ensued.

The next great Leyden figure in the history of clinical teaching was Boerhaave. Unlike Sydenham, who had no academic connections (although he did have some followers in the English academic world, notably at Cambridge), Boerhaave's entire career was in an academic framework. Consequently, Boerhaave's ideas which, in the clinical sphere were derived from Sydenham's, had the acceptance that academic position always affords. Accordingly, Boerhaave became more important than Sydenham in the spread of bedside medicine and its development into the core of medicine in the 19th and early 20th centuries.

Boerhaave was born in 1668 at Voorhout, near Leyden, the son of a minister. He developed a stubborn ulcer on his thigh and, accordingly, was sent to school in Leyden to be near his doctors. Such were his industry and his brilliance that he was allowed to enter the University of Leyden before he was 15 years of age, an early indication of his great potential. His fame as an adult was so great that he was the subject of a 30-page biography by Samuel Johnson in 1739 (Black, 1959). Others also wrote about him only a short time later. Today, we owe our knowledge of Boerhaave to the extensive research and writings of Lindeboom (1962, 1964, 1969, 1970)

By the time Boerhaave began to study medicine in the 1690s he already had a degree in philosophy and was learned not only in its component subjects but also in geography, natural history, Latin, Greek, Hebrew, mathematics, and theology. In fact, he had planned on a career in the ministry but gave up the idea, apparently because he was suspected of having adopted the Pantheism of Spinoza. He received his degree in medicine in 1693, but so great was his interest in chemistry before then that from the beginning his teaching was full of chemical material that, in his opinion, was related to medicine. In 1701 when he started teaching, ostensibly in basic medicine, the students begged him for separate instruction in chemistry. He acted as professor of both subjects without title until 1709, when, after the death of the incumbent, Hooton, he was given the Chairs of Medicine and Botany. In 1714 the Chair of the Practice of Physic also was given to him, after the death of its incumbent, Bidloo (who today is better known as an anatomist). That post involved clinical teaching at the bedside and, hence, was of the greatest importance for the history of bedside teaching. During all of those years he continued his unofficial teaching of chemistry until, after the death of Professor Le Mort in 1718, Boerhaave inherited that chair as well.

In the meantime Boerhaave had started a correspondence with physicians and scientists all over Europe, exchanging information, plant specimens, seeds, and so forth. In his day his great reputation depended in large part on his broad knowledge of the collateral sciences of botany, mathematics, and chemistry, as well as his skill in applying that information to the discussion of problems of medicine as they presented at bedside. Such collateral (or basic) information was largely erroneous or suppositious; however, he was able to use it convincingly in his teaching. One difficulty that arose was that the iatrochemists applied the data of testtube experiments (mostly inorganic) to medicine entirely by means of imprecise conjecture and dubious analogy. Not everyone accepted that. One leader of German medicine, Stahl, rejected those conjectures and analogies and made it emphatically clear that one simply could not detect the findings of testtube experiments in living systems. Nevertheless, Boerhaave took a different approach (Jevons, 1962; Lindeboom, 1972), using the principles of hydraulics and mechanics, together with those of chemistry, to produce a highly convincing system that chemistry pervaded but did not dominate. Regrettably, the system was almost entirely wrong, either as such or in its interpretation of observations. Although it was considered to be a most impressive accomplishment, his version of chemistry in medicine had no lasting effects, except insofar as it stimulated the thinking of Haller, who became one of the greatest physiologists of all time. Boerhaave's first book, *Institutiones Medicae* (1708), contained much in the way of chemical and mechanical explanations of medical phenomena, and although regarded as a work of genius 250 years ago, it is most unimpressive today. Boerhaave did not publish his famous *Elementa Chemiae* until 1732; he was caught in that familiar academic trap of having to explain everything. For example, Boerhaave turned his original chemical thinking to anatomy, taking what was known and concluding that the body had two components, the solids and the liquids. From that he proceeded to devise a classification of diseases based on that obvious fact (Lindeboom, 1970).

There were two distinct features of Boerhaave's medical career-the teaching of chemistry and the teaching of bedside medicine-plus a number of subsidiary items. It is obvious that Boerhaave had to make a decision regarding the extent of their blending. He had to reject the strongly stated opinion of his ideal, Sydenham, who maintained that there was no need to study chemistry, because its content had no place in clinical medicine. Boerhaave also had to reject the equally strongly stated opinion of Stahl, a physician and chemist of enormous prestige, that chemistry, important as it was to learn, should not be involved with medical thinking. Stahl, although best known today as a chemist and the originator of the Phlogiston Theory (one that held back science for years), had no use for anatomy or chemistry in medicine. At that time Stahl was Professor of Medicine at Halle and preferred to deal with the problems of medicine as entirely psychosomatic. He believed, as had Plato, that the soul formed, directed, and controlled the body, the latter serving only as a protective envelope for the former. He was overtly psychotic in the latter years of his life, but his ideas were treated as gospel. At Montpellier, for example, his works were translated and worshipped 50 years after his death in a manner reminiscent of that accorded those of Freud by the more orthodox of his followers today. (The translators and commentators who created that remarkable multivolume work went to considerable length to say what Stahl, often vague and obscure, really meant. In that they resembled theologians who, although worshipping, told God what he could do and think.)

Despite opposition, Boerhaave was influenced into using chemistry by the strong Leyden tradition about the usefulness of blending as much chemistry as possible into clinical medicine. Not only was one of Boerhaave's predecessors, de le Boë, a confirmed iatrochemist, in the Chair of Medicine, but Boerhaave's immediate predecessor in the Chair of Chemistry was Le Mort, who in 1696 published his well-received *Chymia Medico-Physica*. Boerhaave made himself expert in all of the available chemical information, be it true, false, or ambiguous and, in his defense, it must be noted that he made careful selections, rejecting large segments of what iatrochemists accepted. Nevertheless, he retarded the growth of medicine by disregarding the enmity felt between iatrochemists and iatromathematicians and blended elements of both in his teaching. Moreover, those were combined with a certain amount of the unsinkable Galenism that had survived.

When Boerhaave published his medical text, *The Aphorisms* (1709), it, too, was regarded with awe. His pupil, van Swieten, became famous with his translation of that work, which he carried to Vienna. Regrettably, it was most unimpressive and absolutely absurd in certain areas. Since it contained little that was original (King, 1970), Boerhaave only showed himself to be a skilled "blender." The art of mere compilation is not likely to produce a great clinician, and since one aspect of Boerhaave's genius was his ability to compile, select, and organize disparate data and ideas, it is natural to compare him to Hoffman of Halle, one of the greatest organizers of medical thought of his era and Stahl's rival. Indeed, Boerhaave borrowed extensively from him. However great Hoffman's renown, he had no large numbers of students and scholars constantly in attendance; rather, his students were mediocre and did not become creators of great schools like those of Edinburgh and Vienna. In short, being a great compiler and organizer was not then, nor is it now, enough to make a physician a great clinician.

Despite the inadequacies of his theoretical conceptions of medicine, bodily function, and the action of mechanical and chemical factors in the body, Boerhaave must be regarded as the great clinical teacher of his era, because of his brilliance at the bedside. That cannot be established from the clinical reports he published, for he published few. In that he differed from Sydenham who, since he was not involved in the academic teaching of medicine, needed to write only clinical reports, which he did brilliantly with the help of Locke and other friends. He also differed from Sydenham in that he developed a school of medical teaching based on the bedside. A large number of physicians studied under him, and when they returned to their own countries, took with them the concept that medicine had to be taught using the patients themselves.

In effect, Boerhaave founded several schools. When the medical school at Edinburgh was founded, its entire faculty was made up of Boerhaave's students. The influence of Edinburgh on modern medical education and practice was enormous, as will be discussed later. However, the influence of Leyden on Scotland was evident even before Boerhaave became famous in Leyden. Although the influence of Leyden in the establishment and teaching at Vienna and Edinburgh may be recognized, the important role of Leyden's men on medicine elsewhere in Scotland, England, and Ireland is not appreciated widely. Boerhaave had 746 English-speaking students, many of whom went on to distinguished careers in Great Britain and Ireland (Underwood, 1977). The reform of military medical practice in Great Britain was instituted by one of his students, Pringle (Lindeboom, 1969, 1972, 1974). In addition, two Frenchmen must be listed among the distinguished men of Leyden, Boerhaave's men: de Jaucourt, the author of the sections on medicine in Diderot's *Encyclopedie* (see Chapter 6), and la Mettrie, a figure in the Anglo-French Enlightenment of the 18th century. One of the most interesting offshoots of Boerhaave's teaching was the orderly organization of the study of taxonomy, especially with respect to botany, by his student, Linnaeus.

Eighteenth-century Leyden also played an important part in the development of American medical education. A few Americans had studied at Leyden in the 17th century, one of whom was Fuller, physician to the Pilgrims on the Mayflower and in Massachusetts, although he was not a qualified doctor. Several others have been recorded in the 17th century (Guthrie, 1959). In the 18th century the list included Bond and Redman of Philadelphia, the latter also having studied at Edinburgh. Jacob Smith, Professor of Materia Medica at King's College, New York, was a Leyden man, as was John Jones, Professor of Surgery at that institution. Jones also studied at Edinburgh and Paris and served in the Revolutionary War with distinction before settling in Philadelphia. Arthur Lee of Virginia received M.D. degrees at Leyden and Edinburgh, and after a short period in practice in Virginia, he returned to London to study law, subsequently becoming American Ambassador to France. Still another American Leyden man was Wells who, after graduating in 1780, spent most of his life practicing medicine in London and was Physician to St. Thomas' Hospital. He wrote about the connection between rheumatism and heart disease in 1814, several decades before Bouillaud, who today receives the credit for the discovery. Also having an M.D. degree from Leyden was Waterhouse of Newport, Rhode Island. His other distinctions included the following: He was the only professor at the Harvard Medical School at that time to have an M.D. degree, and he introduced vaccination into Boston.

Late in life Boerhaave's illnesses necessitated his giving up a portion of his teaching, until he finally taught no more. At that time his logical successor might have been van Swieten, however, he was not acceptable to the Dutch because he was a Catholic. Maria Theresa of Austria called van Swieten to Vienna, whereupon after taking some of the Leyden faculty with him, he set Vienna on a road to medical greatness that lasted until the destruction of the Austro-Hungarian Empire after World War I.

The death of Boerhaave and the departure of much of the rest of the faculty at Leyden weakened the medical school, and the rise of Edinburgh largely cut off the flow of students from Great Britain, although a few still went to Leyden.

The history of Boerhaave's medicine became the history of medicine in many parts of the world, especially at Edinburgh and Vienna.   However, Göttingen, the Russian schools established by Peter the Great, and several American city universities also must be considered heirs of Leyden.

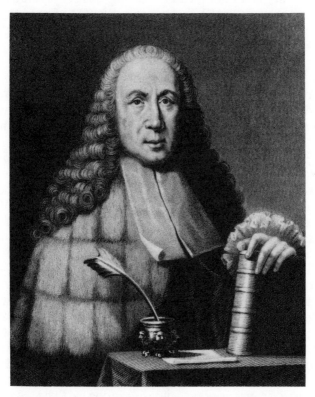

Giovanni Battista Morgagni, 1682–1771

Chapter 3: Gross Anatomy, Normal and Morbid, in the Early Development of Clinical Medicine

THE HISTORY OF CLINICAL MEDICINE is in large measure the history of a search for diagnostic precision and therapeutic effectiveness. The search for aids to diagnosis antecedes recorded history and is still in progress. As far as the search for therapeutic effectiveness, Galenism offered a purported clue in the doctrine of signatures, whereby the shape or color of a plant or plant product was held to indicate its effectiveness in diseases that in some way resembled the remedy. The other principle that underlay medical treatment was the use of procedures restoring the balance of quantities, or distribution, of the hypothetical humors.

In the Middle Ages and Renaissance physicians prescribed strong plant emetics and cathartics, vile and disgusting mixtures of animal products, and repeated bloodlettings, as well as such relatively minor hazards as blistering and scarifying procedures. The physician called to treat an illness in some prominent person always could declare, if the initial treatment was not beneficial, that he needed time to get the results of tests, which in that era consisted in the casting and reading of the horoscope or studying a copy of the Sphere of Life (unless he owned a portable version of the latter). A circle, the representation of the medieval, or perhaps ancient, *Sphere of Life and Death*, played an important role in predicting the outcomes of illnesses (Sigerist, 1942). It perhaps should be regarded as a very early type of mechanical aid to physicians who thought they needed such devices. (The Sphere of Life was a diagram used by *savants* and physicians to record relations between the forces that favor or otherwise determine the character of a person's life.) On the other hand, if a physician was called to see a prominent person wounded in a battle, tournament, or accident, he was forced to undertake effective treatment immediately, especially if hemorrhage still was occurring.   Such a physician might make a fatal error if ignorant of anatomy. Accordingly, by the 14th and 15th centuries military surgery was an actively growing, if mainly practical, art. (For example, Theodoric, an Italian bishop as well as a medical writer of the 13th century, complained that he was unable to keep up with the growing literature on the removal of arrows.) However skillful the military surgeons might have been, they, in fact, needed exact and accurate anatomical knowledge if they effectively were to treat the results of trauma. For those reasons and perhaps others, the study of anatomy played a large part in the initial development of modern medicine.   (Another kind of problem-an occupational hazard of knights in armor who, having been bolted in, could not function normally and hence developed hemorrhoids-also may have had some such effect.   Mandeville, an Englishman trained in France, developed an operative technique for the treatment of that condition.)

This is not to say that an interest in anatomy was purely due to the practical need of treating trauma. To some extent that interest had been manifested by philosophers and psychologists who wanted to be able to develop reasonable explanations about how things worked. For example, after the Greeks discovered the pineal gland (more than 2,000 years ago), they concluded that it must be a valve controlling the flow of memories from the rear cerebral ventricle (where they were stored) to the front ventricle (where they entered consciousness).   There was never any doubt about the existence of a memory valve, for observation had shown repeatedly that a man who had difficulty in remembering something was likely to shake his head or strike it, obviously to loosen the valve that was stuck.   (Although there were no statistics at that time to support the conclusion, it is obvious today that if such studies had been made, the correlation coefficient would have been spectacularly high.)

This is surely not the place to attempt a history of the development of the study of human anatomy. In this respect, Choulant's great work of a century or more ago is of particular importance, because it emphasizes the place of *illustration* in this history.   Others also have written about the earliest dissections, but it simply will be noted that the manual created by dei Luzzi of Bologna in the late 14th century was used widely by students for several centuries, although it was full of Galenic errors.   It was somewhat of a late-comer in the field, since physicians had been practicing human dissections for 100 years before dei Luzzi (Mackinney, 1962).   For example, after studying medicine at Bologna and Montpellier, de Mondeville gave an historic lecture on human anatomy before the medical faculty at Montpellier in 1304 and used the lecture two years later as the introductory portion of his projected five-volume surgical textbook.   Da Carpi, sometimes called "the first modern anatomist," published his commentaries on Mondino's work in 1521 and his own anatomical manual, *Isagogoa Brevis*, in 1522.   It perhaps is ironic that in England in 1532, only a decade or so before the publication of the works of Vesalius, Edwards published his anatomy (O'Malley and Russell, 1961), a work that followed Mondino and was clearly Galenic in inspiration. Edwards, who died in 1542, held the Chair of Greek at Corpus Christi College, Oxford, and then turned to medicine, becoming the interpreter of Galen at Cambridge and a practitioner in both places.   Perhaps his career should be taken as evidence of a classical revival in England which antedated the efforts of Linacre, who usually represented as the prime mover in that effort.

The work of Vesalius not only constituted a turning point in the history of anatomy, but also had important implications regarding clinical medicine and Western civilization in general (O'Malley and Saunders, 1943; Saunders and O'Malley, 1950).   Andreas Wesel, known as Vesalius, was the sixth in line in his family to be connected with medicine.   All were physicians except his father, who was an apothecary, a profession at that time regarded as having therapeutic duties connected almost entirely with the preparation and administration of medicinals.   From the first, Vesalius was surrounded by medical traditions and was able to read and study the medical manuscripts and other works that his family had accumulated.

Born in 1514 Vesalius entered the University of Louvain in 1528, where he pursued the usual classical and humanistic curriculum, although in his spare time he carried out anatomical studies on small animals.   Five years later he began his medical studies at Paris, where the curriculum was thoroughly Galenic.   Vesalius declared himself to be devoted to Galenic concepts and, indeed, on many occasions he later defined himself merely as a corrector of mistaken detail and a reconciler of Galen's data with his own.

There was no actual teaching of anatomy at Paris, and Vesalius taught himself the subject from the bones of criminals and others obtained from charnel houses and cemeteries.   He left Paris without graduating and returned to Louvain when war broke out between the Holy Roman Empire and France.   (As a Belgian, Vesalius was a subject of the former.)   In 1537 he began to teach anatomy to his fellow students at Louvain; moreover, he wrote his thesis and apparently graduated that year.   He then went to Padua and began to benefit from the bedside teaching of da Monte.   Also in that year Vesalius received his M.D. degree at Padua and the following *day* became Professor of Surgery.   He and da Monte became and remained close friends.   Whether or not that was responsible for Vesalius' strong clinical interests is not known, but the pursuit of those interests became an important part of his life.   Another aspect of his life which should not be minimized was the fact that he was a man of considerable aesthetic appreciation, as was shown by his choice of Titian to do the frontispiece of his *Fabrica* (1543) and of lesser artists to do the remarkable engravings for his *Tabulae Sex* (1538) and the *Fabrica*.   He was much more than an anatomist.

In 1538 Vesalius participated in the reworking of the Galenic corpus (*The Institutiones*) and a year later wrote his clinical note, now called the *Venesection Letter*, in which he supported Galenic views.   In 1541 he participated in the production of the complete works of Galen and, finally, in 1543, published his *De Humani Corporis Fabrica*, the great monument of observational science, anatomical illustration, and printing.   He gave a specially bound copy of the book to Emperor Charles V, who apparently deposited it in Louvain, where it was destroyed during the invasion of Belgium in 1914.   In 1544 Vesalius was invited to lecture at Padua, Bologna, and Pisa, but his triumph was tainted by attacks on his work.

When war broke out again between France and the Empire in 1544, Vesalius joined the Imperial Army as a military surgeon. During the siege of St. Dizier he and Paré, a noteworthy surgeon, were on opposite sides. After the siege, Vesalius became Personal Physician to the Emperor, a marked hypochondriac and a difficult patient. In the next years Vesalius made some remarkable clinical diagnoses. At one point, amid opposition from jealous contemporaries, he recommended draining a skull wound of the son of Philip II, thus saving his life. His greatest contribution to surgical practice was the reintroduction of the ancient operation of drainage for empyema. The second edition of the *Fabrica*, published in 1555, contained additional material on physiology. Both editions contained scattered descriptions of changes found in disease, and more than once he recommended post-mortem examinations to determine the nature of disease. He developed a very large practice, but his service with Charles' successor, Philip II, was not a happy one, and he relinquished it all to go on a pilgrimage to Jerusalem. He died at sea.

There is no need to discuss further the development of interest in normal anatomy as a science. Suffice it to say that outstanding surgeons such as de Mondeville, Paré, and Fabricius emphasized the importance of a thorough knowledge of anatomy for surgeons. Fabricius' comment was perhaps the most colorful: "While the young surgeons should apply themselves to the study of Anatomy, they make music, read the owl-glass, drink, fornicate, enjoy themselves or adorn their rooms and waste their time." His book *On The Excellence and Use of Anatomy* epitomized his convictions about the usefulness of the subject (Jones, 1960).

It would be an error, however, to conclude that only physicians interested in the career of surgery pursued anatomical studies. Many physicians regarded anatomical data as the substrate of physiologic understanding and, hence, the understanding of disease. Professors of medicine all over Europe considered knowledge of human anatomy essential. Many members of the Fincke-Bartholin dynasty, all related by blood or marriage, or both, and many others destined to become teachers of medicine in Copenhagen, studied anatomy in Padua, some of them under

Fabricius, the surgeon.   Some also studied at Leyden (Porter, 1963).   Thus, despite the disclaimers of Sydenham and Locke regarding the utility of anatomical knowledge in practice, the new anatomy became a part of medical education, replacing the Galenic errors, both intrinsic and extrinsic (*i.e.*, faulty translations).   Nevertheless, the effect of such studies on the practice of medicine was much more visible in surgery than in other areas.   In the 16th century the introduction of extensive microscopic observations by Malpighi, the phenomenally active practitioner of Bologna, had little effect on the study of anatomy, or on much else, for years to come (Adelmann, 1966, 1975; Belloni, 1967), as will be discussed elsewhere.

A discussion of the history of pathological anatomy (gross pathology) in detail will not be undertaken.   For one thing, Long's encyclopedic account (1965) covers it broadly, if perhaps thinly.   A 1935 address by Welch lists the names that will be the basis of a good part of this discussion.   (It would be well for the student especially interested in illustration in pathological anatomy to read Goldschmid's [1952] perceptive analysis.)   There are many ways in which to discuss the subject of gross anatomical pathology.   Only those aspects that bear on or reflect the practice of medicine and its teaching will be considered. Those philosophical questions relating to the influence of ideas about disease on the orientation of pathologic studies are best left to others (*e.g.*, Mayer [1952]).   The aim in this work is to study how leading medical practitioners used the findings of pathological anatomy.

How did medical practitioners (or at least some of them) know what a post-mortem entailed?   Performing a post-mortem examination implies a fairly accurate knowledge of normal anatomy plus at least a semblance of rational, verifiable concepts of disease.   Regarding the former, if accurate anatomical knowledge was nonexistent before Vesalius undermined the Galenic superstitions, what guided the physicians who performed post-mortem examinations 100 years earlier?   The answer probably is that Galenic anatomy was not totally erroneous.   It is true that its version of the anatomy of the vascular system, especially the veins and the brain, was absurd, and the inner details of some organs such as the heart not much better, but in other respects the Galenic descriptions were not completely wrong. Moreover, to anyone who had seen the intestines, liver, or lungs-even through Galenic eyes-the presence in or on them of gross masses or other abnormal appearances such as shagginess or perforations easily would be recognizable. At any rate, that is what happened even before Vesalius corrected matters. A few practitioners were doing post-mortem examinations definitely as early as the 14th century and telling about them in isolated pamphlets, vocally, or in letters to other physicians, scholars, or government figures. Some of those early reports were preserved only in later collections and, hence, are second-hand.

Regarding the second question-How could the post-mortem findings be explained unless the observers had reasonable concepts of disease?-the answer is that they could not. This is shown clearly by Benivieni in his collection of post-mortem findings in his patients. Although that information was collated some time before Benivieni's death (1502), it was published by his brother in 1507 (Major, 1935). The physician's descriptions of the diseases and the symptoms they caused are recognizable for the most part, though far from perfectly described. However, since his concepts of disease were the humoral concepts of the contemporary Galenism, Benivieni only could describe what he saw, not interpret it. It must be remembered that this was a half-century before Vesalius, who, however strongly he disagreed with Galenic anatomy, still accepted Galenic physiology. Other physicians did much the same as had Benivieni. Paré, Vesalius' contemporary, also wrote reports of his patients who had died and had post-mortem examinations (Hamey, 1960). Fernel and Bartholin published similar works.

By the end of the 17th century, the issue was clear: Pathological anatomy far outranked normal anatomy in importance to physicians. That was expressed clearly by Eustachio in his treatise on the kidney, by Bartholin in his *De Anatome Practica ex Cadaveribus Morbosis*, and most succinctly by Harvey, who said in his letter to Riolan, "The opening and dissection of one consumptive person or of a body spent with some ancient or venomous disease has more enriched the knowledge of Physick than the dissections of ten bodies of men that had been hanged." Bartholin's comments were even more impressive, for he distinguished between the anatomist as scientist (natural philosopher) preoccupied with normal findings and the anatomist as physician interested chiefly in morbid anatomy. There were many writings by others of lesser note.

Such information was to be used by Bonet, who was the grandson, son, brother, and uncle of well-known physicians. Born in Geneva, he had traveled widely when young and had received the M.D. degree at Bologna in 1643. He practiced in Geneva, at that time a melting pot of refugee Protestant scholars from other parts of Europe. His practice was extraordinarily busy, but it became more arduous as his hearing failed. Early in his career he became interested in scholarly pursuits related mainly to medicine and turned more and more to them in his later years. He wrote a clinical guide to physicians and analyzed case material in order to teach them. Moreover, he analyzed the earlier writings of others on the same subjects.

In his *Medicina Septentrionalis* (Northern Medicine), published in two volumes in 1684 and 1686, Bonet presented the ideas of Danish, English, French, and German physicians and philosophers. Many of the data and concepts had been sent to him in letters; others had been published. He also published Latin translations of the monthly memoires of the French Academy of New Discoveries in Medicine from 1680 to 1686. But his greatest work was *Sepulchretum Sive Anatomia et Practica ex Cadaveribus Morbo Donatis* (1679), a compendium of almost 3,000 clinical cases with their autopsy reports, gathered from medical literature of the Western World and including the writings of Vesalius.

The latter book was received with great enthusiasm (Irons, 1942). Bonet's massive compilation was more than a descriptive collection of diseases. It was, both in content and in actual words, a statement of what medicine should be, no longer fixed and based on authority, but fluid and based on bedside observation validated by postmortem study. He wrote,

> There are many things in this Art, wherein for Urgency's sake, it is a piece of Art to depart from Art. For though there be many legitimate and Regular Precepts, yet none are perpetual....For a Rational Physician cures not by Book or Commentary but as Experienced Reason dictates in every affair, and he ties himself to no unalterable rules....Art cannot be confined within so narrow bounds, there is need of Reason to consider all things; for in Cases there is a wonderful variety....There is no Reason without Experience; both Experience without Reason is invalid, and Reason without it is fallacious and captious....Though Reason will not yield to Experience in Dignity; yet in the meantime should Reason halt, let a man stand on Experience, which is the other Leg, and this is often of itself sufficient.

The words may be archaic, but the message is clear; regrettably, its acceptance has not been universal.   If it had, this book would end here.

The idea that post-mortem examinations and associated retrospective clinical correlations might be highly important in medicine had a mixed reception.   However, many prominent physicians adopted it.   Pechlin, originally of Leyden and subsequently Professor of Medicine at Kiel, published his *Observationium Physico-Medicorium* in 1691. Valsalva gathered such material also from his own practice. In 1707 Lancisi, Physician to the Pope, wrote his treatise on sudden death, *De Subitimeis Mortibus*, in which he showed that heart disease and brain disease were responsible.   That was perhaps the earliest attempt to narrow the post-mortem studies to a single area.   Another example of that approach was afforded by Cleghorn's publication in 1751 of his *Observations on the Epidemical Diseases in Minorca*.   Note should be taken also of Clossy, who started in pathological anatomy in Dublin and then crossed the ocean to New York's King's College (later Columbia University) as Professor of Anatomy (Stookey, 1964).   It is ironic that men like Eustachius, Valsalva, and Bartholin, who considered themselves primarily physicians, are known today only because of some anatomical eponym. (This perhaps explains why what purports to be the history of medicine has evoked so little interest among medical students and practitioners.)

In some quarters the idea that clinicopathological correlations might be useful to physicians received a different reception. In Switzerland, Wepfer had been authorized in 1650 to perform post-mortem examinations on all who died in the Schaffhausen municipal hospital, and later von Muralt was given the same privilege in Zurich. However, when von Muralt retired in 1724 the idea was rejected, and his successor, Burkhardt, some years later was threatened with bodily harm if he did necropsies. Finally the tide turned in 1752, when Burkhardt was allowed to restore the previous practice, becoming salaried prosector to a Zurich hospital with no university connections. He accumulated a large amount of clinicopathological material in the next 22 years (Frenk, 1958). Similarly, when in 1745 van Swieten left Leyden to become Head of Medicine in Vienna, he ordered that *all* patients who died in hospitals be examined post-mortem, thereby establishing a practice that contributed to Vienna's rise as a medical center.

Whatever doubts physicians or other persons might have had about the validity of the clinicopathological approach lessened rapidly, although they did not disappear entirely, after 1761. That was the year in which Morgagni published his *De Sedibus et Causas Morborum* (On the Sites and Causes of Disease). The *causes* he referred to were the immediate causes, not the ultimate causes, for there was no great bulk of collateral scientific material with which to establish the ultimate causes. Morgagni wrote the book to correct Bonet's *Sepulchretum* which, because it was too much for any one man to handle, had many redundancies and errors both of fact and attribution. Morgagni modestly indicated that his *De Sedibus* was to a large extent derivative, but modesty was his habit, as was the case when he stated that he had learned all of his medicine from Malpighi and all of his anatomy from Valsalva.

Morgagni was another of the young geniuses who grew up to have a great and lasting influence on medicine.

Born in 1682, by the turn of the century he already had placed behind him several years of poetry composition and essay writing, some of the latter on complex philosophical subjects.   At the age of 16 he began his studies at Bologna under Valsalva, receiving his medical degree at 19, and becoming President of the Scientific Academy at 24. He published his first medical work that year and became lecturer and prosector of the anatomical theatre at Bologna.   At the age of 29 he was called to teach therapeutics at Padua, and at 33 he was Professor of Anatomy there.   His anatomical publications made him famous throughout Europe.   Regrettably, probably only 20% of his total writings have been translated into English from the Latin, and this includes none of his writings on comparative anatomy, archaeology, the classics, poetry, philology, and philosophy.   At one point he wrote 100 clinical cases in Italian, but the rest of his writing remains in Latin, mostly unpublished.   He continued teaching and writing until his death in 1771.

Although his title was Professor of Anatomy, Morgagni was an excellent bedside clinician.   His greatest work, *De Sedibus*, was written when he already had achieved great fame; the book only enhanced it, for it was written in accordance with his belief that post-mortem examinations are useful only when performed by an experienced physician with great knowledge of both normal anatomy and clinical medicine.   The autopsy reports, he maintained, must be accompanied always by detailed accurate clinical reports.   Hence, unlike Bonet, who gave us a formless mass of heterogeneous material, Morgagni produced an ordered, logical body of information (Castiglioni, 1941; Jarcho, 1948, 1961; Klemperer, 1958).   Jarcho (1948) gave us a particularly scholarly and sympathetic discussion of Morgagni's versatility as a scientist and man of letters. Morgagni's *De Sedibus* had widespread acclaim and use, both in its Latin version and in the fine English translation published by Alexander in 1769.

Morgagni gave the study and presentation of clinico-pathological correlations form and meaning; however, he did recognize that in short acute illnesses, the post-mortem findings might be trivial.   In his day there was little information available on the functions of organs and of morbid processes: Physiology and pathogenesis still were expounded in Galenic terms, perhaps modified by the fuzzy nonsense of iatrophysics. Acrimonious humors displaced or made viscid by ill winds or other factors, together with "irritating particles," made up the basis of his ideas about pathogenesis. It is evident that his great work-a landmark-was only a milestone on a long, yet to be traveled road (Jarcho, 1948).

Another milestone, less prominent but not less significant, was created by Baillie in *The Morbid Anatomy of Some of the Most Important Parts of the Human Body* (1793), with its associated atlas published between 1799 and 1803. Baillie was born in Lanarkshire, the son of a minister, who later became Professor of Divinity at Glasgow. His mother was a sister of William and John Hunter. After early education at local schools, he entered the University of Glasgow, but at the age of 18 went to London as William Hunter's house-pupil and then assistant. He entered Balliol College, Oxford, but returned to Hunter's private medical school and museum during his vacations. After his uncle's death, Baillie, still without his degree, became head of the school and commenced to lecture on normal and pathological anatomy. In 1787, having obtained the M.B. degree, he was elected Physician to St. George's, one of the early London teaching hospitals. In 1789 he took the M.D. degree.

Baillie's expertness was recognized early; he received many honors and was Physician Extraordinary to George III. Baillie saw patients or wrote letters 16 hours daily and took no vacations; however, his medical practice grew to such a degree that in 1799 he resigned from St. George's Hospital and gave up lecturing at his institute. He was noted for his gentleness with patients, but was equally well known to respond irritably to foolish comments and questions, although considerate of the intelligent opinions of others. His exposition of clinical problems was at all times clear and precise. His clinical writings, although praiseworthy, do not have the high originality of his observations on morbid anatomy. His great pathology treatise had eight English, three American, and two French versions, as well as one each in German, Italian, and Russian. It was less influential than Morgagni's work, largely because it presented no concepts to explain the origin and nature of what was found; instead it was a straightforward account, organ by organ, of the pathologic findings, with relatively less on the clinical aspects (Rodin, 1973).   In short, it was the first example of a modern textbook of pathology, in which pathology was treated as a separate, but not quite independent, subject.   In that sense it was a landmark.

Both the great Morgagni and the lesser Baillie made contributions that were submerged by the developments of the early 19th century, which will be discussed later. Nevertheless, those subsequent developments were stimulated by such earlier works.

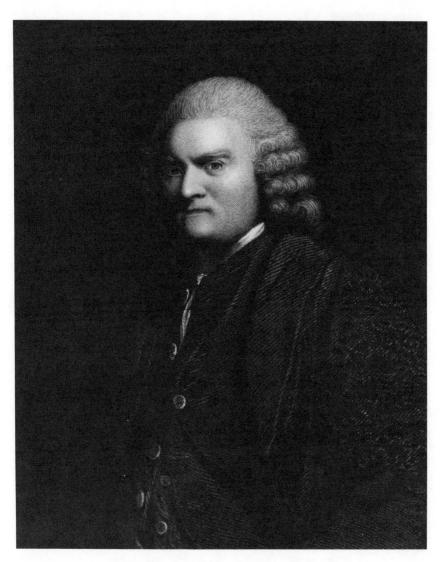

John Pringle, 1707–1783

Chapter 4: Scottish Medicine
During and After the Eighteenth Century

THE DEVELOPMENT OF PADUAN CLINICAL MEDICINE occurred within a university framework and was contemporaneous with progress in the biological and physical sciences in the 16th century. These conditions today would be regarded as the only ones likely to produce such clinical progress. Although the English universities saw great progress in the natural sciences in the 16th and early 17th centuries, however, the medicine they taught was dogmatic and superstitious, and the growth of English clinical medicine had to occur separately from the universities. At Leyden, the remarkable development of clinical medicine also occurred within the university structure (although Boerhaave taught privately for a time), but that clinical development was accompanied by the simultaneous establishment of iatromechanical and iatrochemical superstitions, outgrowths of advances in the natural sciences. Fortunately, those superstitions did not noticeably impair the growth of clinical medicine. It is evident, however, that there was no general correlation between scientific progress and the development of clinical medicine. The inclusion in medicine of the scientific data of the time, if it occurred, could have effects that were either good, bad, or both simultaneously. Similarly, a connection with an established university was no guarantee of good medical teaching-Oxford and Montpellier were notably bad-nor was the lack of such a connection an absolute bar to good clinical teaching.

The situation at Edinburgh exemplified the latter point. Edinburgh medicine was established by Leyden men, at first without the University playing any part in the teaching. In fact, the University's role remained ambiguous in one way or another for almost a century. However, Edinburgh clearly was the spiritual heir to Leyden's university medicine.

Scots had begun to study at Leyden's medical school early in the 17th century. For example, Gilbert Jack studied theology, philosophy, and medicine at Leyden, taking his M.D. degree there in 1611, and he served as Professor of Philosophy at Leyden from 1604 until his death in 1628.   Another early Scottish student at Leyden was Leighton, who received the M.D. degree there in 1617 at the age of 49, after he had practiced medicine in Leyden for some years.   He returned to Edinburgh to practice and became famous, not for medical accomplishments, but for his violent attack on the episcopacy, for which he was fined #10,000 and had his ears cut off and his face branded with the letters "SS" (for "Sower of Sedition"). His son, Robert, became Bishop of Dunblane, Archbishop of Glasgow, and, in 1653, Principal of the University of Edinburgh.   So much for genetics.

The number of English-speaking students of medicine at Leyden before 1700 was large, and of those approximately 25% were Scottish.   In Boerhaave's time (1700-1738) the proportion was higher: 1,919 registered medical students, 659 of them English-speaking (205 Scottish, 340 English, 107 Irish, and 7 Colonials).   Shortly before Boerhaave began his teaching, an event occurred that linked Leyden and Scotland particularly closely: the appointment of Pitcairne in 1692 as Professor of Medicine at Leyden. Initially a student of theology and law, Pitcairne went to Padua and then took his M.D. degree at Rheims in 1680. Shortly afterward he was appointed by the authorities at Leyden to the Chair of Medicine.   Although he remained at Leyden for only slightly more than a year, his service there emphasized the link between Leyden and Edinburgh.

The founding of a Faculty of Medicine at the University of Edinburgh was the hope of Leyden men, and three Leyden men are remembered in that connection: Monro, founder of the great dynasty (Wright-St. Clair, 1964), Pitcairne, and Sibbald (notable also as a distinguished naturalist and Geographer Royal of Scotland). None of the three lived to see his hopes come to fruition.

Actually, the teaching of some medical subjects already had begun under auspices other than those of a university faculty of medicine.   The Royal College of Surgeons established chairs in anatomy and surgery (Guthrie, 1959), and later the Royal Medical Society became a force for education.   Anatomy at first was taught in Edinburgh by the Leyden men, Barthwick and Pitcairne, at the behest of the Barber-Surgeons; but, after 1706 it was taught by Robert Eliot, under the joint auspices of the Barber-Surgeons and the University itself. Botany was taught at the University by Preston, a Leyden man, and later by another, Alsten, who taught materia medica as well and was also in charge of the Royal Garden at Holyrood. Cranford, a Leyden M.D. and student of Boerhaave, was Professor of Chemistry at Edinburgh University. It is evident that anatomy, botany, and chemistry, as taught in Edinburgh before the founding of its Faculty of Medicine, were based on Leyden knowledge and training. When three Professors of Medicine-Pitcairne, Sibbald, and Halket, another Leyden man-were appointed at the University, they did no teaching of that subject. Finally, in 1724 the Town Council, upon the recommendation of the College of Physicians, appointed a professor who was supposed to lecture in medicine. He was another Leyden man, Porterfield, but he, too, gave no lectures. Such early attempts to develop a medical educational organization were clearly more often wishes than deeds.

At last, in 1726, the Faculty of Medicine was formally established at the University. The professors were Monro (*primus*) in Anatomy and Surgery; Rutherford (grandfather of Walter Scott) in the Practice of Medicine, which included bedside teaching; Plummer and Innes in Chemistry and Materia Medica; and Sinclair (or St. Clair) in so-called Institutes of Medicine, a subject that resembled physiology and pathophysiology. Of the five, four had been classmates at Leyden under Boerhaave, and the fifth, Rutherford, also had studied there.

When Leyden began to decline, Edinburgh was ready to take its place as the leading medical school in the Western World. However, before describing Edinburgh's place in 18th- and 19th-century medical education, other notable Edinburgh physicians who had been trained at Leyden but had developed their careers outside Edinburgh's university should be mentioned. They were Stevenson, first President of the Royal College of Physicians; Alexander Dick, another President and also a distinguished philanthropist and administrator, as well as friend of Samuel Johnson and Benjamin Franklin; Pringle, an Englishman and student at both Leyden and Edinburgh, and the founder of military medicine; Rule, first a practitioner of medicine and then Principal of the University from 1690 to 1701; and James Gregory, Professor of Medicine at King's College in Aberdeen (in succession to his father). Gregory's brother John succeeded him at Aberdeen and later went to Edinburgh as Professor of Medicine. In 1772 John Gregory published *On The Duties and Qualifications of a Physician*, a work whose content preceded that of Percival of Manchester, England, another Edinburgh student and Leyden M.D., who coined the term "medical ethics" in his book of that title. John Gregory collaborated with his successor as Professor of Medicine, Cullen. Cullen, in turn, was succeeded by John's son James, another Leyden man. Although Cullen had had no direct association with Leyden, his assistant, John Brown, had studied there.

Francis Home was another Edinburgh man of Leyden background who made important clinical contributions. Born in Edinburgh in 1719, he was apprenticed early to an Edinburgh practitioner and appointed surgeon to a regiment of dragoons in 1742, serving until the end of the War of the Austrian Succession in 1748. While on duty with his regiment in Flanders, he spent whatever free time he had in medical studies at Leyden. He ordered that the troops in the field were to drink no unboiled water. At the war's end he returned to Edinburgh to continue his studies, receiving his M.D. degree there in 1750. His doctoral dissertation presented on that occasion explored the topic of intermittent fevers and became so well known that it was regarded as the standard. In 1752 he joined the Royal College of Physicians, becoming its President in 1776. His *Principia Medicinae* (1758) was used widely in Britain and on the Continent. It contained material on diphtheria, a subject upon which he expanded in 1765, calling his work *An Enquiry into the Nature, Cause and Cure of Croup.* That classic description, a half-century before Bretonneau's celebrated discussion of the same subject, was noteworthy, but it was Bretonneau who gave the disease its name, *diphtheria.* In 1768 Home became Professor of Materia Medica at Edinburgh, the first to hold that chair. (Prior to this, the course was taught with botany.) In 1773 he was appointed to teach the Institutes of Medicine, but for some reason never was given the title of Professor.   His last book, *Clinical Experiments, Histories, and Dissections* (1780), was a treatise on pathology and pathophysiology, in which he mentioned his discovery that the sugar in diabetic urine was fermentable by yeast.   He also wrote learnedly on bleaching and on agriculture, endeavoring to place both on a chemical basis.   He died at the age of 94 (Hume, 1942).

One of the famous Edinburgh alumni of Leyden's School of Medicine was Sir John Pringle, born in Roxburyshire in 1707.   He began his formal education in classics and philosophy at St. Andrews and moved to Edinburgh at the age of 20 to study medicine (Selwyn, 1966).   After a year he left to enter Leyden, where Haller and van Swieten were his classmates.   (Pringle had no high opinion of van Swieten.)   After two years of study he was granted the M.D. degree.   He then went to Paris and, after a short stay there, started practice in Edinburgh.   In 1739 he became Professor of Pneumatical and Ethical Philosophy at Edinburgh.   (Pneumatical philosophy was psychology, the name being derived from *pneuma*, the soul [Altschule, 1965].)   His lectures on moral philosophy, given in Latin, almost had the force and form of sermons.   He continued to practice medicine, however, and in 1742 he was appointed Physician to the British Army.   Although he was away from Edinburgh, he was allowed to keep the Chair in Philosophy until 1745, when he became Physician-General of the Army and resigned at Edinburgh.   He served for six years, both in England and in Flanders, and then began to practice medicine in London, where he soon prospered. Two years later he began to publish material derived from his military experience.   His monograph on what we now call typhus fever explained that so-called "hospital fever" and "jail fever" were the same illness, both able to be prevented by burning the clothes of persons exposed to them.   His greatest work, *Observations on the Diseases of the Army* (1752), discussed such diverse matters as making hospitals immune from military attack, the pathogenesis and epidemiology of hospital cross-infection, and the practice of antisepsis.   (He actually coined the word "antisepsis.") Although not in complete understanding of the living nature of the infectious agents, he did mention that possibility.

He pointed out that putrefaction, which was bad, closely resembled fermentation, which was useful. Many editions of that book were published, both in England and abroad.

In addition to his writings on medical matters, Pringle maintained a voluminous correspondence on music, archaeology, mathematics, electricity, lightning, and the domestication of foreign plants. In 1760 he wrote the first biography of General Wolfe, the hero of Canada. By 1772 he had become Physician to the Queen and President of the Royal Society, and shortly afterward he was given a title and made Physician to the King. His last paper, written in 1775 but published in 1794 (two years after his death), discussed the epidemiology of influenza, demolishing the idea of "an epidemical constitution." All of Pringle's works were models of reasoning based on observation, excluding pure speculation. Like many of his medical contemporaries, he was a skilled musician, an antiquary, and an expert on paintings and prints. In addition, he maintained an interest in ethics and religion, subjects in which he was trained at an early age. Despite, or perhaps because of, those activities in various humanistic fields, he remained the busy, expert clinician.

With the passing of the years, although Scots continued to study at Leyden, the number decreased, and the last, Balfour of Dunfermline, graduated at Leyden in 1842. Before that a number of Leyden men also had reached high position at Aberdeen or Glasgow (Guthrie, 1959). Although the great era of the Leyden men in the early years of the medical school at Edinburgh came to an end, elements of the greatness continued and even grew. Part of the success was the recognized quality of the teaching and emphasis on the bedside approach. At the end of the 18th and in the first decades of the 19th centuries, fully half of the students at the University were enrolled in the medical school; however, the University as a whole also grew in fame. In fact, the whole city of Edinburgh became the center of what has been called the Scottish Enlightenment. The period saw the founding of the *Encyclopedia Britannica* and the *Edinburgh Review*, each of which achieved worldwide fame in its own right. Edinburgh became the premier city of the British Empire: the writings of Hume and others in philosophy, and of Adam Smith in economics; the accomplishments of artists and engineers; the building of Edinburgh New Town; and other evidences of a sustained explosion of creativity.

The development of Edinburgh as the world's greatest center of medical education was part of the phenomenon, but it was also different from the rest in one way: As the crest of creativity in the Scottish Enlightenment passed, Edinburgh's medical greatness persisted in its offshoots in London, Dublin, America, and on the European continent, including such unlikely places as the Russian capital, St. Petersburg.

Catherine the Great played a primary role in extending Edinburgh's influence to Russia. After having her husband, the mentally retarded Czar, killed in July of 1762, she appointed a number of Edinburgh and Glasgow physicians to important posts in Russia, including that of Court Physician. Prominent Scots still residing in Scotland were invited to Russia or were made foreign members of the Imperial Russian Academy, whose president, appointed by Catherine, was a woman, Princess Dashkova. The Princess not only brought prominent Scots into the Academy, but also spent several years in Edinburgh. A number of Russian physicians went to Edinburgh for part of their training, subsequently playing prominent roles in teaching and administration in Russian clinical medicine. Some made clinical contributions that were well received in Western Europe. Although most medicine in the provinces was backward, the medicine of St. Petersburg had elements equal to any in Europe (Appleby, 1985).

There were many great physicians and medical teachers in Edinburgh in the last half of the 18th and first half of the 19th centuries. They included the Hamiltons, Professors of Midwifery, who were untiring in their efforts to make their specialty considered the equal of other medical specialties (Young, 1963). There were the great chemists who were also medical practitioners-Robinson, Cullen, Black, and Hope, "the most popular teacher of science Britain has ever known" (Craig, 1967). There was Duncan, Professor of Materia Medica, known for his writings on medical reform, including his insistence that the hospital and dispensary were not only for patient care, but also for giving practitioners experience and for teaching students the practical aspects of clinical medicine (Chitnis, 1973). A six-bed hospital wing opened in 1729 and it was expanded to become the Royal Infirmary seven years later; nevertheless, private instruction continued to be given. Anatomy was taught by Barclay who, in his private school, reorganized nomenclature and emphasized comparative anatomy (Chitnis, 1973), and by his successor, Knox, who was perhaps the greatest anatomy teacher of his time. Knox's career was destroyed by his seeming complicity in a murder committed by the body-snatchers, Burke and the Harts, in providing a body for dissection (Rae, 1965).

One of the most remarkable physicians of Edinburgh's great period was Whytt; in fact, his reputation today is still excellent. Born in Edinburgh in 1714, he took his M.A. degree at St. Andrews at 16 years of age and entered the study of medicine at Edinburgh. Although wealthy by inheritance at that time, he worked extremely hard and was particularly interested in anatomy as taught by Monro (*primus*). In 1734 he went to London to study under Cheselden and to walk the wards at several hospitals. He then studied under Winslow in Paris and under Albinus and Boerhaave in Leyden. In 1736 he took his M.D. degree at Rheims and a year later received the same degree at St. Andrews. Licensed in Edinburgh, he commenced to practice there. He taught at Edinburgh in both the College of Physicians (where he rose to be President) and, after 1747, in the University (as Professor of the Theory of Medicine). He was an active practitioner and later was designated Physician to the King in Scotland.

Whytt was an excellent clinician, as evidenced by his writings on tuberculosis and meningitis, and more particularly his *Observations on the Nature, Causes, and Cure of Those Disorders Which Have Been Called Nervous, Hypochondriac, or Hysteric*, published in several editions in and after 1765. That work, together with *The English Malady* (written several decades earlier by his fellow Scotsman, Cheyne) was the beginning of regular recognition (in England) of disorders associated with anxiety. Physicians of Great Britain wrote extensively on that subject for more than a half-century (Altschule, 1965). This was more than a century before Hecker, Lowenfeld, and finally Freud took up the subject of *angst* and a century and one-half before journalists convinced themselves that there was an "Age of Anxiety" Whytt estimated that one-third of the population of Great Britain was suffering from nervous disorders. The authors, who at that time wrote in a similar vein, blamed the condition on excessive work or excessive idleness, sexual deprivation or overindulgence, and easy living-plays, novels, and carriages with springs (Altschule, 1965). Whytt's clinical writings on the neurotic disorders were appreciated more fully during his lifetime than were his remarkable neurophysiological contributions. Today he usually is discussed in medical histories as the discoverer of the role of the spinal cord in reflexes, on autonomic function, and on the reaction of the pupil to light, which he described in *An Essay on the Vital and Other Involuntary Motions of Animals* (1751). That book caused Whytt to become unwillingly involved in a then-current controversy in Europe.

Descartes' discussion of cardiac motion and other physiologic processes had eliminated a hypothetical soul as the cause of all bodily function, because the body was a machine. A number of writers violently disagreed with him, pointing out that, as understood at that time, a machine (*e.g.*, windmills, waterwheels, cranks, screw-presses) merely changed one kind of motion into another. A machine, they held, could not create motion *de novo*; only a soul could do that. The vitalistic response to the Cartesian iatromechanistic explanations of physiology included the writings of Stahl, who held that the soul did everything, and other leading Germans, such as Hoffman, whose opinions were not markedly different. The dogmatic systems of Stahl and Hoffman, although accepted by some physicians, left Whytt unconvinced (Neuberger, 1945).

Whytt's book *On the Vital and Other Voluntary Functions of Animals* attacked Stahl's doctrine that an animal soul was responsible for all bodily actions. Whytt held that the involuntary motions of animals were instead "the effect of a stimulus acting on an unconscious sentient principle." That was 67 years before the publication in Germany of Schopenhauer's treatise on the will, a work that ultimately was to start a flood of writings on unconscious cerebral functions. De Sauvages was at that time Professor of Medicine at Montpellier, a stronghold of vitalistic physiology.   When Whytt wrote about the involuntary motions of animals, de Sauvages concluded that he must be a Stahlian vitalist, a judgment that von Haller already had expressed (French, 1969).   The controversy became diffuse and confused and, to us today, not completely intelligible.   Although Whytt believed, in accordance with the religious tenets of the day, that the soul pervaded the whole body, including the heart, he held that it was the entry of blood into the heart, acting on the nerves lining the cardiac chambers, which caused the heart to beat. His emphasis on various stimuli as effectors was a new thing and evidently not accepted by some or understood by many.

In any case, Whytt, in addition to making observations on the physiology of the nervous system, became a member of the group of 18th-century modernists who attacked vitalistic concepts of medicine, but never were able to defeat them.   Those concepts have recurred again and again in different guises through the years.   For some psychosomatic physicians today, the ego is the Stahlian soul. While Whytt was studying reflexes and, inadvertently, preparing the ground for later discussions by others of unconscious thinking, anxiety neurosis, and similar matters puzzling to his contemporaries, others were proceeding along clinical lines more acceptable at the time.   One of them was Cullen.

Cullen was one of the great figures of medicine in the late 18th century.   He was born in 1710 in Lanarkshire, an area that almost simultaneously produced the Hunters and Smellie, the great obstetrician.   Having entered the University of Glasgow for the study of arts and mathematics, he soon turned to medicine and became apprentice to Paisley, a member of Glasgow's Faculty of Physicians and Surgeons.   That was a fortunate step, for Paisley had both a large practice and an extensive library, and Cullen learned much.   At the age of 19 he signed on as Ship's Surgeon on a West Indian merchantman and, after two years at sea, went to London and studied with a leading apothecary for several months.   Returning to Scotland, he spent several years in desultory practice and philosophic reading.   He then went to Edinburgh for formal studies in medicine under the Leyden men then teaching there.   After three years, in 1736, he went into practice in his native town, where he planned to enter into a medical partnership with William Hunter; but, that plan dissolved when Hunter's ambitions took him to London. Cullen finally took his M.D. degree at Glasgow in 1740 and began to teach and lecture there.   In 1746 he made an arrangement with the Professor of Medicine to give a course in theory and practice.   He taught not only medicine but botany, chemistry, and materia medica, all in English, and in 1751 formally was appointed Professor of Medicine.   He also had a chemistry laboratory in which he and his students worked together.   One of his chemistry students was Joseph Black, who became his successor, first in Glasgow and later in Edinburgh.

Cullen also had a huge medical practice, and his rigorous program seemed to be damaging to his health.   He moved to Edinburgh and in 1755 became Professor of Chemistry and Medicine there.   He was the second person to give clinical lectures at the Royal Infirmary, Rutherford having established that method earlier.   In 1757 Cullen persuaded Monro (*secundus*), who taught anatomy, and Whytt, who taught physiology, to join him in the clinical teaching.   The three working together created the bedside teaching that made Edinburgh's fame as a clinical educational center even greater.   In 1760, after the Professor of Materia Medica died, the students persuaded Cullen to take that post also, and he soon produced a course whose notes were sold and circulated widely.

The next years saw a considerable amount of faculty in-fighting, with Cullen and others changing titles.   During that period Cullen had become the most famous physician and teacher in Europe (Johnstone, 1959).   His earliest major publication, *Methodical Nosology* (1766), comprised a classification so rigid as to be artificial, and it did not survive long.   His *First Lines in the Practice of Physic* likewise was marred by excessive preoccupation with rigid theory, especially the theory that diseases of the organs were merely reflections of disordered nervous functions, a doctrine that Hoffman (on the Continent) maintained (Rath, 1959; Johnstone, 1959).   In personal character and behavior he was the opposite of rigid, and his qualities of warmth and sympathy gained him favor among the students.   Paradoxically, it was his very extensive knowledge of medicine that made him want to arrange that material in order and led to his artificial classification.   Also, he felt under great pressure to explain medical phenomena, a pressure many academicians experience and succumb to, becoming theoreticians and even dogmatists.   Perhaps it was the skepticism of his colleagues on the faculty that made his academic career slow and erratic, despite the devotion of his students.

Nevertheless, Cullen's insistence on experience as a guide to medicinal treatment (Crellin, 1971) and his recommendations regarding patient-care demonstrated his expertise as a clinician, for he minimized drastic methods and emphasized regimen and diet (Risse, 1974).   However well he may have transmitted his clinical knowledge in bedside teaching, which could not be written down, he is remembered for his rigid formulations, which were documented.

As the reputation of Edinburgh's clinical medicine seemingly began to fade, first with the poor performance of Monro (*tertius*) as Professor of Anatomy and then with Cullen's death, it was, in fact, maintained by Edinburgh's students who created, together with some others, the clinical medicine of the golden eras of London and Dublin in the early 19th century.   Edinburgh also provided much of the personnel of the armed forces and the East India Company and some of the leading teachers in American institutions.

It is possible also that the decline in Cullen's reputation in the eyes of the world was the result of the peculiar behavior of his former pupil and assistant, John Brown, to whom he had shown much kindness over a period of years.   Brown twisted some of Cullen's theorizing and created his own dogma, known as the Brunonian System. His contemporaries in Edinburgh described him as naive and innocent, but some believed him to be a sophisticated rogue.   Perhaps he was both.   His System held that life was dependent on continuous stimulation by the activity of the brain, the emotions, food, drink, or warmth.   He averred "that the quality of a person's excitability was inborn, although the quantity fell with age" (Risse, 1970). All diseases, said Brown, fell into two categories: too much or too little excitability. The "sthenic" was due to excessive, the "asthenic" to deficient excitability. The remedies he recommended were various procedures or medications that had the opposite effects; for example, the recommended medications included laudanum for the sthenic and whisky for the asthenic states. (He himself succumbed to his own treatment in that respect.)

Brown's system denied the existence of specific diseases, the healing powers of Nature and, in particular, any need for careful study of patients' symptoms (Risse, 1970a,b). Such dogma was ridiculed in Great Britain, although Brunonian activists among Edinburgh students created tensions that precipitated fights with Cullen's followers. Brunonians and Cullenists shoved and struck each other for the good of mankind. (Words like "activist" and "civil disobedience" were not used, however.) In Italy and Germany Brown's dogma was highly successful, both in its acceptance and its destruction of other prevailing dogmas. In France its fate was different. The destruction of organized medicine in the French Revolution permitted some Brunonians to press for acceptance of the dogma; however, its tenets were so completely opposite to those of the French physicians' growing insistence on observation that the Brunonian System soon was rejected (Risse, 1970a). Nevertheless, its adherents on the Continent agreed with Brown when he claimed that he had discovered a universal principle of life and medicine comparable in greatness to Newton's universal laws in physics. That absurd notion did not enhance Edinburgh's reputation as a center of medical scholarship.

The same is perhaps true of the activities of Combe, the Edinburgh phrenologist. Combe, a founder of the Edinburgh Phrenological Society, declared the following (Altschule, 1965):

> The discoveries of the revolution of the globe, and the circulation of the blood were splendid displays of genius, interesting and beneficial to mankind; but their results, compared with the consequences that must inevitably follow Dr. Gall's discovery of the functions of the brain (embracing as it does,

the true theory of the animal, moral, and intellectual constitution of man) sink into relative insignificance.

Combe linked Gall's opponents to the opponents of Copernicus, Galileo, Newton, and Harvey.   However, he wrote *Observations on Mental Derangement,* a good clinical text, but presenting all explanations in phrenologic terms (Altschule, 1965).   Except for some of the words, his explanations sound like many modern psychodynamic works. A   medical   journal   in   Boston,   Massachusetts,   praised Combe's work in almost hysterical terms.   It was in large measure the lecturing, writing, and other efforts of Combe which caused phrenology to be the important force it became   in   mid-19th-century   British   psychiatry   (DeGuistino, 1975; Cooter, 1976).

Although phrenology was born in Vienna, it seemed at first to be a Scottish specialty.   Macnish, a graduate of and practicing physician in Glasgow as well as a writer of   fantasy,   had   met   Gall   in   Paris   while   studying   with Broussais and Dupuytren.   He became an enthusiastic phrenologist and in 1834 wrote in his *Introduction to Phrenology:*

> The phrenological system appears to me the   only   one   capable   of   affording   a   rational and easy explanation of all the phenomena of mind...The   system   is   gaining   ground   rapidly among   scientific   men   both   in   Europe   and America.   Some of the ablest physiologists in both quarters of the globe have admitted its accordance   with   nature;   it   boasts   a   greater number   of   proselytes   than   at   any   previous period.   The prejudices still existing against it, result from ignorance of its real   character.   As   people   get   better   acquainted with the science, and the formidable evidence   by   which   it   is   supported,   they   will think differently.

Among   the   leading   psychiatrists   referred   to   was Conolly, who declared that many people believed to be incurably insane could be cured by the use of phrenology, although how Conolly applied phrenology therapeutically was not stated.   Actually Macnish did some sound work. His *Philosophy of Sleep* was a pioneering study of manifestations and disorders of sleep.   Nevertheless, the Scottish interest in phrenology was remarkable.   A Chair of Phrenology was established in Glasgow.   Lord Glenegly, the Secretary, was petitioned to require phrenologic examination of all convicts before transportation and to take an experienced phrenologist into the public service for that purpose.   Although some outstanding physicians ridiculed phrenology, others equivocated, retreating behind the time-honored statement that the theory probably had some truth and some error, which further study would separate.

Much of the curiosity and creativity that had led to Edinburgh's clinical greatness in the days of the Leyden men seems to have fallen into either the strait-jacket of rigid theory, or into the morass of superstitious dogma. Clinical leadership soon would move elsewhere, although Edinburgh continued to turn out original thinkers.   Thus, although the teaching of anatomy deteriorated at Edinburgh under Monro (*tertius*), 18th-century Edinburgh anatomy was destined to produce one of the great seminal works of medicine, Goodsir's *Anatomical and Pathological Observations*, published with his brother in 1845.

John Goodsir was born in 1814 on the shores of the Firth of Forth, the son and grandson of physicians.   At 13 years of age he entered the nearby St. Andrew's University, where he showed particular interest in natural history.   His family tradition of medical training at Edinburgh was maintained by his matriculation there, after he had been apprenticed to a local surgeon-dentist.   His anatomical studies were pursued under the brilliant Knox.   He completed his medical studies but never took the M.D. degree; nevertheless, he was licensed in 1835 and joined his father in practice from 1835 to 1840.   During that period he maintained his interest in natural history, especially anatomy, as exemplified by his 1839 monograph on the embryology of the teeth.   A year later he returned to Edinburgh and shortly afterward was appointed Curator of the Museum of the College of Surgeons.   His work involved not only the preparation of gross specimens of organs, but also intensive microscopic studies of tissues, and he published much along those lines.   His fame spread, and in 1842 he was made Curator of the University Museum, then Demonstrator of Anatomy and, finally, when Monro (*tertius*) died in 1846, Professor of Anatomy, a chair he held for 20 years.

Goodsir's 1845 publication was a landmark, in that it defined the cells as "the centers of nutrition," and "secreting structures" in health and disease.   The nucleus, he maintained, was the effective portion of the cell.   The whole organism, as he understood it, consisted of single cells, each of which maintained an exact relationship to other single cells or groups of cells.   Virchow in Germany was impressed to a great extent by Goodsir's ideas and dedicated the first English edition of *Cellular Pathology* to him.   Virchow not only appreciated Goodsir, but he actually borrowed his language in places (Follis, 1945). Whereas Virchow reiterated his views repeatedly and had a large following, including many Americans, in Germany, Goodsir was content to spend his life teaching students locally.   He seemed to have no other interests.   One of his vacations on the Continent included 16 hours at the microscope with Kolliker at Wurzburg.   He may have met Virchow at Wurzburg, for Virchow was professor there from 1849 to 1856.

Goodsir's health was poor in later years.   He apparently had syphilis of the spinal cord, which did not seem to have affected his brain adversely.   He was only 53 years old when he died.   In any case, through his 1845 publication and his influence on Virchow, Goodsir must be credited with the creation of cellular pathology in its modern form.   Moreover, he did not make the errors of interpretation which often marred Virchow's work (see Chapter 14).   Goodsir's ideas clarified the way in which the *milieu interieur*, as defined by Bernard, functioned (Holmes, 1963).   However brilliant Bernard's formulation, it still lacked the explanation of detailed cellular function, which Goodsir and his follower, Virchow, supplied by making the cell the functional unit.

The brothers Bell were also original and deserve special mention.   John, the elder, was apprenticed to a physician and took courses at Edinburgh University.   He practiced at the Royal Infirmary but decided to open a school of anatomy in opposition to the University anatomy course run by Monro (*secundus*). He was very successful because he was, in effect, the founder of surgical anatomy in his teaching directed to the practical surgeon. That approach was strikingly different from the prevailing mode. In 1799 he was excluded from the Royal Infirmary, evidently because of the jealousy of powerful rivals, and thereafter gave up teaching to pursue surgical practice exclusively. He became the most famous clinical surgeon in Scotland. The status of anatomy under Monro (*secundus*) and the weaker Monro (*tertius*) deteriorated badly because of poor teaching, whereas Bell's writings on anatomy and surgery were outstanding successes. He illustrated his books with his own drawings and engravings, which were of great beauty (Walls, 1964). (His drawings of scenes in Italy also revealed great artistic feeling.)

Charles Bell was apprenticed to his brother and later assisted him in his private School of Anatomy. When John gave up the school, Charles moved to London, where he led a marginal existence for a time. However, when he published *Essays on the Anatomy of Expression in Painting*, his reputation rose rapidly. In 1812, only eight years after setting up in London, he was able to buy the Windmill Street School of Anatomy, which had been founded by William Hunter in 1765. In 1824 he published *The Nervous System of the Human Body* and later *The Hand, Its Mechanism and Vital Endowments as Evincing Design*. While in London, he was involved in the new Middlesex Hospital Medical School and carried out pioneering work in neuroanatomy and neurophysiology, including the differentiation of sensory and motor nerves (Gordon-Taylor and Walls, 1958). He was unaware of Magendie's earlier work in that area. In 1836 he assumed the Chair of Surgery in Edinburgh and remained in Edinburgh until his death. He wrote the third volume of his brother's *Anatomy of the Human Body* and made the engravings for the illustrations of the second volume. (John himself did the engravings for the first.) Charles was the more famous of the two, both as surgeon and artist, but there was no jealousy between them.

It must not be concluded that the medical school at Edinburgh was completely self-sufficient, since from time to time it welcomed men trained elsewhere. Laycock was one such man. He not only was trained elsewhere, but he contributed ideas to clinical medicine which did not fall into the ordinary local pattern. Born and educated in Yorkshire from 1833 to 1835 he studied medicine at the new University College, London (Cope, 1965). He also went to Paris to study physiology and anatomy. In 1835 he was elected to the Royal College of Surgeons and received his M.D. degree at Göttingen, *summa cum laude*, in 1839, after which he returned to Yorkshire to practice. He became interested in Plato's philosophy, as then expounded at Cambridge, and wrote on the mind-body relationship in health and disease. His 1840 Treatise on the *Nervous Disorders of Women* was based on extensive personal observation.

Laycock also had other interests, and in 1841, in the *Dublin Medical Gazette*, he published a comprehensive plan for state medicine. In 1845 he developed then-current ideas on the reflex so that it applied to mental functions. He was on the faculty at the York Medical School for nine years and then was chosen for the Chair of Medicine at Edinburgh. In many ways his ideas were similar to those of Sechenov in Russia, who also held that thought was reflex in nature (Amacher, 1964). Sechenov was forced to leave Russia to avoid arrest for his materialistic views. (Today his works are joined with those of Wedensky and Pavlov in what is probably the glossiest medical book ever published. The three are now heroes of Soviet science, although two of them lived long before the Russian revolution, and the third despised it.)

In 1859 Laycock systematized his view in *Mind and Brain*, and that work entered the growing pool of writing on the subject of so-called "unconscious cerebration" that Carpenter, Hamilton, and others in Great Britain, and Schopenhauer and Hartmann in Germany were creating. Like so many philosophers in medicine, Laycock seemed dry, cold, and withdrawn, eloquent only in the written, but not the spoken, word. His works-some 300 papers-were expository but not strong on reasoning. His contributions to bedside medicine are neither numerous nor great, but he was an important, if somewhat vague, progenitor of today's psychosomatic medicine. His appointment as Professor of Medicine at Edinburgh suggests that the decline of that institution as a clinical force led to attempted rejuvenation through new approaches-any new approaches-much as occurs today.

Edinburgh provided many physicians to the military services. Since it welcomed dissenters, unlike Oxford and Cambridge, and did not consider wealth and social status important for admission, a number of men from other than wealthy families saw Edinburgh as the place to study medicine and military service the place to obtain security.

Lind was one of the Edinburgh alumni who entered the military. His widespread fame persists today. Born in 1716, he was apprenticed to an Edinburgh surgeon at the age of 15. Lind then became a naval surgeon, serving mainly in tropical waters in the 1740s (Roddis, 1950). He retired to practice in Edinburgh in 1748 and received his M.D. from Edinburgh in 1750, remaining in that city until 1758. He never forgot his experience with scurvy, which at that time killed 4,000 or 5,000 men yearly in the Royal Navy. His famous *Treatise on Scurvy* was published in 1753. In it he described his own observations on its prevention with citrus juice and fresh vegetables, and also reviewed at length - perhaps excessively so - the earlier writings, referring to Woodall's (1639) use of citrus fruits to prevent scurvy. It must be borne in mind that the Dutch and the English India Companies had learned earlier that crews sent on very long voyages had to be protected against scurvy, and they had found out that citrus juice was both preventive and curative (Tickner and Medvie, 1958). Lind's writings on scurvy were criticized for their experimental imperfections and for a time were rejected by some (Meikeljohn, 1954; Hughes, 1975; Wyatt, 1976).

After the passage of several decades, the application of Lind's recommendations by others, particularly Captain Cook, proved their value (Lloyd, 1961; Snell, 1963). Lind's book was received more enthusiastically abroad than in England, and it went through several editions. He had other original interests as well. In 1754 he published an interesting paper on the salts of lead that leached into food from lead-glazed pottery. Three years later he wrote another naval medical text, that one more general than the first. It included not only material on scurvy, but also discussions of malaria and other diseases that occur in seamen. That work likewise went through several editions. A year later he was appointed Physician to the Naval Hospital at Haslar, where he wrote on the infectiousness of typhus fever, the production of drinking water by the distillation of seawater, and tropical diseases in general. His death in 1794 ended a most productive medical career. He seems to have been interested in little other than the health of seamen, and his contributions make him the founder of nautical medicine (Roddis, 1950).

Another Edinburgh graduate who chose a military career was Trotter. He was born in Roxburghshire in 1760, and little is known of his early life. In 1777 and 1778 he is recorded as being a student at Edinburgh, studying anatomy with Monro (*secundus*). He had other interests, and even at that young age contributed poetry to the *Edinburgh Magazine*. He did not graduate but joined the Royal Navy as a surgeon's mate and was mentioned in dispatches after the Battle of the Dogger Bank in 1781. He subsequently was promoted to the rank of Surgeon and served on several vessels. After the war ended, Trotter was not eligible for a pension, so he joined a Liverpool slaver carrying Blacks from Africa to the West Indies. However, he was so dismayed and disgusted with what he saw that on his return to England he participated actively in the attempts then being made to abolish the slave trade. In that connection he testified before a House of Commons Committee in 1790 (Porter, 1963) that on the trip the vessel's master had refused to take on adequate amounts of fresh fruit, and scurvy had broken out among the slaves. Many died of the disease and other causes. It was not until the vessel arrived at Antigua that fresh fruit finally became available.

After the revolting experience on the slave vessel, Trotter resumed his studies at Edinburgh. Just before Cullen was to give his lecture on scurvy, Trotter wrote to him about his own experiences. Cullen magnanimously stated that he "never came to that chair so badly prepared" in his reading on the subject but that he would use the material which he "had just received from a gentleman present that was the cause of his making his declaration." Cullen then gave his lecture without referring to Trotter again.   Trotter published his *Observations on Scurvy* in 1786, which was translated into German in 1787.   The revised edition appeared in 1792 and was reprinted in America the following year.

In Edinburgh from 1787 to 1788 Trotter studied materia medica, medicine both practical and theoretical, and botany, all taught by its famous faculty.   He received the M.D. degree in 1788 and rejoined the Royal Navy at the end of that year, serving at sea until 1793, when he was appointed Second Physician to the Staff of the Naval Hospital at Haslar.   A year later he was appointed Physician to the Channel Fleet and served during its "glorious first of June" victory over the French.   In 1795 he achieved fame by quickly terminating a serious outbreak of scurvy in the Fleet.   He published further observations on scurvy in various places, including his *Medicina Nautica* (1797). Trotter held that fresh vegetables impart something to the body that "fortifies it against the disease."   He emphasized that fresh vegetables were far superior to lemon juice in that respect, a fact that is mentioned little today.   (He was wrong, however, in concluding that citric acid was the active material.)

Trotter wrote extensively on reorganizing the naval medical service, recommending teaching conferences and pathology services at Haslar.   In 1801 he recommended a presentation to Jenner for his introduction of vaccination. Trotter retired from the Navy in 1802 and did his best writing after settling in Newcastle-on-Tyne, adjacent to the new medical school there.   He had a large practice, but still was able to produce his remarkable *Essay on Drunkenness* ("a disease of the mind"), two pamphlets on protecting miners from gases, and his epoch-making *A View of the Nervous Temperament* (1807).   That is one of the great writings in the English language on illnesses that today are called psychosomatic.   In it he emphasized that in wartime boredom is at least as likely to cause those symptoms as the fears and anxieties produced by combat.   The book went through several editions and is his monument. His role as reformer of naval medicine is recognized less widely, but here, too, he was outstanding.

Despite its declining reputation, Edinburgh continued to supply Great Britain with fine practitioners, although London and Dublin were to become outstanding as educational centers by the early part of the 19th century, partly because of the rapidity with which they adopted innovations that were developing in France.   One sign of dissatisfaction within Edinburgh was the recurrence of teaching organizations separate from the University.   Over the years extramural teaching sprang up in Edinburgh, and in 1841 an attempt was made to combine the private medical schools by creating Queen's College.   The attempt failed, although the University recognized the extramural courses in 1855.   A new medical school was founded in 1895, but it lasted for only a half-century and then was absorbed into the expanded University (Guthrie, 1965).

As Edinburgh grew mainly out of Leyden, the medicine in some other cities was almost exclusively out of Edinburgh, Philadelphia being a prime example of the latter.   All members of the first Faculty of Medicine at Philadelphia were Edinburgh graduates: Morgan, Shippen, Kuhn, Rush, Wistar, and Physick.   The story of how they succeeded in making the medical school of the University of Pennsylvania a partial replica of Edinburgh, despite their jealousy and quarreling, set a pattern for the development of academic medicine in America.   Two great men of New York also were Edinburgh men: Bond and Hosack.

However, unlike the other major seaboard cities of pre- and postrevolutionary times (New York, Philadelphia, Newport, and Charleston), Boston physicians who wanted European training mainly went to London.   Only about 20% of those men had any of their training in Scottish universities.   No reason for that difference has ever been established (Cash, 1979).

For the most part, Americans who had taken part or all of their training in Edinburgh-some of whom had earned the M.D. degree-practiced along the East Coast. One exception was McDowell, famous for his surgical removal of the ovary in 1809.   He was an Edinburgh student, who made his mark in rural America and lived to become internationally famous.   The few who crossed the Appalachian Mountains included Samuel Brown, Virginia-born, who returned to Virginia to practice.   After a time he moved to New Orleans and then to Huntsville, Alabama. Finally, in 1799, he settled in Cincinnati, Ohio, as the first Professor of Anatomy at Transylvania College, where he presumedly exemplified the Edinburgh ways and ideals.

Another Edinburgh man who came to America was Dunglison, who began inland but made most of his career in Philadelphia. His notebooks of his course with Home at Edinburgh have come to light (Jones and Gemmill, 1967) and described the clinical training of students at the Royal Infirmary, mainly under Home, Rutherford, and Hamilton. The meticulous history-taking and examination made almost entirely by inspection were described in detail. In selected cases the sugar and urea in the urine were measured. In the clinical history, a careful inquiry into causes-"predisponent, hereditary, or exciting"-was made; the effects of treatment noted. The student saw the patients daily, and the professor made rounds twice weekly, discussing diagnosis, prognosis, and clinical course with the students. Of the nine patients described in the notebooks who died, eight were examined post-mortem, an examination that was considered highly important. In treatment, the usual bleedings and administration of cathartics and blistering agents were performed with restraint. Home is quoted in one place as being skeptical of the effects of treatment: "Perhaps the medicines may have had some effect in bringing the disease to a more speedy termination but in all probability it is owing to the natural course of the fever...."

Dunglison left Edinburg before receiving his M.D. degree. He studied for a time in London and Paris, and then was awarded the degree in Erlangen (Bavaria) for a thesis. In 1825, at the invitation of Thomas Jefferson, he went to the University of Virginia at Charlottesville as Professor of Anatomy and Medicine. However, he was required also to teach surgery, theoretical medicine, physiology, pathology, materia medica, and pharmacy. He transferred to the University of Maryland and then to Jefferson Medical College in Philadelphia. The year 1837 saw the publication in Philadelphia of his *The Medical Student; Or Aids to the Study of Medicine*, a frank discussion of some problems of medical education. He wrote (on page 164),

In respect to the best method of profiting by the *Clinical course*, a great deal will depend upon the method adopted by the professor-as to the plan the student should pursue. Too often, perhaps, the clinical instructor selects the singular and the striking, rather than the common and more useful cases; and it has fallen to the lot of the author-as it must have done, more or less, to every one-to have had his attention directed chiefly to cases, during his period of hospital attendance, which he has rarely or never met with since. The object of the clinical professor should be to select mainly those cases, that must necessarily present themselves to all in their ordinary course of practice; to inquire aloud into the history of the case, and, at a fitting opportunity, to explain the etiology, semeiotics, diagnosis, prognosis and treatment adapted for the particular case, and for the class to which it belongs,-attracting the attention of the student to the more prominent points. With these views, acute cases should be first considered, as being most common and urgent; and afterwards the more chronic. The young student is generally disposed to be over active in his treatment, and, if one remedy does not appear to be producing all the effect he anticipated, he is apt to fly at once to another; but if the professor be judicious, the student will soon learn that infinite mischief may be done in this manner, and that more reliance has to be placed upon the recuperative powers of the system, than he may have been disposed to imagine. It will be well for the clinical pupil to keep a journal of such cases as may merit the trouble; and never to permit an occasion to slip for verifying or disproving, by dissection, the views which he or his teacher may have been led to form of the precise nature of fatal maladies.

Except for differences in the use of some words 140 years ago, this paragraph might have been written this morning.   Dunglison was certainly a prime factor in the establishment and maintenance of Philadelphia's preeminence in clinical medicine. As late as the 1850s Edinburgh methods still were being followed eagerly in Philadelphia medicine (Penman, 1978).

The remarkable comments by Dunglison become even more remarkable when we realize that earlier he had come to be considered America's leading physiologist on the basis of his lectures at the University of Virginia and his publication of a popular physiology textbook.   He was regarded so highly as a physiologist that in January of 1833 he was invited to join Beaumont in some of the latter's experiments on digestion several months before Beaumont's definitive report on the subject was published.   That was at a time when teachers of what are today called "basic sciences" were expected to be expert physicians as a matter of course, and their sciences were considered collateral or accessory (Numbers and Orr, 1981).

Another fine Scottish medical school-at Aberdeen-produced some notable graduates.   The Gregories, both fine clinicians, were so recognized in their lifetimes, the younger, James, being instrumental in the organization of medical teaching at Edinburgh.

Among the Aberdeen men who should be remembered for specific contributions to clinical medicine is Alexander Gordon, a graduate of the University there and a medical practitioner in that town. Although others previously had noted that puerperal fever might occur in epidemics, Gordon recognized the infectious nature of the disease, as Holmes in Boston a half-century later acknowledged in his writings on it.   Further discussion of Gordon's work can be found in Chapter 13.

Another Aberdeen alumnus who is known today to at least a few is Cheyne, who practiced for the most part in London.   His writings on anxiety and hypochondriasis were read widely.   Together with Whytt's writings on what today is called neurosis, they comprise an early formulation of an important clinical concept, fully appreciated 200 years ago, but now hailed as a recent discovery (Altschule, 1977.)

IN 18TH-CENTURY ENGLAND medical practice developed differently from that of Scotland, where the leading physicians were Leyden men, or Edinburgh or Aberdeen men who had been trained by Leyden alumni. A few English physicians in the provinces were graduates of the old English universities, and there were also some Leyden men. More numerous were those English or Scottish, who had been trained at Edinburgh. However, only men who had taken courses at Oxford or Cambridge could practice medicine in or near London. Accordingly, London medical practitioners had to have had a period of residence at one of these universities, no matter where they had received their main training. That requirement did not apply to surgeons, who could practice as members of the Barber-Surgeons Guild.

The developments in Edinburgh stimulated the growth of medical education and practice in London along lines of clinical and post-mortem observation, but London had no university at the time, and the need for medical training led to a unique development-the teaching of medical subjects in private medical schools and in hospitals. The reader will recall that at Edinburgh, before the creation of the Faculty of Medicine, some portions of the medical curriculum had begun to be taught at the behest of professional organizations of physicians. In the 18th century this occurred in London as well but largely was overshadowed by the development of private medical schools that taught some of those subjects. During that period medical schools began to be created at English hospitals, and they soon proliferated; however, those hospital schools had no university connections for some time.

The generally depressing centuries of medicine at Cambridge have been discussed well (Langdon-Brown, 1946); however, there were some men who tried to improve the situation. The most notable 18th-century Cambridge graduate was Heberden, the elder. (His son of the same name was also a physician.)   The elder Heberden was born in London in 1710 and entered St. John's College, Cambridge, at the age of 14.   He received his M.D. degree in 1739, after having studied medicine at Cambridge and also in one of the London hospitals.   It was probably his training at the hospital that encouraged him to develop clinical interests.   Nevertheless, he remained in Cambridge, where he practiced and also lectured on materia medica.   He became recognized as a clinical scholar and had several translations from foreign texts published at his own expense.   In 1748 he left Cambridge for London, where his practice continued to be successful and received a number of honors, including the Presidency of the College of Physicians. His practice, according to such laymen as Cowper and Samuel Johnson, was characterized by notable kindness and great skill.   His careful clinical notes were published as *Commentaries* shortly after his death in 1801, but his most notable writing was on the subject of angina pectoris (1768).

Heberden's *clinical* description of angina pectories was based on 20 carefully observed patients described in his case reports, although he said he had seen 100.   His ideas about angina pectoris led to a controversy with Parry, who maintained that angina pectoris was merely a kind of fainting spell attended with unusual anxiety, due to calcification of the coronary arteries.   Parry based that conclusion on studies of only three patients, who were observed to become pulseless during the attacks (Livesley, 1975).   In two of the patients the attacks were prolonged and may well have represented myocardial infarctions.   He properly related the disorder to coronary artery sclerosis, a finding that his friend Jenner had called to his attention. Heberden did not consider the syndrome a manifestation of heart disease, because in his cases the pulse remained unchanged.   Both men clearly were wrong to some extent and right to some extent.

Heberden also wrote perceptively about many other medical disorders, including chicken pox, night blindness, and arthritis.   Moreover, throughout his life he continued to show interest and competence in the classics.   Samuel Johnson called him "*Ultimus Romanorum*, the last of our learned physicians," and in Germany he was known as

"Medicus vere Hippocraticus."   When Heberden refused to
scarify Johnson's massively swollen legs to let the fluid
out, Johnson called him *"timidorum timidissimus."*   Johnson
enlisted another physician to do the procedure; however,
he remained sick.   At various times he was bled and given
purgatives and squills; in fact, after being given digitalis,
he lost 14 pints of urine.   At post-mortem, severe emphysema was observed, signifying that he evidently had died
of *cor pulmonale* (McHenry, 1976).

An English physician wrote of Heberden, "No other
person, either in this or any other country, has ever exercised the art of medicine with the same dignity, or contributed so much to raise it in the estimation of mankind."
In evaluating Heberden's work and influence, proper emphasis must be given to his studies in a London hospital
and his practice in London after 1748.   Certainly his medical writings, aside from his early lectures in materia medica, were more typical of a London doctor than of a traditional Cambridge one.   Heberden had collected his notes
for his son, who published them after his father's death.
The son was a recognized classicist, as well as a distinguished physician in his own right.   Although he received
his M.D. degree at Oxford, he took his clinical training at
St. George's Hospital in London.   He became Physician to
George III and treated him for, among other things, his
psychiatric disorder, using a simple form of supportive psy-
chotherapy (Cantu and Cantu, 1967).   Young Heberden disagreed with the treatments recommended by the other attending physicians and was the only one for whom the King
asked.

The younger Heberden subsequently had many other
psychiatric patients.   Like Pinel's treatment, Heberden's
was "to sooth, to cherish, to comfort a mind worn by disease and disappointment, to encourage it by indulgence, by
amusement, by conversation, by company, by reading, by
the exercise of its own faculties."   As a classicist, he
knew and approved of the ancient recommendations of So-
ranus in such cases: mild use of restriction, physical
treatment, personal contact with the physician, and environmental manipulation.   Psychiatric treatment, Heberden
said, should have as its aim giving a new direction to the
mind.   He held that prevention was likely to be more suc-

cessful than treatment, and to that end he recommended a balanced, self-disciplined life, with special attention to study and religion.   In his writings young Heberden regularly referred to ancient writers, foreshadowing modern psychiatric thinking by distinguishing between mental states due to disorders of feeling (now termed *affective*) and disorders of thinking (now termed *delusional*).

Another Cambridge alumnus who prospered in London was Baker.   Born in Hampshire in 1723, he was educated at Eton and at King's College, Cambridge, taking his M.A. in 1749 and earning his M.D. in 1756 at Cambridge.   After trying country practice for a time, he moved to London. Elected a Fellow of the Royal College of Physicians, he became President in 1785 and was also Physician-in-Ordinary to the King and Queen.   He was among the physicians who attended the King in his mental illness during and after 1788.   Baker was an amateur of literature and enjoyed the society of literary and artistic characters, including Gray, who dedicated his *Elegy Written in a Country Churchyard* to him.   Sir Joshua Reynolds was among his patients.   Baker wrote Latin "with purity and elegance" but was not above composing doggerel rhymed couplets when the occasion required it.

Baker's friend, the Leyden alumnus Huxham, lived in Devonshire and wrote about the epidemic of colic there which seemed to occur at the same time every year.   In addition to the gastrointestinal symptoms, Huxham noted in his treatise *De Morbo Colico Denmoniensi* (1739) that wrist drop also occurred, together with muscle pains and weakness, and then the final fatal paralysis.   Huxham was also the author of highly respected clinical studies in fevers and scurvy.   In 1747, before Lind's writings, he recommended that sailors with scurvy be given fresh vegetables. Huxham echoed the prevailing lay opinion that Devonshire colic was due to drinking large amounts of "rough" cider. In 1707 Musgrave, an Oxford M.D., had described the disease as a form of arthritis.   After referring to both Musgrave and Huxham in his classic monograph, Baker pointed out that Devonshire colic was indistinguishable from lead poisoning.   His appreciation of the symptoms of lead poisoning had been stimulated by the writings of Tronchin in France in 1737, who wrote about what he called *Poitou colic,* which in his opinion was caused by drinking water brought in through lead pipes.   Baker's essay on Devonshire colic, first published in 1767, stated his belief that lead which was poured to fill cracks in the cider-making apparatus was the source of the metal traces in poisoning. He analyzed samples of the cider for lead and demonstrated its presence.   The response to his publication among the apple-growers can be imagined (McConaghy, 1967), but the fact that Devonshire colic was actually lead poisoning was accepted within a decade.

Nevertheless, the source of the lead remained unproved, since a number of workers could not find the metal in all of the presses used.   Baker also had suggested that cheap glazed pottery used by the poor could be the source, as Lind had mentioned earlier.   In fact, another physician, Hardy, proved that it was (Waldron, 1969). Hardy's writings were more general and also referred to the epidemic of lead poisoning in ancient Rome, discussed by Paulus Aeginata.   (The Roman aqueducts were made of stone, but the pipes into the houses were made of lead.) Hardy also mentioned the use of lead salts to keep wine from "turning," an observation that led some to conclude that the so-called "gout" seen in the great wine drinkers of the time was, in reality, lead poisoning.   In any case, the relationship between cheap glazed pottery and lead poisoning as discussed by several physicians two centuries ago was known to only a few scholars until practitioners in recent years heard about it as a great discovery of modern medical science.

Another Cambridge man of interest was Glynn, who was born in Cornwall and educated at Eton and Cambridge, where he took the B.A. and M.A. degrees, and, in 1752, the M.D. degree.   He practiced in Surrey for a short while and then returned to Cambridge, where he remained for the rest of his life.   Despite his often abrasive behavior and sarcastic wit, he was successful in practice.   A devoted follower of Heberden's precepts, he was methodical in history-taking and careful in clinical reasoning.   Beginning in 1749 Glynn began to give lectures similar to those of Heberden, but at irregular periods, since in the 20 years after 1750 there were never more than 10 medical students in residence at Cambridge in any given year.

Actually, he moved more in literary than medical circles of Cambridge and won a prize for his poetry. He is to be remembered as a small-town doctor as competent as any, but different from many others in his attempts to emulate specifically the clinician he admired, though separated from his direct influence.

Some of the English university-trained medical men of the 18th century came to think more and more like modern clinicians, basing their practice of medicine on the appreciation of the way in which disease expresses itself in the symptoms of the sick. Symptomatology became the focus of thinking, and theoretical explanations, whether valid or fanciful, became secondary. These men escaped the blighting effects of traditional Oxford and Cambridge medicine.

Human nature being what it is, it is not surprising that some of the university men continued to become physicians who adopted the iatromathematical superstition in order to explain scientifically what they observed clinically. That preoccupation with the notion that explaining everything was essential-however fragmentary, antefactual, or erroneous the scientific data may have been-did not keep some of them from being good physicians. Jurin exemplified this. Born in 1684, he entered Cambridge University in 1702, taking his B.A. and M.A. in 1705 and 1709, respectively. He became a schoolmaster, gave public lectures on science, and translated Latin classics. Resigning his school post, he reentered Cambridge and took his M.D. degree there in 1716. (He had studied at Leyden at times in the interval.) Jurin became active in the College of Physicians and in the Royal Society, ultimately becoming President of the first and Secretary of the second. He was also Physician to Guy's Hospital from 1725 to 1732. He had a very large practice and became known for his enthusiasm for inoculation to prevent smallpox. He was regarded during his lifetime as one of London's leading medical practitioners; today he is best known for his expert knowledge of Newtonian physics and for his attempt to use it, rather than the Cartesian system, to explain bodily functions. Jurin studied the heart as a pump and also investigated the attraction that capillaries have for fluids, concluding that the heart alone could not circulate the body's blood supply and that the small blood vessels must play a part through a kind of attraction. His calculations were criticized by a number of men, including the iatromathematician Keill, then in practice in Northampton after taking the M.D. degree at Cambridge. The physiological controversies between these two Cambridge men consumed much paper, but both were good physicians.

A second group of English physicians consisted of men trained at Leyden, one of whom, Mandeville, was atypical, at least as a physician practicing in London. Although not an Englishman, he must be included among the Leyden graduates who became well known in London. He was born around 1670 in Dordrecht in the Netherlands, of a medical family. After several years of studies at the Erasmus School in Rotterdam, he entered the University of Leyden and received the M.D. degree there in 1691, six years later. For reasons not known today, he settled in London in 1695. Here his career in the practice of medicine seems to have attracted little attention, except that he was cited by the College of Physicians for practicing without a license, for he had no Oxford or Cambridge degree. He had not applied for one, but practiced anyway. He himself admitted that he was a slow and often uncomprehending physician, although as an admirer of "the great Sydenham" he was a severe critic of the academic medicine of Oxford and Cambridge. In fact, most of his writings were nonmedical and scathing criticisms of one thing or another, delighting in perverse opinions. He cynically declared great spending to be the creator of prosperity (an opinion that would make him popular in American politics today). Mandeville held that philosophers were hypocrites, whereas prostitutes were useful socially. He wrote cynically about free thought and religion, virginity and marriage, and private vice as the precursor of public good. His views were criticized severely in writing by many individuals and some official bodies, but that seemed to have little effect on his loud and overbearing behavior. He was the life of a tavern club to which Benjamin Franklin once was taken, but did not return, because of his (Mandeville's) views on society and people and his vigorously expressed cynicism.

Mandeville was considered to have an excellent literary style-for a foreigner. In 1711 he proved it when he published his *Treatise of the Hypochondriach and Hysteric Passions*, not as a technical medical text but as a work for educated laymen. It consisted of exchanges involving the hypochondriacal husband, the hysteric wife, and the long-winded physician. No psychiatric social worker was included, as that species had not yet come into existence, and there was no child psychiatrist in the transaction, as there would be today. One might ask what purpose Mandeville's Leyden medical education had served. His influence, if any, on London's medical practice is not evident today, but his book on hypochondriasis and hysteria has been preserved (having gone through several editions in the 18th century) and is worth reading.

Several of the English Leyden alumni became famous practitioners in England. One, Mead, functioned as a physician in London, and another, Cadogan, settled in Bristol, at that time "the greatest, richest, and best port of trade in Great Britain, London only excepted," according to Daniel Defoe. Both had interesting but markedly different careers in practice; neither taught.

Mead was born in Stepney in 1673 (Winslow, 1935). His father, a nonconformist preacher there, had been ejected from his parish after the Restoration of Charles II and was forced into exile in Holland in 1683. He remained in school in England until 1689, after which he studied in Utrecht for three years. He then went to Leyden where he studied botany under Herman and physic under Pitcairne, the Scot. Boerhaave was a fellow student. However, Mead took his degrees of Doctor of Philosophy and Physic in Padua in 1695, after which he returned to Stepney and commenced his practice of medicine there. In 1702 he reported some elementary but courageous experiments on himself with snake venom. The following year he was appointed Physician to St. Thomas' Hospital and gave anatomy lectures at that school. Four years later Oxford conferred the degree of Doctor of Physic on him, and a few years later he was elected to both the College of Physicians and the Royal Society. In 1714 Radcliffe, Physician to William III and the leading practitioner in London, retired and turned over his practice to Mead. The affection that the two evidently had for each other was somewhat unexpected.   Radcliffe was ignorant of books and was rude and arrogant in manner, whereas Mead was a courtly and polished scholar.   In 1722 King George I asked him to study the use of inoculation for smallpox, and he did so using condemned criminals.   The results of that study became instrumental in the introduction of inoculation in England.

Mead became the leading physician in England, having as a patient George, Prince of Wales, who later became King George II.   In 1747 he published his *Treatise on Smallpox and Measles*, and in 1751 his most important work, *Medical Rules and Admonitions*, provided a summary of his extensive clinical experience in his practice in high society.   In personality he was warm, friendly, and generous.   He is said to have persuaded Guy to build the hospital that bears his name, specifically for the care of the poor.   A patron of the arts and sciences and a linguist, Mead opened his table to the learned and cultivated of all countries.   He carried on a constant correspondence with Boerhaave about clinical and chemical matters and was a friend of the poet Pope, the astronomer Halley, and Isaac Newton.   He is said to have earned and spent more money than any physician before him.   Although an outstanding humanist, he nevertheless believed that all vital phenomena followed physical and chemical laws, as was then the belief of iatrochemists.   However, he also believed that the sun and moon influenced the human body and caused or modified disease through Newtonian mechanics.   His treatise on the subject, published in 1704, was plagiarized boldly by Mesmer, who, in the opinions of at least early French revolutionists and of some of today's American psychoanalysts, was a genius.

The results of Mead's methods of treatment, which have not been recorded, are out of the reach of our evaluation.   One of his major contributions was *A Discourse on the Plague* (1720), written a few years after the great plague of Marseilles.   In that book Mead described the spread of the plague as consistent with contagion, an idea then unacceptable to most physicians and theologians: "Contagion is propagated by three causes, the air, diseased persons, and goods transported from infected places....I have been thus particular in tracing the Plague up to its first origin, in order to remove, as much as possible, all objection against what I shall say of the causes, which excite and propagate it among us.   This is done by contagion." Furthermore, he ascribed the failure of some persons to contract the disease, when exposed, to vital resistance and noted the apparent effects of anxiety, doubt, and dejection in aggravating the effects of infection.   He urged the isolation of the sick and recommended that the statistics of the disease be kept by experts and not, as was customary, by ignorant old women of the community. In short, although a physician untrained in modern epidemiology, he was able to formulate a concept of infectious disease that, however primitive and incomplete, had much merit.   His legacy included a great number of contented patients, who had recovered in some way unknown to us, and a host of encouraged literary and artistic persons. However, except for his book, there is no evidence that he made any lasting impression on medicine.

Another example of a Leyden alumnus who felt constrained to develop his powers of observation is Cadogan. Born in 1711, he entered Oriel College, Oxford, in 1727, as a "servitor," a student who paid his way by doing chores. He then went to Leyden in 1732, receiving the M.D. degree in 1737, and began his practice in Bristol (Rendle-Short, 1960, 1966).   He married and had his only child, a daughter, in 1747.   During that year he also was elected Physician to the Bristol Infirmary.   The birth of the child stimulated his interest, heretofore only theoretical, in the practical aspects of child care and rearing, and he wrote his remarkable *An Essay Upon Nursing and the Management of Children* in 1748, in the form of a letter to the Governors of the Foundling Hospital.   The hospital had been established by Coram, a retired bachelor sea captain, who had been horrified by the sight of abandoned children in London, where in some parishes all of the children born in a given year died, and in others only a few survived. Cadogan's letter probably had been commissioned by the Governors, and at any rate they voted to publish it.   One of the physicians of Bristol was Conyers, also an alumnus of Leyden, who claimed that Cadogan had plagiarized a work of his; but, inspection of both works does not support that view.

Cadogan's book made recommendations about diet and clothing (denouncing swaddling), and against the routine use of cathartics. The book was used widely, and several editions were printed. In 1749 Cadogan was made a Governor of the Foundling Hospital, shortly before another famous person, Handel, also became a Governor. Cadogan left Bristol and moved to London in 1752, where he served on two occasions as Physician to the Foundling Hospital during illnesses of Dr. Conyers. However, without an M.D. degree from Oxford or Cambridge he could not practice legally in London. He returned to Oxford to take his degree in 1755 and also was given a Cambridge M.D. degree by royal mandate. In 1762 he joined an Army expedition to defend Portugal against Spanish attack. John Hunter was one of the surgeons in that force. After seven months of service, Cadogan became ill and had to be relieved. He returned to practice, though on half pay, and in 1771 wrote his famous *A Dissertation on the Gout and All Chronic Diseases Considered as Proceeding From the Same Causes.* In his view almost all chronic diseases were psychological in origin, being caused by "indolence, intemperance, and vexation." He, therefore, advocated activity, temperance, and peace of mind and recommended avoidance both of strong drink and of strong medicine, and a generally bland balanced diet. The response was ferocious abuse from many physicians (Rendle-Short, 1960). His two works-on infant management and gout-tell us all that is known of his ideas about treatment. They were sound and far from sensational, although when they were written they seemed so. Here again we see a practicing physician who, trained in an institution where bedside observation was encouraged, was able to make contributions to medicine based on his own experience thereafter.

Mention also should be made of another Leyden man, Sims, born in County Down, Ireland, in 1741, the son of a dissenting minister. Sims studied medicine in London, Edinburgh, and finally Leyden, where he received the M.D. degree in 1764. He practiced in Tyrone for a time and then moved to London, where he joined the Medical Society in 1773 and was elected President in 1786, holding

that post for 22 years.   The Society was initially
bankrupt, poorly run, and on the point of dissolution, but
during his tenure it became well established and prosperous.   That improvement probably was not entirely due to
his own efforts, for at a crucial point the Society was
given a large house by Lettsom for its meetings and its library.   Sims' tenure was not a complete success, however,
for a group dissatisfied with his management organized the
Medical and Chirurgical Society of London, from which the
Royal Society of Medicine traces its descent.   Sims' medical writings were in no way notable, but he did collect a
large library, which he later sold to the Medical Society
of London.   On the other hand, when appointed in 1774 to
give the first oration of that Society, he did make a memorable comment about the dogmatist: "living in a narrow
cell, hedged in on all sides by his system, his timorous soul
dares not look beyond it, lest he might chance to spy anything which should create in him a doubt of his darling
hypothesis."   On a later occasion he wisely stated that
"the chit-chat at the patient's bedside is often neglected
and condemned by young practitioners who think it beneath
a man of science; yet, I will venture to affirm, that it is
often of as much importance as all the medicines that can
be administered, and that there is no old steady practitioner who has not saved many patients by it."
    Sims was described as a "good-humored pleasant
man, full of anecdote, an ample reservoir of good things..."
Another physician said that he was "a man of learning and
great good humor, but strangely tinctured with vanity
about his person which he thought irresistible...It was not
till late in life that he succeeded in obtaining the hand of
a young and fair lady, who, strange to say, was not *blind*
but deaf!"   Perhaps his preoccupation with books kept him
from marrying earlier, or perhaps it was the other way
around, but in any case his library became a useful re-
source.   That he used it is proved: He had "a most reten-
tive memory, but when that failed in any particular, he referred to a book of knowledge in the shape of a pocket-
book, from which he quoted with oracular authority."   Sims
is an example of a man who, despite the best of education, became in no way distinguished as an original thinker.

He probably never would have been remembered were it not for his activities in a medical society.

Two other alumni of Leyden, one English and one Irish, played interesting roles in English medicine of the 18th century. One of them, Clifton (M.D. Leyden, 1724; also M.D.[Hon.] Cambridge, 1728) wrote on the history of medicine, severely criticizing the medicine of the past and stating that progress would ensue only if "three or four persons of proper qualifications should be employed in the *Hospitals*...to set down the cases of patients there from day to day, *candidly* and *judiciously*, withough any regard to private opinions or publick systems, and at the year's end publish these facts just as they are, leaving every one to make the best use of 'em he can for himself." He was ahead of his time.

William Black was born in Ireland but received his M.D. at Leyden. He was licensed to practice in London in 1787 and also published historical writings in medicine, which were translated into German and French. He, too, was critical of the medicine of the past and stated that improvements in medical knowledge became important-and recognizable-only if they improved treatment (Neuberger, 1950).

Although a group of Leyden men in their English practices could not be distinguished from other 18th-century English practitioners, that was not true of one Leyden alumnus in practice in England, John Hall, who was especially interesting. After taking his M.D. degree at Leyden in 1770, he practiced in London. In 1785 he published *The Medical Family Instructor* and then, in 1805, produced a remarkable work, *Effects of Civilization on the People in European States*. That was in large part a discussion of the untoward consequences of industrialization. The work, which was cited by social reformers for decades afterward, proved, among other things, that workers received not more than one-eighth of what was produced by the value of their labor because of exploitation by the capitalists of that period. Hall was evidently a man of high principle and strong character. Imprisoned for debt in what he considered to be an unfair verdict in a court suit, he refused to let his friends pay the debt, and he died in prison.

Despite the fact that Edinburgh alumni practicing in London had no distinguishing features as a group, one alumnus who achieved great fame in London practice was Fothergill, a Yorkshire-born Quaker. Apprenticed to an apothecary at the age of 16, he subsequently entered the medical school at Edinburgh. Monro (*primus*) noticed his abilities and hired him to help revise his work on osteology. Fothergill graduated in 1736 and then studied at St. Thomas' Hospital in London for two years. He began his practice in 1740 and rapidly became successful in it. He wrote a book on diphtheria that enhanced his fame. Botany was his hobby, and vast sums of money were spent on his garden of exotic plants, a garden excelled nowhere in the world and equalled only by the Royal Gardens at Kew. He became known for aiding Quaker and non-Quaker medical students, including the Americans Shippen, Morgan, and Rush of Philadelphia, and Waterhouse of Newport, Rhode Island.

A patron of artists and scientists, he commissioned a collection of 500 natural-history drawings, purchased after his death by the Empress of Russia. His expressed opinions about almost anything were firm, and he obstinately believed in the organization of society as it was: royalty, quality, and commoners. Although Fothergill wrote and spoke in favor of American independence, he criticized the Americans for disagreeing with his ideas of society and their bad manners. He was a busy letter-writer, not only concerning his collections of plants and other things, but also regarding the affairs of the Quakers in Pennsylvania, the disgraceful character of the French, the founding of schools for Quaker children, and other aspects of his high-mindedness. His medical writings included clinical descriptions of tic douloureux, (probably) migraine, and epidemic influenza. Of great importance in his rise to fame was the demonstrated success of the mild treatments he recommended, in contrast to the then-prevalent drastic procedures. Among physicians of the time his insistence on observing patients and ignoring traditional theories was also noteworthy.

Withering was another Edinburgh graduate of English origin who returned to England to practice. He was born in Shropshire, descended from physicians on both sides.

(His maternal grandfather had delivered Samuel Johnson.) He seems to have had an average childhood and adolescence except for his skill with the flute and the harpsichord. He had considerable personal charm, an attribute that later opened many doors.

He entered Edinburgh to study medicine, but also greatly enjoyed the culture of the city. He adapted well to Scotland, learning to play the bagpipe and becoming an enthusiastic golfer. His teachers at the medical school were Monro *primus* and *secundus* in anatomy and surgery; Cullen in the practice of medicine; Black in chemistry; and Whytt in neurology and psychiatry. Curiously, Hope's course in botany evoked no interest in Withering; indeed, he found the study of botany "disagreeable." However, he developed a friendship with Pulteney, the historian of English botany and the biographer of Linnaeus. Withering spent his vacations with Thomas Arnold, the psychiatrist, and William Hunter, the London lecturer on anatomy. He took the M.D. degree in 1766 with a thesis on diphtheria, which he subsequently elaborated to include his observations on scarlet fever. He later published separately his *Sore Throat of Scarlet Fever*, considered one of his most important writings.

After a short Continental trip he started practice in Stafford, where the death of the local physician had created a need. Withering became the first attending physician of the newly opened Stafford Infirmary. His practice was sluggish, and he expanded his interests in natural history. Shropshire was noted for the luxuriant growth of the purple foxglove, which attained the height of five feet; but Withering's interest in botany remained low, until he met Helena Cooke, one of his first patients, who painted wildflowers. During her convalescence in the spring of 1768, they spend a good deal of time together searching for rare specimens for her to paint. He soon began to collect flowers, herbs, rocks, and crystals, and he enjoyed reading to her on the beauty of nature, as described in the works of Horace and Tasso. He himself drew well.

Withering participated in local music and became popular with his playing of the flute and, peculiarly, of the bagpipe. After four years of an old-fashioned romance, he and Helena were married. A few years later, in 1775, he was asked about a local family remedy for dropsy, which was the secret property of an old Shropshire woman who had cured a number of people whom the physicians had been unable to help. The remedy was a mixture of almost two dozen herbs, but he wrote, "it was not very difficult for one conversant in these subjects to perceive that the active herb could be no other than foxglove." He carried out experiemnts using foxglove in animals and began to collect clinical data on its effects. Earlier that year his friend Erasmus Darwin had written to him concerning an opening for a physician in Birmingham (this, too, brought about by the death of the local physician). Withering moved there and soon was so successful and well liked that he aroused Darwin's jealousy, for his practice became the most remunerative in England outside of London.

In 1776 his two-volume work on the botany of Great Britain, organized after the manner of Linnaeus, was published and was the first scientific treatise on British plants in the English language. It became very popular and grew with every subsequent edition. Also in that year he first showed signs of having tuberculosis. Nevertheless, in addition to medicine and botany, he actively pursued interests in chemistry and geology. When his book on scarlet fever was published in 1790, he stated that he thought that disease contagious and spread by "animalcules capable of generating their kind." Withering then decided to publish his data on the foxglove, after using it clinically for ten years. His results with the plant had made him famous much earlier, but he wanted to state explicitly the conditions and drawbacks of its use. When his illness forced him into inactivity, he was able to finish his *Account of the Foxglove*. During his inactive period he also wrote several nonmedical works. His stubborn illnesses drove him to the warmer climate of Portugal in 1792 and 1793, but the trips were disappointing, perhaps because, instead of resting, he devoted his time to studies in medicine, botany, mineralogy, climatology, and even air-conditioning. Later he had to spend most of his time in bed, but he continued to read, write, and even see patients. He died in 1799 at the early age of 58 (Moorman, 1942).

Much of Withering's life revolved around his friendship with Erasmus Darwin, the grandfather of Charles Darwin. Darwin observed the effects of the use of the foxglove as recommended by Withering and wrote about it five years earlier than Withering, without bothering to indicate the source of his observations, but the two remained friends (Musser and Krantz, 1940). Darwin was another 18th-century English physician of mixed Edinburgh-Cambridge background. He was born in 1731 and, after preliminary education, entered Cambridge in 1750. He graduated in 1754 after having written some poetry there, and then went to Edinburgh to study medicine. One year later he took the M.B. degree at Cambridge and, after further study at Edinburgh, started to practice. His life was distinguished by the great multiplicity of his interests. For example, he invented a carriage in which he might read and write while being driven; however, there was an accident which left him with a damaged kneecap and a bad limp. His friends included Watt, Wedgewood, and many others whose monthly scientific meetings led to their being called the Lunar Society. When his first wife died after 12 years of their marriage, he began to write passionate poetry to the mother of several of his young patients. There is no record of what her husband made of it, but after a time he was obliging enough to die, and Darwin married the widow.

Darwin was a great talker and felt competent, as well as impelled, to discuss almost any topic. A Mrs. Schimmelpenninck recorded her horror and dismay at his blunt speech and radical views. He strongly recommended temperance, but on one occasion was found swimming in the river fully clothed, full of good spirits of various sorts, after which he stood in a tub and made a rousing speech on prudence and sanitary arrangements. He wrote large works on natural history: *Zoonomia*, *Phytologia*, and *Plan for the Conduct of Female Education in Boarding Schools*. His great masses of peotry are now (fortunately) largely inaccessible but were described by Coleridge as "glittering, cold, and transitory." He was reported by a Miss Seward to have stolen some of her verses, as well as to have committed other discreditable actions, but her comments evidently were occasioned by his having encouraged, but then having failed, to marry her.   At any rate, she subsequently retracted her accusations, still unmarried.

Darwin also invented a cure for insomnia, which consisted in lying on a rotating millstone.   The fact that he could sleep despite the grinding roar must be taken to be a remarkable placebo effect.   His procedure is considered by some today to be the forerunner of the centrifuging of mental patients, an early form of shock therapy (Altschule, 1965).   Through all of the complications of his daily life, he still was the kindly, sympathetic physician, charitable to all except those who tried to talk while he was talking, as on the occasions when he and Samuel Johnson met.   Erasmus Darwin is remembered less for the product of his brains than that of his loins.   Two of his sons were physicians: The first, an Edinburgh man, cut himself doing a dissection and died of it.   The other developed a successful practice and also became the father of Charles Darwin.   One of Erasmus Darwin's daughters married a Galton, and she became the mother of Francis Galton, whose writings on free association so enthralled Freud.

Another famous English Edinburgh man was Parry, born in Gloucestershire in 1755 and educated at the famous dissenters' academy at Warrington, Lancs.   At the age of 18 he began his studies of medicine at Edinburgh. After a few years he went to London to continue his medical education at the hospitals, subsequently returning to study at Edinburgh.   He obtained his M.D. degree in 1778, went to Bath to practice, seldom leaving the town throughout the rest of his life.   He was Physician to the Bath General Hospital and also developed a large private practice.   A meticulous notekeeper, he collected a vast amount of clinical data which his terminal illness prevented him from publishing *in toto*.   His friendship with Jenner led him to study angina pectoris, while other writings described manifestations of thyroid disease, megacolon, and the effects of disease on the arterial pulse.   He was deeply interested in agriculture and animal husbandry, and spent much time in improving the breeds of sheep in England.   With other physicians in Bath, he lived an active, interesting, and effective life as a practicing physician, but his hobbies were in large measure for the benefit of

the agricultural, rather than cultural community. A physi-
cian-son tried to carry on his work, but did not exhibit
the fertility of mind of the father.

Lettsom is included here not because he made lasting contributions to the practice of medicine, but rather
because his career exemplifies several aspects of it. Lettsom, an English Quaker, was born in the Virgin Islands in
1744. At six years of age he was sent to England for
schooling and entered a Quaker academy run by Samuel
Fothergill, the preacher. At the age of 17 he was apprenticed to a surgeon in Yorkshire, and at the end of his
five-year term, he was sent by Samuel Fothergill to his
brother, John Fothergill, in London. There he entered the
medical school of St. Thomas' Hospital and soon became
known as an outstanding compiler of clinical notes. In
1767 he went to the West Indies to take over his inheritance, the most valuable portion of which was 50 slaves,
whom he promptly freed. He went into practice, earning
#2,000 in six months, and returned to London hoping to
live a life modeled on that of John Fothergill. Lettsom
entered the medical school at Edinburgh in 1768, studying
under Cullen, and the next year went to Leyden, where he
received the M.D. degree. Returning to London, he started
to practice in 1770, married a wealthy woman, and benefitted from John Fothergill's recommendation, for Fothergill
was then in the process of closing his London practice.
He started a library, a museum, and a botanical garden after Fothergill's model. Despite his huge practice, his ex-
penditures for those and other worthy purposes soon caused
him to be in serious financial difficulties. He evidently
had not acquired Fothergill's practice of frugality, perhaps
because he was a relaxed, or relapsed, Quaker. He is
known for having been a founder of the Royal Humane Society, the Royal Sea Bathing Society at Margate, and the
Medical Society of London. He wrote against intemperance, for the keeping of bees, on the introduction of the
mangel-wurzel, on the reform of prisons, on the general
relief of distress, and on the use of vaccination. (There
is no record that he slew dragons or rescued virgins.) He
is known also for the rhymed couplet, not only satirical
and unkind, but not in conformity with his reputation,

which his name evoked:

> I pukes, I bleeds, I sweats 'em
> and when they dies I Lettsom.

Lettsom exemplified several things.   He was an alumnus of Edinburgh and Leyden who established himself in London, although not originally from that city.   He tried to follow a model afforded by a great man and did not succeed totally because of his lack of greatness.   His indiscriminate doing of good works is perhaps typical of habitual do-gooders.   Despite those human weaknesses, or perhaps in a measure because of them, he was believed by his patients to be a good physician.

A most interesting alumnus of Edinburgh and Glasgow was Currie.   His life is a remarkable account of triumph over hardship, with illness-rheumatic heart disease-triumphing at the end.   Also of interest was his contribution to clinical practice, seemingly small at the time, but soon to reveal itself to be of great importance.   Currie was born in 1756 in Dumfiresshire, the son of a minister.   His early education trained him in Latin and Greek, but he began to think of studying medicine.   In 1771 he visited Glasgow with his father and became fired with the notion of going to America.   He went to Virginia but did not prosper there and, in addition, developed a recurrent febrile illness.   Upon the death of his father in 1774, he inherited some money, which he declined and turned over to his penniless sisters.   His business enterprises in America continued to do poorly, and he went to live with a relative who was a physician in Richmond, Virginia.

Currie's earlier interest in medicine now revived, he decided to go to Edinburgh in 1776 to study in preparation for a medical career in America.   However, after three days at sea, the vessel on which he was a passenger was captured by a privateersman in the service of the then-rebellious American colony.   Deprived of all of his goods, Currie was left to wander on the Virginia shore.   In the next few months he was twice drafted into the army and twice bought his way out of it.   He set out in another vessel for Great Britain, was captured again, and that time was put into an open boat.   He and his companions, ill with fever and dysentery and buffeted by a hurricane, made their way for 150 miles to the West Indies.   Hoping to repair his fortunes, Currie undertook to purchase supplies for the English admiral in charge of the station, who refused to repay him.   Ruined financially and subjected to fevers and other illnesses, he nevertheless started for England again.   Severe storms and two narrow escapes from shipwreck notwithstanding, he finally arrived there in 1777, whereupon he entered the medical school at Edinburgh and soon became known for his superior performance. In September of 1778 he developed rheumatic fever.

Despite that illness, he studied hard-philosophy as well as medicine.   Promised a medical appointment in the West Indies if he could get his M.D. degree quickly, he transferred to Glasgow and was given his degree in 1780. He went to London in connection with his promised appointment, but found that it had been given to another; nevertheless, he had planned to go to the West Indies and booked passage.   However, the vessel was delayed and, hearing of an opening in Liverpool, he settled there to practice medicine.   In spite of his reverses and illnesses, he was never depressed or bitter.   He started his practice in October of 1780 and soon was elected Head of the Dispensary.   Currie had literary hobbies and, with some others, founded a literary society, of which he became president.   He and others in the society also became active advocates of abolition of the slave trade.   He maintained his medical interest in fevers and in 1792 made the highly important recommendation that the thermometer be placed under the tongue for greatest accuracy (Shapiro, 1963). His many case reports in which the body temperature was so measured constitute an important pioneering effort.   In 1804, his health beginning to fail, he moved to Bath.   His condition worsened, and in 1805 he died of valvular heart disease.

In addition to the previously discussed men-all graduates of one university medical school or another-there were some outstanding London physicians who had no formal training at all, except as apprentices and in "walking the wards" at hospitals.

Cheselden was one of an impressive line of London surgeons (Power, 1912).   Like some others of his era he

never took a degree, nor in fact did he study at any recognized medical school.   He was born in Leicestershire in
1688, and little is known about his early education.   He
may have been apprenticed to a local surgeon.   In 1703 he
went to London to study with Cowper, then at the height
of his fame as an anatomist.   He also was apprenticed to
a surgeon at St. Thomas' Hospital.   By 1711 he was
teaching anatomy, his course consisting of 35 lectures
given four times yearly.   That course was given for 20
years, sometimes in the Hospital, sometimes in his home.
In 1714 he was in some trouble with the Company of Barber-Surgeons for carrying out dissections in his home without their permission.   Cheselden was elected to the St.
Thomas Hospital staff in 1718 and was made Principal Surgeon the next year.   From that time he lectured both in
anatomy and in operative surgery.   He invented an operation for bladder stones, which, on one occasion, he performed in 54 seconds.   His *Anatomy of the Human Body*
was used widely, although its text was sparse.   His *Os-
teographia* also had little text, but the illustrations that he
drew were remarkably beautiful.   In 1744 he was instrumental in the separation of the Surgeons from the Barbers.
He became Surgeon to Queen Caroline and Surgeon to St.
George's Hospital when it was founded, and received many
honors.   A notable sportsman, his chief interest was box-
ing, but like other leading physicians of the time he also
mingled with artists, writers, and scientists.   One of his
hobbies was architecture, at which he became expert,
drawing the plans for the bridge at Putney and for several
other structures.   In addition to all of that he had a very
busy practice, being widely liked for his geniality and gai-
ety.   His patients found him kind and tender-hearted, but
today he is remembered primarily as a teacher of many of
England's great physicians.

Pott is another example of a man who, despite having had no formal training whatsoever, became a leader in
clinical medicine.   He was born in London in 1714 and at
the age of 15, after early years of poverty, was apprenticed for seven years to Nourse, Assistant Surgeon to St.
Bartholomew's Hospital.   The fee required was #210.
Nourse gave a course of lectures in anatomy in his own
home, and Pott's duties included preparing the subject.

He showed great aptitude for that work and was recognized for it. His professional life seems to have been his entire life. He brought his mother and his half-sister to live with him. He was admitted to the Barber-Surgeons Company in 1736 and, therefore, was allowed to practice. When the Barber-Surgeons Corporation was dissolved in 1745, he naturally joined the Surgeons Corporation, and they elected him and John Hunter lecturers. In 1761 Pott became an examiner for the Corporation and soon afterward was Master of it. Having been made Assistant Surgeon at St. Bartholomew's in 1744, he later rose to higher rank.

In his practice he made notable changes in wounddressings which reduced their damaging qualities. In January of 1766 he was thrown from his horse and suffered a compound fracture (with the bone protruding through the skin) of the lower leg. He insisted upon lying on the cold pavement until he could purchase a door, hire two men to affix poles to it, and have them carry him the long distance to his house. Immobilized for a long time because of "Pott's fracture," he wrote the first of a long series of works on surgical diagnosis and technique. His name became associated with Pott's disease of the spine. He lectured to the students of St. Bartholomew's, first privately at home, later publicly in the hospital. Among his many honors were election to the Royal Colleges of Surgeons of Edinburgh and Ireland. He is an outstanding example of on-the-job training and of how it is possible to grow in stature while affiliated with the same hospital for more than 50 years.

As noted previously, private medical schools played a prominent part in medical education in London. The size, quality, and time of existence of those schools covered wide ranges that will not be discussed at this time. Suffice it to state that their total educational contribution was very large. Only the most famous will be considered: The "Great Windmill Street School," its name derived from its location, founded by William Hunter, an alumnus of Glasgow and Edinburgh.

William Hunter was born near Glasgow in 1718 and entered the University in 1731 to prepare for a career in the church by studying Latin, Greek, philosophy, and logic.

He stayed until 1736 and, having decided against the church career, chose medicine instead.   (Fourteen years later, having become famous elsewhere, he was granted the M.D. degree by Glasgow [Beekman, 1944; Illingworth, 1967].)   In 1737 he became Cullen's resident pupil and then studied medicine at Edinburgh University from 1740 to 1741.   Afterward he practiced in London, probably with Dr. James Douglas, and also at St. Thomas' Hospital.   In 1746, still without his degree, he began to give private lectures in surgical anatomy to some naval surgeons.   Two years later, after studying at Leyden and Paris, he lectured and practiced surgery and obstetrics in London, and in that year was appointed to the staffs of two hospitals (*sans* degree).   His practice was limited to obstetrics, and that, together with the fees from his teaching and his salary as Professor of Anatomy at the Royal Academy, made his a wealthy man.

He spent #20,000 in developing his main hobby, a museum of anatomical specimens (some injected), coins, old manuscripts and books, and natural-history specimens.   His museum was enlarged by the addition of Fothergill's at a cost of #1,200.   His teaching influenced the careers of many physicians from different countries, and his anatomical discoveries enriched that subject.   Upon his death his school and museum passed to his nephew, Baillie.   In the early 1800s Brodie and Bell, both leaders of London surgery at the time, joined the School, which was purchased by Bell in 1812.

John Hunter, William's brother, became one of England's greatest surgeons.   Unlike his elder brother's boyhood, John's was characterized by a love of sports and marked laziness and indifference to scholarship.   He left grammar school prematurely.   In that respect the permissiveness of his parents made it impossible for him ever to become a well-educated man in the atmosphere of that period.   At about the age of 17 he stayed for a time in Glasgow, helping his brother-in-law, an expert cabinet-maker, and seeming to enjoy acquiring manual skills.   At the age of 20 he went to London with the idea of assisting his brother William in his dissections, and was put to work on the arm muscles.   He was so enthusiastic, adept, persistent, and conscientious at that work that the next year he was able to supervise students. He was also very helpful in another way-he was extremely popular with the body-snatchers.

John enjoyed convivial company, in general, and the theater and its habitues, in particular. In 1749 his brother William secured permission for him to study under Cheselden at the Chelsea Hospital. In 1753 he was teaching anatomy in the Surgeons' Corporation, and a year later he enrolled formally as a surgical pupil at the medical school of St. Thomas' Hospital. Although he enrolled at Oxford a year later, his presence was recorded only for a month. He became a partner in his brother's school in 1758, but had little enthusiasm for public speaking and proved to be a poor lecturer. However, he was an excellent dissector and made many contributions to anatomical knowledge. Possibly because of fatigue or failing health due to overwork, he joined the Army in 1761, serving in several campaigns during which he made studies in blood-clotting, war wounds and, in fact, anything of interest that offered itself. Returning to London in 1763, he started practice as a surgeon and also took house-pupils for a fee of 500 guineas each. (One of his later students was Jenner.)

His attempts to develop a school were unsuccessful because he was a poor lecturer, but his studies in human and comparative anatomy, and the museum he developed from them, brought him increasing fame. He soon began to keep live exotic specimens as well and seemed intent on working hard as a surgeon only to make the money necessary to develop and maintain his collections. Through it all he managed to write and publish profusely. In 1773 he began a revolutionary course of lectures on the principles of surgery. Still a poor speaker, he became accustomed to settling his nerves with laudanum before his lectures. Although his classes were small by the standards of the time, they included Cooper, Abernathy, and others destined to become leaders in surgery. He began to suffer from angina pectoris in 1773, but he continued his anatomical work, built a new museum building, and gained new honors, including that of Surgeon to George III. In 1792 his assistant and brother-in-law, Horne, began to give the lectures, while Hunter busied himself with the writing of his work on infection and trauma.   He did not live to finish it, dying during a dispute with staff members of St. George's Hospital about regulations regarding teaching. The autopsy showed severe coronary artery calcification; the mitral valve also showed calcification.

Despite his coronary artery disease of 20 years' known duration, he was able to work very hard for long hours, starting his day at 4:00 or 5:00 A.M. and ending at midnight.   Although a good companion in social groups, he was often arrogant, overbearing, and irritable at work. Ceremony bored or angered him.   In his work he was a genius who could abide neither those less intelligent than himself, nor those unappreciative of his great attributes. Nevertheless, he was candid about himself.   Throughout his highly productive life he manifested little interest in books, and his phenomenal knowledge was based solely on his own investigations, observations, and clinical experience.   The permanent influence of his teaching on subsequent clinical practice is so great as to be impossible to detail (Oppenheimer, 1946a,b, 1949; Gloyne, 1950; Beekman, 1954; Thomas, 1958; Morris, 1959).   He is an example of a country boy-unsuited to formal education and too stubborn to pretend to submit to it-who became so stimulated when he encountered the opportunity to make observations and experiments, working with his hands and his mind together, that he made contributions far greater than those of men with formal educations.   Hunter became one of the greatest practitioners of his age-certainly the greatest surgeon-despite the lack of booklearning and university education.   He is notable also for having been able to work incredibly hard for at least 20 years with coronary artery disease-dying not as the result of overwork, but rather in an emotional episode.

The name of Jenner is mentioned in almost every general history of medicine because of his role in the popularization of smallpox vaccination.   However, his medical career is also important because it exemplifies the process of becoming a doctor and practicing medicine in 18th-century England.   Jenner was born in Gloucestershire in 1749, the son and grandson of clergymen, and spent much of his free time as a youth collecting fossils and other objects of natural history that abounded around Gloucestershire.   He was apprenticed to a surgeon in Sudbury, and then, in 1770, entered John Hunter's home as a resident pupil. Although he was there for only two years, the two men became close friends and later often wrote to each other. His time with Hunter solidified his interests and gave him the concepts and techniques needed to pursue them.   In 1771 he was employed by Sir Joseph Banks to prepare some of the specimens collected by Captain Cook in his South Sea voyages.   During the time of his residence in London he pursued his studies at the Medical School of St. Thomas' Hospital, returning to his birthplace in 1773 and starting his practice, which grew rapidly.

Nevertheless, Jenner found time to study birds and plants, to write poetry, and to play the flute and violin. He often sent specimens of one kind or another to John Hunter.   His first scientific paper, *The Natural History of the Cuckoo*, was published in *Philosophical Transactions*. Part of the account seems to have been imaginary or hearsay, but in the main it was accurate. He was one of the founders of a group that met to read medical papers and then dine; in fact, it was at one of the meetings that he presented his observations on angina pectoris, heart disease, and cowpox, among other things.   Although he also wrote some strictly chemical papers, he made it plain early in his medical career that at his best he was a good clinical observer.   His practice grew so rapidly that he gave up obstetrics and surgery.   In 1792 he received the M.D. degree from St. Andrew's.   Two years later he was stricken with severe typhus fever, and during the long convalescence he developed his ideas about vaccination.

Jenner had known since boyhood that for some time the milkmaids of Gloucestershire recognized that cowpox protected them from smallpox.   The physicians who heard that evidently regarded it as mere folklore.   However, a farmer of Dorsetshire, Benjamin Jesty, in 1714 inoculated his wife and two sons with cowpox, and they did not contract smallpox even when inoculated with it.   In 1791 Platt, a tutor in a household in Schonwade, Holstein, learned (from milkmaids) about the protective effects of cowpox and inoculated his employer's three sons with the cowpox. When a smallpox epidemic occurred in Schonwade in 1794, those three children were the only ones to escape infection.   In May of 1796 Jenner vaccinated a young boy with cowpox serum and the boy developed the disease; however, when he was inoculated with smallpox material six weeks later, he did not develop the disease.   There is nothing to indicate that that experiment was subjected to peer review by human-studies committees, or to questioning by people today quaintly called "consumers of medical services."   Jenner's original report remained an unpublished manuscript, but he did publish a more extensive report in 1798 in the form of a small illustrated book.   His work was contradicted by a number of persons, and in 1800 and 1801 he published further data.

The idea of vaccination spread slowly.   Among those who favored it was Waterhouse, Professor of Physic at Harvard, who had written an article in the *Columbian Sentinel* (March 12, 1799) with the title, "Something Curious in the Medical Line."   In 1800 Jenner was asked to vaccinate the entire 85th Regiment of Foot, as well as their wives and children; however, since they all were infected with scabies, the idea was dropped.   The following year the Royal Navy successfully was vaccinated and Jenner soon was deluged with congratulatory messages from many parts of the world, some as far away as Russia.   Parliament voted him #10,000 to compensate him for loss of income during his studies.   It was probably the letter by Baillie to the government that had the greatest effect.   A Jennerian Distribution to promote vaccination was formed, and in 1808 that was replaced by the government's National Vaccine Establishment.   In 1813 Oxford granted him the M.D. degree.

It is evident that Jenner was a country practitioner whose interest in sick people and in the phenomena of Nature made it possible for him to make one of the greatest discoveries ever made in the field of public health.   He was not a scientist.   The discovery was only one of his important discoveries, albeit the one that most quickly made its great value known.

Thomas Young was an English physician of the 18th century whose professional life exemplified some problems that still plague medicine.   On the one hand, his contributions to medical science were outstanding; on the other hand, he was not satisfied with his medical education, wandering from place to place and, finally, after entering practice, was not successful.   Owing to the way in which medicine was organized at that time, his early professional years were years of accomplishment, but his mature years were disappointing.   Young was born in Somersetshire in 1773, a son of a prosperous Quaker merchant.   He was highly precocious and became a fluent reader by the age of two, reading omnivoursly thereafter.   His interests from the first were remarkably wide, and later in life he wrote not only on medical subjects but also on such subjects as calculation of motion of a body projected from the moon, the deciphering of Egyptian hieroglyphics, and the natural history of the cricket.   However, as he himself states, biographies bored him and he could not become much interested in the details of people's lives.   Perhaps that was a warning that he would not become a good medical practitioner.

Young visited his uncle, a prominent London physician, on several occasions and, in 1791, decided to study medicine.   The next year he commenced to study at Hunter's Great Windmill Street School and in 1793 also began to study at St. Bartholomew's Hospital.   In that year, at the age of 20, he gave a paper before the Royal Society in which he stated his hypothesis on the role of the eye's lens in accommodation.   Home, professor at Edinburgh, disagreed; but subsequent studies by Young showed Home's objections to be invalid.   In 1794 Young began to study medicine at Edinburgh but, dissatisfied with his teachers, went to Göttingen.   He graduated from the University there, visited several other cities in Germany, and then returned to England.   In order to gain the right to practice in London he entered Cambridge in 1800 and gave a remarkable lecture there in which he reported his experiments on wave motion in light and sound.   He gave another remarkable lecture in 1801 on his theory of color vision, a theory adopted by von Helmholtz in Germany some decades later.   Young continued to do work on the lens in accommodation.   Although his use of the principles and data of physics to elucidate medical problems was well in advance of his time, his medical practice was unsuccessful; however, his reputation as a medical scientist enabled him to get an appointment as Physician to St. George's

Hospital.   He wrote and lectured on medical subjects, despite his unease in that work; clearly, he lacked confidence in his clinical capabilities (Behrman, 1975).   Today he would be heading a clinical department at some American university hospital, despite his clinical inadequacies. The story of his professional life exemplifies one of the unsolved dilemmas of modern medicine: where to place and how to define properly the role of a physician who is not much interested in patients as people.

The private medical schools discussed earlier in this chapter began to decline after a time, owing largely to the fact that each was created and maintained by a single outstanding person.   When that person left, the school deteriorated, if no equally outstanding successor was found. Nevertheless those schools had a great effect on the practice of medicine in 18th-century England, not only because of the men trained in them, but because of their role in the development of some of the hospital medical schools (e.g., Middlesex and St. Mary's).

The hospital medical schools of England gave medical teaching and practice a distinctive quality, and it is appropriate to discuss their development.   When Henry VIII dissolved the hospitals of his era, his action was part of the dismantling of the Roman Catholic establishment in England.   In the long run that did more good than harm to medicine, for it placed the responsibility for hospital care in the hands of the secular authorities who had the support of wealthy benefactors (Gale, 1967).   By the mid-18th century, a large number of competent graduates of Edinburgh, Glasgow, Aberdeen, and Dublin-with some from Leyden and other Continental schools-had begun to practice in London.   In that century these and other men at London's five hospitals instituted formal teaching in medicine.   In order of establishment these hospitals were Guy's, St. Bartholomew's, St. Thomas', St. George's, and the London (Newman, 1957; Singer and Holloway, 1960).   Before the end of the 18th century six other hospital medical schools had been established in London.   Medical schools also were established at Manchester, Birmingham, Sheffield, Leeds, Newcastle, Bristol, and Liverpool, with others, which did not succeed, at Hull, York, Nottingham, Exeter, and Bath (Wetherill, 1961).   At Liverpool, for example, the prominent members of the 19th-century staff were alumni of Edinburgh or Glasgow (Cohen, 1972). Free dispensaries also were important in teaching (Cope, 1969; Paynter, 1957). (The detailed histories of the great English hospitals have been covered extensively and are highly interesting, but not essential for us here [Brockbank, 1952, 1965; Dainton, 1962; Anning, 1963; Clark-Kennedy, 1962; McInness, 1963; Ober, 1973; Medvie and Thompson, 1974; Handler, 1976].)

The statistics show that the London hospitals had far more surgical than medical students (Zimmerman, 1963). This is explainable in several ways. Whereas most of the nonsurgical practice of the leading physicians consisted of house calls, with the apprentices, house-pupils, or assistants accompanying the teacher, much of the surgical practice was in hospitals. Perhaps because of that situation, each hospital physician was allowed only two students, whereas hospital surgeons were allowed many more. And finally, even though a man's hospital training might have been surgical, his subsequent practice need not have been so. That was the case for a number of London physicians. Nevertheless, in France, if not in America, England's medical leadership in the 18th century was considered to be in the field of surgery (Huard, 1968). The hospital medical schools emphasized bedside medicine in all its practical aspects, and theory was minimized in the teaching. These schools became the main factor in the growth of clinical medicine in England, as evidenced by the contributions of their physicians in the late 18th and in the 19th centuries. English medicine of the 19th century was taught mainly in the hospitals. London, the largest medical center in the country, had no university at all until well into the 19th century. Hence the physicochemical superstitions that had stultified teaching at Leyden and Edinburgh (as well as the continental university medical schools) had less influence at the English medical schools.

The medicine-related science of 18th-century English medicine was anatomy, and that was predominant until the explosive rise of chemistry and physiology in the 19th century. Since the anatomical contribution to medicine, in contrast to surgery, was largely post-mortem, anatomy's role in functional considerations could be only inferential.

The absence in relative terms of a strong scientific component in medicine was beneficient to some extent, since the patient was the only tool with which the physician could work.   That kind of patient-oriented medicine, established at Padua, Leyden, and Edinburgh, reached its full development in the London medical scene.   The growth of medicine based on patient-doctor interaction-replacing medicine based on theory-became increasingly rapid, most notably in London.   However, events in France in the 18th century had begun to move in the same direction.

The development of medical education in English hospitals in the late 18th and early 19th centuries was due to several factors.   The failure of Oxford and Cambridge to function as centers of modern medical education has been noted.   Another factor was the change in the Poor Law, which required that the parishes provide medical care to the sick poor.   There were only seven provincial hospitals in all of England in 1700, but the number increased more than fivefold before the end of the century (Thomas, 1980).   The parishes sent their sick poor to nearby provincial hospitals.   Over 100 parishes sent their sick to the Radcliffe Infirmary at Oxford and paid for their care there.   The hospitals in London received patients not only from among the local population, but also from nearby rural parishes.   Thus England was served by several dozen local hospitals, all smaller than the gigantic institutions built in France and Austria.   The English local hospitals, staffed by men engaged in the treatment of patients and with little time for, or patience with, theories, became centers of clinical teaching, thereafter giving English medicine its character.   Garrison's comment that the physicians of earlier eras must have been doing something correct is supported by English 17th-century experience: When England's hospitals were opened in response to requirements of Poor Law, the mortality rates improved (Thomas, 1980).

Clearly the English physicians of 300 years ago were not practicing 20th-century medicine and could not begin to imagine its large scientific content.   This raises the possibility that today's so-called "scientific" physicians are doing something different from what they think they are doing.   The aspects of medical care which are responsible for clinical improvement may be different in different cases and certainly are not related to current scientific theory.

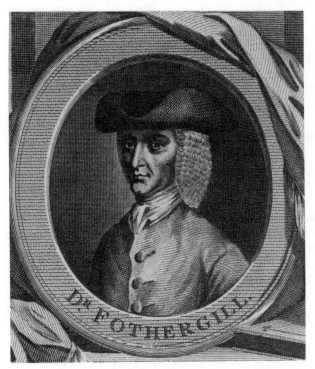

John Fothergill, 1712–1780

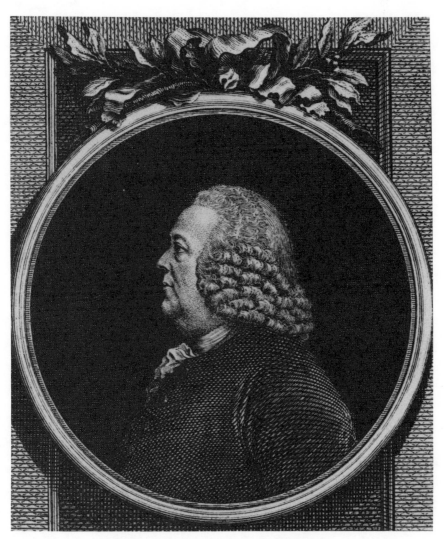

Gerhard Van Swieten, 1700-1772

Chapter 6: Medicine in Eighteenth-Century Vienna.
Notes on Göttingen and Spain

MEDICINE IN 18TH-CENTURY AUSTRIA was important in the development of modern clinical medicine for several reasons. In
the first place, it was the lineal, if not the spiritual, heir
to Leyden medicine as it was developed under Boerhaave.
Although it was true that the Leyden emphasis on the phenomena exhibited by patients as opposed to the phenomena
listed by dogmatic systems did not receive an unmixed
welcome in 18th-century Austria, patient-oriented medicine
replaced theory-oriented medicine, after a time. For the
half-century that preceded World War I, Vienna became
the most important center of clinical teaching in the
world.
       Changes were bound to occur in Leyden medicine
when the Boerhaave era came to an end there: The possibility of finding another Boerhaave was slight. The existence of a position does not guarantee the existence of a
man to fill it. After de le Boë and Boerhaave, Leyden
needed another great clinician with prominent qualities of
leadership. There were many good clinicians in Leyden in
the early 18th century, but the man who had outstanding
qualities of leadership as well was not acceptable. He
was van Swieten, a Catholic in a country that had suffered cruelly at the hands of a Catholic country, Spain.
There may have been questions about his orthodoxy-there
were rumors that he was a Jansenist-but this did not affect the thinking of the non-Catholics, who were not influenced by variations in the degree of Catholic orthodoxy in
maintaining their apprehension and dislike.
       Although an authoritative biography of van Swieten
has yet to be written, the main facts of his life in Leyden
are fairly well known (Brechka, 1971). Born in Leyden in
1700, his parents, five siblings, and some other relatives
having died by 1712, he found himself in the care of two
guardians, one of whom was a physician. Van Swieten en-

tered the University of Louvain, the nearest Catholic University, in 1714.   At that time, Catholics in the northern republican Netherlands could practice their religion and their commercial pursuits, as well as study in the universities; but, they legally could not hold office.   The southern Netherlands remained Catholic and by 1714 had been ceded to Austria by the Treaties of Utrecht and Rastatt-Baden. Van Swieten stayed at Louvain for only 18 months.   In 1717 he entered the University at Leyden, where he received the M.D. degree in 1725.   He lived for a time in the house of an apothecary and joined the Apothecaries' Guild.

Van Swieten studied medicine at Leyden when Boerhaave was at the height of his career.   Soon after graduating, van Swieten began to lecture on materia medica, but his teaching was informal and unpaid because, although Catholic and Protestant students equally were welcome, only Protestants were admitted to the faculty.   Van Swieten complained that his nine years of teaching pursued in this way rewarded him only with the Faculty's jealousy, and in 1734 he was forbidden to lecture to students, even privately. Nevertheless a group of men, including Boerhaave, Linnaeus, and other scholars and scientists, continued to meet with him for frequent discussions.   After Boerhaave's death in 1738, clinical teaching in the hospital ceased, and the laboratories, museums, and libraries stagnated.   However, van Swieten took over and maintained his old professor's extensive professional correspondence. He also had a large and successful medical practice and remained active in the Church.   When prevented from teaching orally, he decided to teach by the printed word, and he started the *Commentaries on the Aphorisms of Boerhaave*, which later made him famous.   For 20 years he had taken down Boerhaave's words in shorthand, and he interspersed that material with an astonishing array of apt quotations from the medical literature of the Western World, largely Great Britain.   The first volume was published in 1742, and the remaining work took 30 years to complete.   Several editions were published.   In the meantime, van Swieten worked in his chemical laboratory and with his botanical collection; but a great change occurred in his life in 1745, when he went to Vienna at the invitation of Maria Theresa.

When Maria Theresa took the throne of Austria-Hungary in 1740, she found herself the ruler of a shaky kingdom. Her friend, Frederick the Great of Prussia, attacked Austria because, as he said, "The Army was ready." Silesia was lost, and her country's morale suffered. Her husband, Francis of Lorraine, was no help as an administrator, so she planned to strengthen her position through her only sister, the wife of Francis' brother. The idea of a double dynastic connection with Lorraine was important to her, but when her sister became ill and died, the plan died with her. Actually, the Austrian situation at that time was not all bad, since Austria, with the help of a Hungarian force, had beaten the Turks, and recently had come through the War of the Spanish Succession.

Austrian medicine, however, had fallen behind that of Leyden-formerly an Austrian possession-and needed to be modernized. In fact, the situation had become so poor that the M.D. degree had not been granted in Vienna since 1703. Maria had come to know van Swieten when he treated her sister and had been impressed greatly by his qualities as a physician (despite her sister's resultant death). She asked van Swieten to accept the posts of Physician to the Royal Family, head of all physicians in Austria, and Director of Medical Education. He did so in 1745 and by 1749 instituted reforms, such as the reorganization of the medical faculty at Vienna, and the opening of medical schools and strengthening of others in Austria and Italy, part of which Austria then ruled. In 1754 van Swieten invited his colleague at Leyden, de Haen, to head the hospital teaching. De Haen wrote extensively about clinical medicine, using mainly English and Scottish sources (Neuberger, 1942, 1943; Lesky, 1965, 1976), and particularly was known for his admiration of Sydenham, emphasizing the case method, including post-mortem data, in clinical teaching. (He also became famous for his clinical use of the thermometer.)

Nevertheless, both van Swieten and de Haen proved to be curiously rigid, de Haen especially so, as shown by his belief in witchcraft. Van Swieten banned Jewish physicians, however well qualified they might have been, not only from having Christian patients (as was true everywhere in Europe), but also from having Jewish patients. De Haen, for his part, was opposed violently to inoculation in the prevention of smallpox, although he was shaken badly by Maria Theresa's narrow escape from death by that disease.   Both men rejected Auenbrugger's great discovery of percussion in 1763.   Nevertheless, clinical medicine based on clinical phenomena was established as the official way, albeit in an old-fashioned and dogmatic manner.   To van Swieten, Boerhaave was the ultimate unchangeable authority.

When van Swieten died in 1772 he was succeeded by Storck, who was much more progressive.   For example, Storck believed in evaluating medications as they affected patients, not theoretically, and also was known for having introduced a number of plants into medicine, notably members of the atropine family.   (The atropine group had been used for some time in witchcraft and for hallucinogenic purposes.)   Later, de Haen was succeeded as Director of the Clinic by Stoll, another progressive praised both as a great teacher and a beloved physician.   He favored the use of inoculation and had long been practicing percussion privately with Auenbrugger and other friends.   A curious situation existed: Dutch physicians who had been moved to Austria to modernize its medicine did so, but at the same time made it unprogressive.   When they left the scene, native Austrians replaced them and led Austrian medicine along the road of progress, at least for a time.

In 1765 the widowed Maria Theresa invited her son, Archduke Joseph, to share the Imperial Throne with her, which he did, becoming Emperor Joseph II.   A year earlier he had appointed Brambilla of Pavia (then an Austrian possession) to the post of *Leibchirurg*, translated as "Personal Surgeon."   In 1778 Brambilla was appointed Chief Staff Surgeon and, in 1779, Sole Superintendent of the Army Health Service.   Brambilla then proceeded to give the Army Health Service something approaching university status, and spent much care and effort in recruiting instructors for it.   A special building, the Josephineum, was constructed for it and opened in 1785.   Brambilla gave the future instructors special grants and sent them to study at the foremost foreign teaching hospitals, especially those of

London and Paris. The first of those instructors was a Czech named Hunczovsky, who on his return wrote a treatise on medicine and surgery as practiced in the English and French teaching hospitals (Belloni, 1972). That account supplemented his letters to Brambilla, which were written before that. Among other things, the work contained a highly sophisticated discussion of Pott's account of Pott's disease of the spine.

The foreign-trained physicians did much to give Vienna its high standing in the 19th century. In 1784 Joseph II built the Allgemeine Krankenhaus, the huge general hospital used for teaching in clinical medicine and pathologic anatomy. Moreover, he established a 1,200-bed military teaching hospital, complete with libraries and laboratories, and also passed the Act of Tolerance, admitting Jews to universities. He continued to send Austrian physicians abroad-particularly to Great Britain-for study, and instituted reforms of insane asylums and prisons. When the progressive Stoll had to retire, Joseph appointed an excellent successor, Johann Peter Frank. Frank took the Chair at Vienna in 1795 and also was made Director of the General Hospital there.

Frank was a most unusual physician for his time, for he was much in advance of it. Born in 1745, his early life seemingly destined him for that of a good, but not outstanding, physician. In 1784 he was still physician to the Prince-Bishop of Spires; however, the first three volumes of his remarkable work on the responsibilities of the state toward the people's health were published. He was at once offered chairs at three institutions, but went first to Göttingen as Professor of Clinical Medicine. Supported by the King of England, Göttingen was the great teaching center that had been made famous by von Haller. Frank taught not only medicine, but physiology, pathology, forensic medicine, and public health. Not satisfied with conditions there or the climate, he went to Pavia (in Austrian Italy) in 1785. Although the school was improved in the time of Maria Theresa, it needed more work and, encouraged by the Emperor Joseph II, Frank made the necessary changes, which included instituting hospital ward rounds for the students. In 1786 he was made Director General of

Public Health of Austrian Lombardy and the Duchy of Mantua.

He continued to teach medicine, but also exhibited marked administrative capacity. The Spring of 1790 was a gloomy one for the Austrian empire, and Frank chose that time to give his famous address, "The People's Misery: Mother of Diseases," in which he emphasized the importance of the rural masses, the most useful citizens of the state. He exposed their poverty, malnutrition, miserable housing, and lack of clothing and fuel. That, he said, was a result of exploitation, since farming in the Empire was actually highly productive and profitable. Frank called for a redistribution of the products of agriculture, more in the interests of public heath, than those of justice. He was not a social revolutionary, but merely a good physician (Sigerist, 1941). When Emperor Joseph II became ill, he was fearful that revolutionary ideas would spread through Europe from France, and as a result abolished most of his own reforms. He was succeeded by his brother Leopold II who, encouraged by Metternich, continued the reaction that Joseph had started, which forced Frank to resign in 1804. Stifft became the new Chairman of Medicine. Frank went first to Vilna and then to St. Petersburg in 1805 as Physician to the Czar; but, later he returned to Vienna.

Frank was a competent but not outstanding bedside clinician, and for a time, he adopted the Brunonian superstition, as did other physicians in northern Italy. He gave it up when he went to Vienna, where it was not popular. On the other hand, he was an outstanding pioneer in the field of social medicine, which later led to his downfall during the Metternich reaction in Vienna. Frank had little lasting influence on Viennese clinical medicine, although his contributions to our understanding of public health remain memorable.

Frank and his son, Joseph, were friendly with Beethoven, who had left Bonn in 1792 to live permanently in Vienna. Beethoven had shown great interest in a well-known singer, Christine Gerhardi, but she did nothing to encourage him and instead married young Joseph Frank, who was a competent composer. Beethoven consulted the elder Frank with respect to his deafness and other ills.

The Viennese man who made large and lasting changes in clinical medicine was Auenbrugger, born in 1722. Although his official contemporaries in Vienna did not appreciate his work, today Auenbrugger ranks high with respect to his influence on the practice of medicine. After his preliminary education, he entered the Medical School in Vienna, studied under van Swieten, and received the M.D. degree in 1752. For the next ten years he was on the faculty. He was Assistant Physician at the Spanish Hospital in Vienna, where he became Chief Physician in 1762, holding that position briefly, and resigning as a consequence of the sort of professional (or perhaps personal) dispute that has been enlivening Viennese medicine since its resuscitation 250 years ago. He entered private practice and did well. Early in his adult life he became interested in music: His two daughters were highly talented as singers and pianists, and the family had Sunday afternoon musicales to which many of the cultured were invited. Salieri (teacher of Beethoven), Schubert, and Liszt became Auenbrugger's friends. Salieri had come to Vienna from Italy at the age of 16, and when only 24 years old, he was engaged as Court Composer, serving in that capacity for 50 years. Auenbrugger wrote the libretto for Salieri's *Chimney Sweep*, a comic opera first performed in 1781 (Rosenberg, 1958). Although Maria Theresa made it a favorite, Mozart considered it trash.

During his service at the Spanish Hospital, Auenbrugger studied percussion in many patients, checking his interpretations against autopsy findings. He also injected water into the chest of cadavers and observed the changes in percussion note which resulted (Sigerist, 1936; Jarcho, 1961). As a child, and the son of an innkeeper, he was accustomed to watching men tap the sides of casks to ascertain the degree of fullness. In 1761 he published *Inventum Novum ex Percussione Thoracic Humani*, received mainly with indifference and occasionally with derision. (In 1778 Cullen expressed doubt about its value [Jarcho, 1959].) Forty-five years after its publication it was made popular in Paris by Corvisart. The book was translated into English in 1824 and into German in 1843 (Sigerist, 1936); and, a flood of papers and other discussion of it followed (Bishop, 1961). This standard story of total neglect followed by total acceptance probably is not accurate, since a favorable review of the first edition (1761) appeared in a London newspaper that very year. The review seems to have been written by Oliver Goldsmith, then a writer on medical subjects for that and other newspapers. However, Goldsmith's favorable and learned review seems to have impressed no one at the time. Auenbrugger's death in 1809 came after the importance of his discovery finally was recognized.

Several other Austrian physicians of the period had a prolonged effect on the course of clinical medicine, for better or worse. One whose influence was for the better was Prochaska, born in Lipsitz, Moravia, in 1749, who studied at Vienna, especially under de Haen in medicine and Barth in anatomy. Starting as an anatomist, he became an expert in this field and began publishing in 1778. His studies were based not only on injection methods but microscopy as well. However, in 1786 Emperor Leopold II ordered that microscopy be omitted from the study of anatomy, thereby threatening the development of microscopic anatomy. On the other hand, Leopold created a chair in physiology, and Prochaska became the first professor in 1791, having been forced to develop in this direction because of the Emperor's decree regarding microscopy. The change in emphasis was beneficial to him, since by 1784 he had already begun his brilliant studies in reflex functions, which he expanded subsequently. Regrettably, as his work continued into the 19th century, it fell under the influence of *Natur-Philosophie*, a powerful superstition at the time, and suffered because of the introduction of vague yet rigid speculation. Nevertheless, he was recognized then, as he is today, as a pioneer in reflex studies.

Another of Vienna's physicians who achieved fame did so in quite another way. Mesmer, first a student of theology and philosophy at Vienna and then of medicine, he received the M.D. degree in 1766 at the age of 32, after which he married a rich young widow and began to practice in Vienna. The pair seem to have given some wonderful parties in their house and its grounds: In fact, Mozart created an opera for one of the parties and had it performed in the garden. Mesmer was influenced by the ideas of a Swiss Jesuit, Father Hell, who believed that all ills, whether of the flesh or the soul, could be dispelled by magnetism. Mesmer's reputation as a physician suffered, and in 1782 he left Vienna to start a practice in Paris. He and his followers established centers for magnetizing illness out of the body, and they also promised erotic bliss. Mesmer did well as a practitioner. The controversy surrounding mesmerism produced much literature after he published his firmly stated views in 1779.

Gall deserves a mixed press, although for the most part comments about him today are adverse. He was born in Swabia in 1758, and as a schoolboy showed great interest in physiognomy. When he began his medical practice he was a cranioscopist, that is, one who diagnosed abnormalities by palpating the head. Unfortunately, this nonsensical approach to medical practice overshadowed his excellent studies on the *inside* of the skull and on other parts of the nervous system (Lesky, 1970).

It can be understood why 18th-century Vienna was unable to become an heir to Leyden. Vienna had elements from Leyden grafted onto its own system-a system that depended on the whims of emperors for its structure. Although Maria Theresa, who brought Leyden to Vienna, did not interfere, her successors did; and their fondness for peculiar superstitions served to confuse the serious clinicians who tried to follow the ways of Sydenham and Boerhaave-not to mention van Swieten and de Haen. (These last two were in themselves too rigid to be the leaders of a completely successful change. The superstitions referred to here were the Brunonian system accepted by Johann Peter Frank, the *Natur-Philosophie* by Prochaska, and the personal nonsense systems of Mesmer and Gall.)

Nevertheless, Vienna had entered the modern medical world, albeit lamely. It would have to suffer serious setbacks until, after the middle of the century, it was able to realize its full potential for greatness. In short, although Vienna was the lineal heir to Leyden, it was not the spiritual heir. When Viennese medicine came to develop along clinical lines, it was not because of Leyden's tradition *per se*, but because of Leyden's tradition as expounded by Scottish, English, and French physicians at the turn of the century and later.

A Note on Spanish Medicine

That politics makes unexpected bedfellows is clearly true regarding the reform of medical practice in Spain in the 17th and 18th centuries. The fact that the Netherlands, Austria, and Spain were parts of the Hapsburg Empire determined the course of medicine in Spain. Galenic medicine-until then the only medicine in Western Europe-was overthrown in Spain in the late 17th century due to the influence of de le Boë and other Netherlanders at Leyden (Pinero, 1974). The subsequent influence of Boerhaave was equally strong, not only with respect to medical teaching but also to medical theory. Because of Boerhaave's influence, iatrochemistry became the one acceptable dogma. The leaders of this movement in Spain (given the euphonious and expressive name of *novatores*) were most active in Madrid, Valencia, Saragossa, and Seville. Among their other innovations was the founding at Seville of the *Regia Sociedad de Medicina y otras Ciencias*.

The decline of Leyden's influence after the end of Boerhaave's tenure was followed by the temporary rise of Maria Theresa's Vienna as a medical leader. Prominent Spanish physicians now followed the lead of van Swieten and his group. Spanish clinical medicine became established mainly in the Chair of Practical Medicine of the University of Valencia, the Royal School of Practical Medicine at Madrid, and the Royal School of Clinical Medicine at Barcelona. Translations of the works of well-known Viennese and other European authors were made, and excerpts from such works were included in Spanish medical writings. Published works of Spanish physicians in some cases were referred to in the writings of Viennese or German physicians. This was not always felicitous, as when Johann Peter Frank discussed Casal's 18th-century pioneering description of pellagra as a description of leprosy. However, Spanish medicine's entry into the mainstream of European medicine was a welcome addition.

A Note on Göttingen

Like Vienna, another German-speaking medical school was a beneficiary of Leyden's excellence. This was Göttingen, in Hanover. The Hanoverian dynasty was established in England in 1714, with George I, Elector of Hanover, becoming King of Great Britain and Ireland. His court, much of which he took with him from Germany, spoke English poorly or not at all. His son George II maintained the ties between England and Hanover in a very material way. On the one hand, he brought Handel to live and work in England, where he created masterpieces, great as well as popular. On the other hand, in 1734 George II founded and endowed in Germany the Göttingen University, which was given the name Georgia Augusta. The Chancellor of the University, von Munchhaussen, appointed von Haller, a Leyden alumnus, Professor of Medicine. Von Haller also was required to teach anatomy, surgery, and botany. Werlhof, Court Physician to George II and famous as a poet and also as a clinician (for his description of *purpura hemorrhagica*), was the man who had suggested von Haller. While at Leyden, von Haller had been friendly with English students there, including Pringle, and after obtaining his M.D. degree, he went to London in 1727 and joined a group of young physicians who frequented the coffee houses together with authors, poets, and scientists.

There von Haller was introduced to Cheselden of St. Thomas' Hospital and Sir Hans Sloane of the Royal Society, and he spent much time in the surgical department of St. Thomas'. After his arrival at Göttingen in 1736, he built an anatomical theater, a botanical garden, and a lying-in hospital, as well as founding a journal and a learned society. His teaching attracted students from all over Europe, and its emphasis was clinical-pathological-physiological correlations. In 1739 he was made Physician-in-Ordinary to King George II as well as an English State Councilor. His anatomical studies were widely influential, for he taught the first of the three Meckels, and Meckel, in turn, taught Monro (*secundus*) later of Edinburgh. Ill health and homesickness finally drove von Haller back to

Switzerland, but from the beginning of his career, he was one of the great links between medicine at Leyden and medicine elsewhere.

Von Haller's contacts in England attracted some English physicians to Göttingen, not all of whom were happy there.   When Thomas Young, dissatisfied with Edinburgh, transferred to Göttingen, he admired its library but found the professors dogmatic and cold.   Although he previously had criticized medical teaching in Great Britain, he concluded that he could have learned all of what was known in medicine in London.   Nevertheless, for many years physicians from Great Britain considered Göttingen as an alternative place for medical learning.

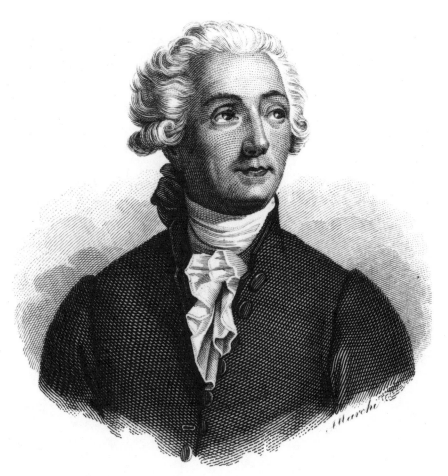

Antoine Laurent Lavoisier, 1743-1794

FRANCE WAS DESTINED TO CREATE one of the greatest clinical centers that ever existed - Paris medicine - in the first half of the 19th century. The story of this explosive development can be plotted clearly, but its beginnings can be understood only on the basis of certain events of the early 18th century - events that not only foreshadowed but actually defined much of what occurred in the 19th century. Moreover, there were happenings in the 18th century that indicated certain other trends involving the medical doctrine of vitalism, and although these trends never totally came to fruition, they did leave their mark.

Medical education in France was, from its medieval beginning, a university process, and it remained so thereafter. The outstanding medical school of the Middle Ages was in Italy, at Salerno, and after the destruction of that city by military action, the best of then-available medical education developed at Bologna, in Italy, and at Paris and Montpellier, in France. Bologna set the example for the other Northern Italian cities pursuing the road of natural sciences. (The later role of Padua in stimulating and directing medical education in Europe already has been discussed.)

The two French cities - Paris and Montpellier - at first developed along lines that were different from Italy as well as each other. The University at Paris was one of rigorous booklearning and its outgrowths in logic. In the 13th century Paris was the city not only of Albertus Magnus, the greatest biologist of his era, but also of his pupil, Thomas Aquinas, one of the greatest philosophical theologians of any era. Montpellier, on the other hand, was shaped in large part by Arab and other Mediterranean influences. Its acceptance of material from these sources made Montpellier a remarkable center for medical education in the later Middle Ages, so much so that by the 12th century it was famous throughout Europe for its physicians and medical teachers. At that time John of Salzburg wrote that many students who failed in philosophy at Paris went to Montpellier to study medicine. The liberal atmosphere that prevailed in Montpellier was demonstrated by the Edict of 1181, which permitted all medical teachers regardless of national origin or religion to function there. This edict was intended to recruit Jewish and Christian physicians who had been forced out of Moslem Spain by the fundamentalist Moslem sects that had gained control there. In addition, Jewish physicians trained at the Jewish medical schools in southern France at Lunel, Arles, and Narbonne influenced Montpellier teaching either in person or by their writings.

In general, teaching at Montpellier received a severe setback when, after the success of the crusade against the Albigensian heretics of Southern France, the University was placed under strict ecclesiastical control. This did not make much difference to the study of medicine, because it was all booklearning at Montpellier or Paris: No attempt was made to base medical teaching on what patients exhibited, and none was to be made in any systematic way until after da Monte introduced the concept at Padua in the late 16th century. The inadequacies of medical teaching at the universities in France were proclaimed from time to time by outstanding medical practitioners - much as was happening in England then and later. From time to time an outstanding physician came to the fore, particularly in anatomy and surgery, to give medical training a semblance of validity, but medical education as a whole stagnated in France until the 18th century. If anything, developments in sciences other than anatomy and botany only continued to stultify medical teaching, as was the case when Cartesian physics helped to create the iatromathematical dogma that participated in the imposition of the then-available data of physics and chemistry on medicine. It is of historical interest that the most progressive medical schools - in Leyden and Northern Italy - were the most eager to adopt iatrochemistry and iatromathematics and to establish them as dogmas. The Universities of Paris and Montpellier continued to rely on booklearning (from selected books) in medical teaching.

In the 18th century, however, several new factors arose, which, by the end of the century, were to cause drastic changes in French medicine. It must be emphasized that these factors were present decades before the French Revolution; but later, they were to be considered manifestations of new directions in thinking, reaching full development during and after the Revolution.   At Paris, the earlier institution of anatomical studies was followed by extended teaching of anatomy and surgery to a degree that made Paris attractive to students of medicine.   An unexpected development was the extension of chemical methods to botany, resulting in the study of the medicinal value of plant extracts.   French pharmacy became famous and was to maintain its leadership for a long time, and although French medicine clearly was awakening, its stimulation was to come largely from outside sources.

One stimulus grew out of the strong influence among the *intelligentsia* of a philosophy that was an outgrowth of Locke's ideas.   This philosophy, called *sensationism* (or by some *sensism* and by others, deplorably, *sensationalism*), held that all knowledge came only through the sense organs.   It created a bias favoring observation, and hence clinical, as opposed to theoretical, medicine.   The fact that Locke, who was popular in France, had been a close associate of Sydenham automatically made Sydenham's approach to medicine the one to follow.   Locke had stated it in a simple form - the sensationist philosophy - and, in France, Condillac first, and later Cabanis and de Tracy, developed it.   The hypothetical primacy of sensation in all mental processes led to the primacy of observation as the basis of medical study: A sound conclusion thus developed from an unproved hypothetical formulation.   Cabanis, in particular, insisted on the importance of bedside clinical teaching, and this idea came to play a leading part in the reform of medical education later instituted by the Revolution.

Another factor in favor of this approach was the writings of Jaucourt, a Leyden alumnus and a pupil and (forever afterward) admirer of Boerhaave.   Jaucourt's influence was important, for he was one of the three creators of the *Encyclopédie*, although his name usually is omitted, with all credit given to the other two, Diderot and D'Alembert (Schwab, 1958).

Jaucourt was a most unusual man. He had immense learning in history, the classics, law, politics, biology, and the nature of humans. A nobleman descended from an illustrious family, he was friendly with most of the intellectuals of the day. His contributions to the *Encyclopédie* were numerous and large, encompassing medicine and its history, botany, and related topics. The editors of the *Encyclopédie* made it a practice to insert sharp criticisms of government and society into various technical articles that censors were not likely to read, much less understand. Jaucourt inserted criticism with remarkable skill and wit in his articles. In fact, he completely rewrote the then-accepted Judeo-Christian version of history and was not punished in any way for it. His importance to the history of medicine lies in his admiring description of Leyden medicine: It made bedside medicine the standard to be adopted.

However, Leyden medicine was iatrochemical and iatromathematical in theory, and its supporters persistently attempted to explain biological and clinical phenomena on the bases of inorganic chemistry and theoretical Cartesian concepts of physical laws. Many physicians and others would not accept this kind of biology and medicine. There were strong reactions, initially from vitalists - van Helmont at first, and later Stahl and others. The vitalist reaction that occurred in France developed in Montpellier, which became the seat of French vitalism in the 18th century at the time when Paris was adopting materialism. The concepts advanced by different Montpellier professors of medicine contained different details, but they all agreed that living matter was distinguishable from nonliving matter by a vital principle, or force, or soul: Living material became alive because of this force. The concept maintained that observed vital phenomena never could be explained completely by physics and chemistry.

In Germany Stahl was one of those who maintained that the matter of the body was inert and that it required the action of a vital force to give it living qualities. At a time when the prevailing medical theory in Europe was mechanical, the introduction of Stahl's ideas into France by de Sauvage's early teaching at Montpellier in 1734 created an uproar. It soon became evident that many believed the mechanistic theories then extant to be unsatisfactory. One of these antimaterialists was de Bordeu, a student of de Sauvage who had taken his medical degree at Montpellier in 1744 (High, 1976; Moravia, 1978). In 1778 Barthez, who received his Montpellier degree nine years after Bordeu, advanced his own version, *Nouveaux Eléments de la Science de l'Homme* (Haigh, 1977). All three of these men were professors of medicine at Montpellier at one time or another, with Barthez, a lawyer, philosopher, editor, and soldier, the most broadly educated of the three. He had served for a time as Consulting Physician to the Army in Westphalia before taking the post at Montpellier, and afterward became Physician to King Louis in Paris. All of this vitalist discussion was swept away by the Revolution, however, the issues remained unresolved. There was a widespread belief in the mid-18th century that vitalists were really talking about the soul in a form disguised by words - indeed Stahl, their leader, invoked the soul specifically. Since the Revolution was not only anticlerical but specifically antireligious, any antimaterialistic views implied in the teachings of the King's physician, Barthez, clearly had to be uprooted.

In the meantime, the influence of the Leyden example was beginning to be felt in France. Famous men, such as Desault, the surgeon, and de Rochefort, the physician, practiced observation and teaching that involved both the bedside and the post-mortem room. (Among other things, de Rochefort used electricity therapeutically and described applying it to the head in a young woman with a grief reaction.) The Faculty of Medicine in Paris was in a state of decline during the latter half of the 18th century; in fact, it did not grant the M.D. degree after 1785. Whatever bedside teaching that was being conducted in Paris was independent of it, as when de Rochefort introduced it at his hospital. He previously had antagonized the Royal Society in Paris and had been removed from the Faculty; but, when he became a Staff Physician at the Charité he introduced bedside teaching and strengthened this teaching with an emphasis in pathological anatomy. His friend Corvisart succeeded him in 1788 and continued this kind of teaching enthusiastically.   Desault did the same for the practice of surgery at the Hôtel Dieu in 1787, despite the opposition of the nuns who ran the institution.   In addition, the incredibly bad hygienic state of the hospitals in the early 1780s came under scrutiny by the King's ministers; some wanted hospitals to be abolished, while others argued for reform.   Change was slow, until the Revolution began.

In many respects the Revolution seems to have been spontaneous, but in medicine the stage was set in large measure by a group of thinkers and writers who established many controversial ideas in mid-18th-century France.   At first - before and at the beginning of the Revolution - the ideas of these men seemed to be directing the future, but subsequent events reduced many of the concepts to mere slogans.

In addition to armchair philosophers such as Condillac, Helvetius, and Cabanis there were some less rational and more fanatical types who contributed to the French version of materialism existing in the mid-18th century. One of them was Diderot's friend Thiry, Baron d' Holbach, whose *The System of Nature or Laws of the Moral and Physical World* was a most extreme expression of materialistic thought.   He borrowed extensively but selectively from Hobbes, Locke, and de la Mettrie, which gave him the confidence of apparent scholarship, but was actually blind dogmatism.   Voltaire called the book "the bible of materialism," because of its dogmatism and comprehensiveness.   (D'Holbach seemed to have a weakness for any dogma, for he translated Stahl's writings on phlogiston into French.)

An even more unreasonable materialist was de la Mettrie, born at St. Malo in 1709.   As a youth de la Mettrie was considered to be a talented poet, and he intended to make literature his career.   His father objected, and the youth began to study theology at Rheims.   Soon afterward he became interested in medicine and left Rheims for Leyden, where he became a student of Boerhaave and translated some of his works into French, publishing them several years later.   Returning from Leyden in 1735, he began his practice, but soon signed on a French Indiaman and traveled to India and China.   Returning to St. Malo, he married and reestablished a practice, subsequently leaving for Paris for five more years of medical study. During that time he wrote several clinical papers, as well as one on the subject of prolonging life. He had serious quarrels with some of the leading professors, including Astruc, and left Paris to join the army. He seems to have had some sort of a neurotic disorder at the Siege of Freiburg, after which he wrote *The Natural History of the Soul*, a treatise on psychosomatic disorders. After his commanding officer was killed at Fonteney, de la Mettrie lost his position and returned to Paris. Evidently he was soon on bad terms with his colleagues, for he wrote his bitter *Doctors' Politics* and thereupon was expelled from the medical society. He returned to Leyden and in 1748 anonymously published *L'Homme Machine*, a fiercely materialistic document. His anonymity was short-lived, and he was expelled from Leyden. Through the intervention of Maupertius, the famous St. Malo astronomer who was then Director of the Berlin Academy, de la Mettrie was invited to the court of Frederick II. He died in 1751 after attending a dinner given by the French ambassador. Throughout his adult life he was a hyperactive rebel who succeeded in alienating almost everyone. Diderot called him "frivolous," adding the epithets, "dissolute," "impudent," "buffoon," "flatterer," and "ignorant," among others; however, Diderot did not hesitate to use some of his ideas. Some of de la Mettrie's more temperate statements were "man is but an animal" and "the body may be considered as a clock." He believed that thought was merely a property of organized matter and advised physicians in trouble with their patients to blame everything on consultants, a most modern idea. He not only held these views, which was his privilege, but he sarcastically attacked those who did not, which was not.

Trembley of Geneva was quite a different kind of man, who was to have a much more shattering effect on the enemies of materialism. The proponents of vitalism were forced to give up or change their ideas as a result of his work (Baker, 1952). He was an invertebrate biologist and an expert microscopist, but also was interested in philosophy, religion, politics and, above all, education. Trembley's ideas on education were espoused later by the reformers Pestalozzi, Frőbel, and Montessori. His general approach to life was that of a humane liberal. However, his biological work had anything but gentle effects. For example, in his work on the *hydra*, he showed that no matter how much of the organism was removed, it always would regenerate completely, and that when it was divided, each part became a complete individual. This experiment so completely upset the then-current notions of the individuality of the organism and the nature of life forces that it became a cornerstone of French materialism.

The prominence of French science in the late 18th century often is not recognized today. In fact, from 1770 to 1800 France was the scientific capital of the world (Shryock, 1957). All of the branches of science not only were being studied, but were being developed - and in some cases created - by French men of science. Most of this activity was exclusive of the universities, for there was a barrier between research and teaching (Huard, 1970). During this period, which was interrupted temporarily by the Revolution, the men of science pursued their interests and were not affected visibly by the developing political crisis. Also at this time French medicine was coming to life. It is noteworthy that the phenomenal accomplishments of science were not the primary cause of the rebirth; rather, it was the result of the recognition by some French physicians that medicine could advance only through patient-oriented studies (much like the model created at Leyden).

The suddenness with which the French Revolution began, its explosively rapid spread, and its violent destruction of the social system have never been explained satisfactorily (Coates *et al.*, 1954). Nevertheless, some of the Revolution's manifestations greatly affected medicine. For one thing, the Revolution destroyed privilege, the factor that controlled a man's advancement in medicine as well as in everything else (Vess, 1975). In no revolution before or since have ideas played as great a role as they did then, at least initially. The 17 physicians in the National Assembly were noted not for excellence in medicine but for radicalism in political and social matters. Large numbers of medical students participated in the storming of the Bastille. Many physicians wore radical dress and were leaders in political affairs, including the activities of the Jacobin Club (Vess, 1975). However, when the commotion subsided, a few men were notable. After the zeal for abolishing privilege in France had resulted in the closing of all medical schools and the dissolution of all academies, the rulers of the country were forced to reconsider. The large number of men wounded in wars at the borders and in the internal revolts made it necessary to have many new physicians. A massive epidemic of venereal disease followed: Passionately patriotic young women enlisted as soldiers and disabled more men than did bullets. However, the French Revolution will be discussed only insofar as it bears on the practice of medicine at that time and subsequently. Such a discussion does not require a deep understanding of the Revolution, even if that understanding were possible, which it evidently is not (Coates *et al.*, 1954).

The philosophy that dominated liberal thinking in the mid-18th century came to be called "Ideology" at the end of the century. It perhaps was stated most explicitly by de Tracy, who wrote, "It consists in observing facts with the greatest care, inferring from them only the most certain conclusions, in never giving to hypotheses the status of facts, in undertaking not to write truths unless they are naturally linked together without gaps, in admitting frankly that we do not know, and constantly preferring absolute ignorance to every assertion which is merely probable." This extreme approach never could be fulfilled by anyone needing to utter two or more sentences at a time (although parts of it might be). It appears that portions of this system did appeal to French clinicians for several reasons: because of medicine's general revulsion against authority during the century preceding the period under discussion; because it was a current fashion; because of the examples of Sydenham in England and the Leyden school and its disciples in many places; and perhaps because Diderot's *Encyclopédie* endorsed its application to medicine.

De Tracy was more than a mere troublemaker, as were many of the materialist philosophers of the period. His ideas contained much that was original, either as such or in application, and it was he who, in 1796, proposed the term "idealogy" to signify the science of ideas. He used the word "ideas" to designate the units learned by sense perception, rather than the abstract concepts of things, which was the description used by Plato and his many followers in succeeding centuries.   De Tracy intended Idealogy to be the basis of a theory combining natural science, political science, and morals in an organized entity, not the analog of metaphysics or psychology.   Its basis was to be entirely materialistic and secular, and its derivatives were freedom of thought and individual liberty.   Yet, it could be thoroughly concrete and practical.   (One concrete expression of de Tracy's philosophical system was his proposal to depose Napoleon in April of 1814.)   After the Bourbon restoration and the resultant repression, de Tracy's works became a principal expression of liberal thought; as such, they came under attack by the Government and its supporters.   However, Idealogy began to lose ground for other reasons: Other materialist or liberal philosophies became increasingly popular (as new or so described), and by the year of de Tracy's death, 1836, Idealogy had ceased to be an effective force.   Idealogy's original basis of materialism became attenuated as specific ideas themselves were given increasing emphasis.   When Comte's philosophy - with its tenet that the chief motivational forces in behavior were passions, biases, and feelings - achieved its position of dominance, Idealogy, with its conviction that ideas (as it conceived them) constituted the only such force, rapidly lost many of its supporters.

Nevertheless, Idealogy was a strong, if vaguely directed, force in the medicine of the French Revolution, and years later social philosophers felt that they had to refute its arguments.   Long after de Tracy's death, Karl Marx felt so constrained because de Tracy had the idea that property was an expression of the personality and that the abolition of property would lead to equality only with respect to unhappiness.   Hence, de Tracy believed, poverty and inequality were inevitable.   Although de Tracy held that the value of any object was due solely to the amount of labor put into it (one of Marx's oft-expressed beliefs), he maintained that only the capital applied to the creation of an object could be considered to be a truly creative force.   Marx concluded in his usual strongly worded style that de Tracy's expression of the high general value of political and social liberalism was merely a device by which a wicked bourgeois hoped to have his reactionary views accepted by right-minded, but gullible, liberals. Dogma creates paranoia, or perhaps the reverse is the case.

It was not only his personality, but also his ideas that made de Tracy unwelcome among persons with conservative leanings. Long after his disagreeable personality was forgotten, his ideas continued to evoke attacks from the right and the left. Only an original mind can be the focus of a following and at the same time the object of attack by opposite kinds of extremists. He received few attacks from physicians, for although early spokesmen for medical reform in the medicine of the Revolution claimed to be "idealogues," they brought forward nothing specifically derived from Idealogy which had any definitely medical effect on clinical practice, whatever effects it may have had on making medical care widely available.

The high-minded, if at times naïve, rhetoric of the "idealogues" - expressed in Diderot's *Encyclopédie* and elsewhere - played a prominent part in the early plans of the Revolution: Poverty was decried, and the right of the poor to medical care was taken for granted (Rosen, 1946, 1959; Weiner, 1970). The Constituent Assembly in 1790 and 1791 acted upon these principles: It appointed two committees, one for the extinction of poverty and the other for the promotion of health. (It is worth noting that the latter viewed home care as preferable to hospital care.) The two committees were headed by physicians: the first one by Guillotin, a deputy of the Assembly and professor of anatomy, physiology, and pathology at the Faculty of Medicine; and the second by Thouret, not a deputy, but invited to participate because he was the founder of the Royal Medical Society and friend to the politically powerful La Rochfoucauld-Liancourt. The two committees were soon in conflict, with personal accusations briskly exchanged (Weiner, 1970). As time passed, the inspiring rhetoric of the Constituent Assembly ultimately became subordinated to politics (as usual); that is, dog eat dog, and when deemed necessary, persuasion by terror. One result was the pamphlet by Babeuf, a blueprint that mapped out how a small but well-organized group of conscienceless conspirators could succeed in taking over a country. (Babeuf's pamphlet was superfluous, for the Jacobins already had done it.) The progressive radicalization of the revolutionary governing bodies forced some liberal physicians to withdraw from politics, while others, like Marat, rode the tide (Vess, 1975). A considerable number were executed for not being sufficiently radical.

The French Constitution of 1791 enunciated the principle that all education had to be reorganized in accordance with the changes that had occurred, either by mandate or spontaneously, in French society. In 1792, however, when the radical elements came into full power, the universities, learned societies, and teaching organizations were abolished. Medicine also was affected: There was to be no more teaching or licensing in the manner of the old society. The resultant chaos was ameliorated partially by the fact that several provinces set up unofficial examination boards, but more importantly, the Universities of Montpellier, Paris, and Strasbourg illegally continued to issue licenses to those who had passed their (still) traditional examinations. This disregard of the bureaucrats in the capital characterizes many of the actions traditionally taken by universities in Western Europe and America, which permitted them to carry out their functions. On the other hand, there were still other factors that demoralized medicine. The hospitals not only lost their endowments, but also, since most of them were run by religious organizations, lost their personnel also (Vess, 1975). The situation deteriorated due to the increased need for physicians, which was occasioned by the ill-advised declaration of war on Austria in 1792 and by the widespread internal disorders consequent to resistance to the Revolution itself. The number of military physicians, which should have been increasing, fell markedly. The crisis was apparent, and quick action was essential. Although many participated in the planning leading to that action, two men are most noteworthy.

Lavoisier, although not a physician, was drawn into medical matters early in his scientific career. The present discussion properly falls into three parts: (1) his role in public health, prison reform, and respiratory physiology; (2) his exposure of Mesmer's quackery, both during and after the reign of Louis XVII; and (3) his role in medical education under the revolutionary National Convention before his execution.

His early career (1763-1771) was devoted mainly to geology and mineralogy, hydrology, meterology, and lighting. During his field studies he became very much aware of the poverty and misery of the peasants. In 1772, during the course of his studies on combustion - which were to destroy Stahl's "phlogiston theory" - he reported observations on respiration in animals. In 1777 he explicitly stated that combustion was associated with the uptake of oxygen, and in 1783 he and Laplace described the elaboration of heat during both combustion and respiration. When Lavoisier demonstrated oxygen absorption and carbon dioxide production in respiration, and pointed out that the phenomenon was, in fact, nothing but slow combustion, he created a new branch of physiology. His subsequent studies on ventilation involved him in the prison and hospital reforms then in progress. During the administration of Necker as Director-General of Finance (1776-1781), there was a growing concern within the government regarding the prisons. Lavoisier's report was the result - incorporating recommendations on a wide variety of hygienic matters as well as a classification of the inmates - and as a consequence of the report, King Louis in 1780 issued orders that were described by prison-reform experts of the time as among "the most humane and enlightened." Also in that year a commission, including Lavoisier, was ordered to investigate the deplorable state of the hospitals of Paris. Here, too, the recommendations were sound and humane, and in 1787 the King ordered the construction of four new hospitals to be built using guidelines recommended by the Commission. Much of the report was related to material written about English hospitals and compiled by Lavoisier's brother-in-law (Duveen and Klickstein, 1958).

Lavoisier's second main connection with medicine was as head of the commission studying Mesmer's medical claims. Resultant unfavorable reports were printed in 1784 and then reprinted in *Journal De Médicine* in the same year.   Nevertheless, today Mesmer is regarded by some psychoanalysts as a pioneer in their profession.

Lastly, Lavoisier played a part in the reorganization of the teaching of science and medicine after the Revolution, and he was well prepared for these tasks. He was a disciple of Locke, Rousseau, and Condorcet in educational matters in general and, hence, comfortably in sympathy with the provision of the Constitution of 1791, which required the establishment of a system of universal free education.   In fact, before the Revolution, Lavoisier had established a free school for the poor children who lived near his estate.   Condorcet's view that the sciences were more important than the classics was in harmony with Lavoisier's ideas.   The Convention created a group to carry out these plans, with Lavoisier and de Fourcroy, among others, as members.   Lavoisier was appointed to draw up its report, the first of which was entirely his work (Abrahams, 1958); however, he did not live to see these and other educational plans carried out.   The medical aspects of Lavoisier's plans - dated August of 1793 - are most interesting, and in December of 1794 a law was passed legally re-establishing the three medical schools that had functioned illegally.   Further regulations were instituted in 1796 which, in most respects, conformed to Lavoisier's ideas about increasing the size and stability of the faculties, enlarging the scientific content of the curriculum, and the addition of work on preventive and forensic medicine.   Conditions of admission were defined.

It remained for de Fourcroy to carry out these ideas.   He was especially important in this respect because he was a physician and because for years the two had been closely associated.   For these reasons de Fourcroy played an outstandingly important role in the reconstruction of education in general and medical education in particular.   Although he was active in public life for many years, very little is known about him.   He was born in 1755, descended from a noble family whose fortunes had declined.   His father was an apothecary.   His educational record during his childhood was mediocre, and at the age of 16 he became a clerk in a government office at a small salary, which he supplemented by giving private lessons in writing.   By accident he encountered Vicq-d'Azyr, who was soon to become a famous anatomist. For some reason the young government clerk made a very favorable impression on Vicq-d'Azyr, who persuaded the family to let young de Fourcroy study medicine. As a student de Fourcroy greatly impressed members of the Royal Society of Medicine at the University, and relations between the two groups remained bad for years. The Society wanted Ramazzini's pioneering work on occupational diseases translated from Italian into French, and de Fourcroy, although still a student, was chosen to do it. De Fourcroy's Introduction and commentaries on Ramazzini's work were original and progressive. He completed the work needed for the M.D. degree between 1778 and 1780; however, the de Fourcroy family could not pay the 6,000 livres, which was the fee for the examination. De Fourcroy applied for the money from a fund for impoverished students maintained by the Faculty of Medicine, but since he had been associated with the Royal Society of Medicine, the Faculty's rival, his application was rejected. Some members of the Society then raised the money, and he received his degree in 1780; however, the Faculty refused to admit him as *docteur régent* and, hence, he was forbidden to teach in any medical school. He never practiced medicine, but he did become one of the Society's most active members, submitting original papers in chemistry to the Academy of Sciences. He began to lecture in chemistry at the Lycée, a private school and was appointed Professor of Chemistry at the Jardin du Roi in 1784. He was a remarkably eloquent lecturer.

Because all of his scientific work was based in chemistry, he soon was recognized as one of the greatest chemists of any era. The application of chemistry to medicine became one of his aims, and he stated, as did many chemists before and after him, that medicine should be based entirely on chemistry. His dozens of research projects on the chemistry of body fluids, kidney and gallstones, and animal tissues were interesting, but afforded little that was useful to physicians. Although a large part of the chemistry was alleged to be medical, much of it was wrong because the use of inaccurate or grossly incorrect methods produced the data used to provide physiologic explanations, which also were likely to be erroneous. Most of the findings of these studies, however, important to chemistry, were irrelevant to medicine. Some of the chemical data were misinterpreted, as was the case when de Fourcroy had tubercular patients breathe oxygen in high concentration, after which their condition worsened, and he recommended that patients with tuberculosis should avoid fresh air. On occasion, he missed an important conclusion: After isolating urea - an important contribution - he found that it could be transformed into ammonium carbonate, but failed to point out the relationship between inorganic and organic substances. (It remained for Wohler, 30 years later, to point out this relation after converting ammonium carbonate to urea.)

De Fourcroy believed that it was difficult for physicians in practice to benefit from the latest scientific knowledge (which he refused to acknowledge as fragmentary and often wrong), because such data were not to be found in medical journals. Therefore, in 1791 he started a new journal with the pretentious title, *La Médicine Eclairée par les Sciences Physiques*. It contained abstracts, letters, and original articles written by physicians, surgeons, and pharmacists, and de Fourcroy claimed that this was probably the first time that the three branches of the healing art had worked so closely. Publication ceased before the end of 1792, at which time de Fourcroy's political activities increased. For example, in 1792 he was active in "cleansing" the learned societies of counterrevolutionaries; some of these men had left the country (temporarily, they hoped), but many were still there. Scientific societies were abolished in 1793, and de Fourcroy supported this action. He was a member of the Committee of Public Instruction and then, after the fall of Robespièrre, of the Committee of Public Safety. When the medical school in Paris was re-established, he was appointed its Professor of Chemistry. De Fourcroy was the main author of reports on education after Lavoisier's execution, and he made original administrative contributions; for example, the licensing law of 1803 was his work (Heller, 1978). He became a member of the Convention in 1792 and the Director of Public Education under Napoleon; however, he fell out of favor with Napoleon in 1809, shortly before he died of a stroke.

De Fourcroy survived the many changes in regime that occurred during the Revolution, perhaps because he participated in the persecution of the counterrevolutionaries. Later, when Lavoisier, his teacher, mentor, and friend was being tried, de Fourcroy, who was by then a man of power in the government, remained silent. When Lavoisier was condemned to death, de Fourcroy finally spoke up, not to point out the injustice and inhumanity of the verdict, but only to state that Lavoisier was a very useful man. Robespièrre warned de Fourcroy to be silent or he, too, would lose his head; de Fourcroy complied. However, eventually it was Robespièrre and not de Froucroy who was executed. Lavoisier was a victim of the French Revolution because it had no need for *savants*; today's revolutions take a different stand. Thus a few decades ago, when Sauerbruch, after decades of brilliant surgical practice and teaching, became so senile as to be a danger to his patients, he not only was permitted but was encouraged to continue in his incompetence by the revolutionary government of East Germany. As its Director of the Academy of Sciences stated, "In the coming struggle of the proletariat, in the clash of socialism and capitalism, millions will lose their lives. In the face of this fact, it is a trivial matter whether Sauerbruch kills a few dozen people on his operating table. We need the name of Sauerbruch" (Thorvald, 1962). (It is evident that political humanitarians are often dangerous to human life and dignity, but always can justify their acts.)

His unpleasant personal characteristics should not negate de Fourcroy's work in the theoretical and practical aspects of chemistry, which prove him to be a great scientist. Despite the fact that he never practiced medicine, he clearly knew enough about its nature and problems not only to help repair the chaos induced by the do-gooders in power, but also to propose changes that would make French medicine much greater than it was before the Revolution. Although his contributions to the reorganization of education were outstanding, he was refused the title of "Grand Master of the University" by Napoleon. This action, reminiscent of the refusal of the Faculty of Medicine to give him the title *docteur régent*, is curious; however, we do not know enough about de Fourcroy to explain it.

While Lavoisier and de Fourcroy occupied themselves in reforming the medical curriculum and administratively restoring education so that it could function much more effectively, the philosophy of medicine was not neglected. Here the name of Cabanis is outstanding. An idéalogue, he built upon the writings of Jaucourt in the *Encyclopédie*, but interwove his own ideas. Cabanis was the medical member of the Idealogues' group of philosophers, all of whom were followers of Condillac's sensationism. Cabanis was born in 1757 in a small town in southwestern France. His father was a lawyer but also was interested in scientific agriculture. Young Cabanis was sent to Paris at the age of 14 and, after preliminary studies, graduated in medicine there at 23. Early on he met the leaders of the Enlightenment in the salon of Mme. Helvetius, becoming both friend and physician to Mirabeau and participating with him in the early phases of the Revolution. Prudently remaining out of sight during the Terror, he came forward again after Robespiêrre's execution. Although he drafted the proclamation endorsing Napoleon's seizure of power in November of 1799, he was denied political preference and returned to medicine. His writings were concentrated on the reform of hospitals and medical education, certitude in medicine, and the physical and moral nature of man. Although he wrote a clinical book on catarrh in 1803, his most famous works dealt with the reform of medicine. He was professor of Hygiene and later of Medical History and Clinical Medicine at Paris. Cabanis died in 1808 at the age of 51. Like many other physicians of his period, politics occupied much of his time, and his reformist writings were praised widely. In the spirit of the sensationists, he wrote, "the true instruction of young doctors is not received from books but at the sickbed." In fact, at the very beginning of the Revolution, he advocated the establishment of clinical teaching, something that one of his professors, Dubrueil, already had established at the naval hospitals at Brest and Toulon. Combined with his progressive views on medical education, he still retained a belief in Galenic temperaments and was uncertain of the role of pathological anatomy. He admired that great dogmatist Stahl, because he had declared physics and chemistry unnecessary for an understanding of medicine.   On the other hand, he wrote, "Better no theory than one contradicting proved facts."   His rejection of physics and chemistry led him to doubt the usefulness of Harvey's discovery.   (Thomas Jefferson had expressed the same belief.)   Cabanis spoke strongly in defense of medicine in his book *On the Degree of Certitude in Medicine*, which was intended to refute the views of Rousseau and the Jacobins, who wanted to dismiss it as quackery.   His influence persisted despite his early death, and the empirical sensationist view of medicine prevailed (as it would have without him).

It was the French genius for organization, encouraged particularly under Napoleon, which permitted the remarkable developments that made French clinical medicine the greatest in the world in the first decades of the 19th century.   However, it should be remembered that no system will work well without competent people.   When people are more than competent, they will use the opportunities afforded by a good system to develop in new directions.   This is exemplified by the French clinical medicine of the Napoleonic and post-Napoleonic periods, whose developments were not prevented by turmoil of political change and conflicting philosophies.

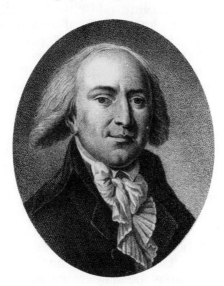

Antoine Francois de comte de Fourcroy, 1755-1809

BY THE TIME OF NAPOLEON'S ASSUMPTION of the dictatorship of France, its medicine had passed through the phase of functional disintegration, resulting from the urge of its leaders to destroy every vestige of the *ancien régime.* The realities permitted cooler heads to prevail, although some (*e.g.,* Lavoisier's) did not remain in position in every sense of the word. The reorganization of medical services and medical teaching planned by the revolutionary committees was intended to produce large numbers of medical personnel, and it succeeded. However, there was also a need for new ways of structuring the growing volume of medical data.

Clinical medicine began to change after the Sydenham-Locke formulation was adopted by Leyden, Edinburgh, London and, to some extent, Vienna and some other areas. The rate of change accelerated with the spreading acceptance of the idea that knowledge of anatomy, both normal and pathologic, was critical in *clinical* practice. A further acceleration, almost explosive in intensity, started in France in Napoleon's time; it is difficult to say why it happened at that time in France. Travelers' accounts document the high enthusiasm among physicians and their great eagerness to experience and learn about clinical matters, using live patients as well as cadavers. Although enthusiasm alone can accomplish much, more than that is required, and that *more* cannot be explained convincingly: Why, for example, did Napoleon's physician, Corvisart, resurrect percussion after it had been buried in Vienna a half-century earlier? Why was auscultation discovered in France rather than Edinburgh, London, Dublin, or Leyden? These events clearly were part of a revolutionary change in attitudes and habits, but what caused them? The answers to these questions become more obscure, since these explosive events were not part of a uniform change. A scientific revolution - exemplified by the works of Lavoisier, de Fourcroy, Berthollet, and Vauquelin - had made chemistry a particularly French science years before the political Revolution occurred and decades before the French revolution in physical diagnosis developed. Moreover, other revolutions in medicine were in progress. The work of Baillie in London had focused attention on individual organs as the sites of diseases that caused specific symptoms. Baillie's revolution, most noticeable in England and France, eventually fused with the revolution in physical diagnosis then developing in France; but, surely, it had no relationship to the political events in France, or anywhere else for that matter. In short, there was a succession of clinical revolutions and, although the rates of and characters in their development must have been affected by political, social, and economic events, these revolutions were independent of each other. A distinction must be made between the clinical revolutions on the one hand, which were primarily procedural and conceptual and, on the other hand, the merely technical revolutions, much like those currently engulfing medicine.

Another basic issue deserves comment. In the 17th and 18th centuries the hospitals in France were huge, each having hundreds of beds and several times that many patients. The new hospitals planned late in the reign of King Louis were improved, but still were very large. That was not the situation in England, where as early as the 17th century, Sir Francis Bacon, then Solicitor General, had taken a strong stand against large hospitals. The situation began when Sutton, an extremely wealthy coal dealer and money-lender, died and left a large sum of money to support an institution for the care of the sick poor in London. The will came before Bacon, and he recommended that King James I disallow it (Shepley, 1967). Bacon wrote, "Some number of hospitals with complete endowments will do far more good than one hospital of exorbitant greatness." By placing hospitals in areas where there is the most need, "the remedy may be distributed as the disease is dispersed...Chiefly I rely upon the reason that in these great hospitals the revenues will draw the use, and not the use the revenues, and so through the mass of their wealth they will swiftly tumble down to a mis-employment" However, the French (and the Viennese) believed differently.

In fact, very large hospitals were useful, particularly if one needed to train many physicians quickly, as was the case after the Revolution. The combination of the availability of a very large number of patients together with new methods of diagnosing their illnesses soon made French clinical medicine the world's leader. Similarly, in surgical services a large patient population permitted the development and teaching of techniques. However, those circumstances did not favor the enhancement of the relationship between a doctor and his patient, which raises clinical medicine to its highest level. Nevertheless, the development of "hospital medicine"-the term coined by Ackerknecht (1967)-rapidly led to the acceptance of the value of percussion and auscultation. These procedures, when used by a physician in his examination of his patient, prolong and enhance the interaction that constitutes clinical medicine. Thus French medicine, while demonstrating little concern for the doctor-patient relationship manifested in English practice, nevertheless led to the growth of just such a relationship. In fact, the period in which percussion and auscultation developed must be considered, because this contribution of French medicine was incorporated into London practice and later reached America.

The accomplishments of the clinical revolution in France spread to England and Ireland rapidly, to Vienna less rapidly, and to Germany irregularly. (Within Germany indifference was the rule and opposition common.) The reverberating waves of clinical information among England, Ireland, and France led to a reorganization of nosology along clinicopathological lines. Until the mid-19th century, German-speaking writers played only a small part in this development. The clinical revolution in France - initiated in the reign of Napoleon I - lasted throughout the short Bourbon restoration, the liberal period of Louis Philippe, and the very brief life of the Second Republic. It diminished under Napoleon III, except for continued brilliance in the clinical area of neurology and the laboratory science of bacteriology.

The French medical renaissance, which began prior to the Revolution, accelerated and changed its character in several phases during and after it.   The revision of its administrative status was outlined previously; however, the successive phases in the changes in its clinical aspects must be noted.   Here the history of the early phase is dominated by several people, two of whom were Pinel and Bichat.   (It is my opinion that the name of a third, Corvisart, is the most important.)

Pinel was the son and the grandson of physicians but originally was not planning a medical career.   He was born in 1745 in a small village in Southern France.   After several years of being tutored at home, he was sent to a religious institution known as the Oratorian College at Lavaur.   The bishop, struck by Pinel's high intelligence, persuaded him to take minor orders; however, after four years Pinel left the College and priesthood and entered the University at Toulouse to study mathematics and medicine. There he studied from 1767 to 1774, received a master's degree in mathematics, took the M.D. degree, and then, evidently because he considered the medical teaching at Toulouse to be inadequate, entered the medical school at Montpellier, where he studied for two more years, receiving an M.D. degree there also.   Having become interested in mental disease because of the violent death of a psychotic friend, he began to study the subject intensively and took employment at a private asylum in the 1780s. His experience there convinced him that the best treatment was what was then called "moral treatment," a sympathetic, considerate psychological treatment, and in 1789 he wrote an article on insanity.

After the Revolution, through the influence of the still powerful Idéalogues, he was appointed to the faculty of the new medical school in Paris, first as Professor of Hygiene and then as Professor of Internal Pathology.   He also was made Physician to the Bicêtre and then the Salpetriêre.   Pinel became known as one of the leaders of psychiatric reform, together with Daquin in France, Chiaruggi in Italy, and Tuke in England (Woods and Carlson, 1961; Grange, 1963; Risse, 1969); but at the time he was more famous in other ways.   However great were Pinel's contributions to the classification of psychiatric disorders and their treatment, his influence on general medicine is of primary interest.   Beginning in 1778 he busied himself with the translation of Cullen's *Institution of Medicine* and Baglivi's *Opera Omnia*. In addition, he assumed the editorship of the *Gazette de Santé*, a journal that published many papers (some by Pinel) on Mesmerism, concluding that it was a form of suggestion. He also wrote reviews, abstracts of foreign works, and papers on zoology, anatomy, and blood-letting.

His works in general medicine demonstrated his admiration of the Edinburgh school. He translated not only Cullen, but also his own case histories in his *Médicine Clinique* (1802), which followed the Edinburgh model. From 1795 to 1822 he taught primarily general medicine. His political fortunes varied; and, because of his influence with the leaders of the Revolution, he was able to save Condorcet and others from the Terror. After the restoration of the Bourbons in 1814, he was left undisturbed; but, he was dismissed during the great purge of 1822. He died in 1826.

In his nosographic writings Pinel followed Sydenham's concept of classifying diseases by symptoms. He opposed theorizing and, like a devoted Idéalogue, favored direct observation of phenomena. His following among physicians was an important factor in the acceptance of bedside teaching among them, and his insistence on bedside observation, combined with his admiration for pathology (as taught by Morgagni) and his belief in the value of numbers, made him a powerful teacher. Although he may be regarded as the father of the statistical study of clinical medicine, his greatest contribution, according to his contemporaries, was as a classifier. *Nosographic Philosophique* (1798) was regarded by his contemporaries as his greatest work, and his classification system came at a time when many physicians, scientists, and sociologists still were highly interested in organizing information (some of them more interested in classification than in discovery). Since his classification was based primarily on symptoms alone, it was largely inadequate because it only described reality in those sections where data of pathological anatomy were available. Today Pinel is famous as a student of mental disorders, as well as a great influence on bedside teaching in general medicine.

Bichat was born in 1771, the son of a physician who had studied under Barthez and had taken his degree at Montpellier.   Young Bichat evidently absorbed some of what his father had learned at Montpellier, for his writings showed strong influences of the Montpellier vitalist theories (Entralgo, 1948; Haigh, 1973).   Since there were no officially functioning medical schools when Bichat began his studies in 1791, he studied in Lyon privately with Petit, the well-known surgeon and anatomist.   He remained there for two years and then in Paris entered into a similar relationship with Desault, the surgeon who introduced bedside teaching into the Hôtel Dieu.   Desault thought highly of him and took him into his house to live.   When Desault died in 1795, Bichat collected and edited his works throughout the next three years, during which time he gained a reputation for his private lectures in anatomy, surgery, and physiology, while continuing his surgical practice.   In 1799 he became Physician to the Hôtel Dieu (subsequently called "Grand Hôpital de l'Humanité," a change made by the revolutionaries, which had no evident effect on its characteristics).

During that time Bichat wrote *Treatise on Membranes*, previously a favorite subject of Bordeu at Montpellier, and also *Physiological Studies on Life and Death*, another subject much discussed at Montpellier.   In the latter work he defined life as the sum of the forces that resist death, but he neglected to define death.   His statement, however majestic in its pretentious triviality, was not original.   Rather, it was based on one of Stahl's ideas-one that was admired widely, or at least quoted. Thomas Percival, in his *Essays Medical and Experimental* (1790), wrote that "Stahl supposes two opposite principles of propensities in the human frame: one constantly and uniformly tending to corruption and decay; the other to life and health."   Although this seems loftier than Bichat's version, it was made even more impressive by Freud, who wrote about Eros and Thanatos as the "Life Force" and the "Death Wish," respectively.

Bichat was regarded in France as a most profound philosophic thinker.   He maintained his sense of realism, however, with 600 post-mortem examinations performed in less than six months.   He compiled this data in *General*

Anatomy Applied to Physiology and Medicine and in the first part of *Anatomie Déscriptive*. His frantic pace ended abruptly in 1802, when he died after a short illness, presumably tuberculous meningitis. Despite the massive amount of work he did in great haste, he was regarded as a modest, generous, warm-hearted person, opposed to the controversy and personal invective pervading Parisian medicine. He was the most beloved teacher of medicine of his time, influencing many who came after him.

Bichat's contribution to medicine relates not to his work on life and death-which today seems empty and pretentious-but to his initiating the concept that organs should be studied in parts. Up to that time, when an organ was diseased, it was believed that the whole organ was affected; however, Bichat showed that organ membranes could be considered separately from their organs as sites of disease (*e.g.*, pleuritis, pericarditis). His discussions became vague and irrational because he could not forbear to seek for *vital forces* to discuss. Despite his often far-fetched reasoning about *sympathies* and other imaginary physiologic functions, he was capable of sound physiologic experimentation, such as transfusions. Like any confirmed vitalist, he insisted that the laws of physics and chemistry did not apply to physiology. He refused to use the microscope, but nevertheless considered himself justified in proposing a classification of tissue types. This was a way-station on the road to cellular pathology, which in itself was a mixture of shrewd conceptualization overloaded with unfounded conjecture. But perhaps his main contribution was emphasizing that one could not reason effectively about disease from the symptoms alone: "The symptoms, corresponding to nothing, will offer but incoherent phenomena. Open a few corpses, and immediately this obscurity, which live observation alone could never have removed, will disappear."

In terms of the development of clinical medicine Bichat was more a polemicist than a contributor of usable data. Aside from his stirring exhortations to follow his vitalistic ideas and his inevitable attractiveness to historians of medical theory, there is little to recommend his works. Bichat-like the nosographer Pinel-built visually beautiful structures that were devoid of mentally satisfying foundations.   These two men were among the last of the great dogmatists in general medicine.   (The supply of lesser, more localized dogmas shows no signs of diminishing.)

In considering the teaching clinicians of the immediate post-Revolutionary France, it must be concluded that the greatest was Corvisart, whose accomplishments were accorded only a few sentences, or even fragments of sentences, in the great histories of medicine-those of Castiglioni and of Garrison-of the 20th century.   Nevertheless, Corvisart perpetuated the pioneering leadership of de Rochefort and Desault in clinical practice and bedside teaching and made famous Auenbrugger's revolutionary percussion method, now known and accepted throughout the Western World.   His pupil Laennec was another creator of modern clinical medicine, although he expounded no theories and espoused no dogmas.   At most, he voiced agreement with the philosophies of both the sensationists and Voltaire and, at a time when most of the leaders of Paris medicine were highly critical of each other, he engaged in no polemics.   He had none of the delusions of grandeur common in Parisian physicians of the time and wrote, "Medicine is not the art of curing diseases; it is the art of treating them with the goal of cure, or of putting the diseased person at ease and calming him."

Corvisart was born in 1755 in Champagne and was the son of a lawyer.   In 1782 he became *docteur régent*, a title that carried with it the right to teach.   At first he worked with the surgeon Desault and taught anatomy and surgery.   Later he worked in medicine under de Rochefort at the Charite and succeeded him as physician there in 1788.   Because he had refused to wear a wig, he previously had been refused a post at the Necker Hospital.   He became Professor of Clinical Medicine at the newly reopened medical school in Paris, which was renamed the Ecole de Santé, and a few years later was appointed professor at the Collège de France.   In 1804 Corvisart gave up all of these posts to become Physician to Emperor Napoleon I, with whom he was on terms of relaxed intimacy, but not familiarity.   When Napoleon fell in 1815, Corvisart gave up medicine entirely, never speaking of it again.   He died in 1823.   He remained proud, stoical, and dignified, and although his nonprofessional life was devoid of family affection, he was not withdrawn. A *bon vivant*, he made his prim student Laennec uncomfortable. He was a skeptic at a time when skepticism was no longer fashionable.

However admirable his personal qualities may have been, he is recognized for his great work in the development of clinical medicine. When he translated Auenbrugger's book *Inventum Novum* into French in 1808, he could have taken more credit than he did, for his additions and comments essentially made it a new book. (The original work was ignored for nearly a half-century after its publication.) During the next two decades the book's use was widespread. The comments, aphorisms, and other additions reveal the extent and high quality of Corvisart's knowledge of clinical medicine. His more famous *Maladies du Coeur* (1806) was generally like that of Morgagni's *De Sedibus* (which Corvisart admired greatly), except that it was more coherent because its scope was limited to one organ and its diseases were arranged systematically. The much larger amount of clinical data, including the findings revealed by palpation and percussion, skirted the emphasis from the post-mortem to the *in vivo* status. Nevertheless, the post-mortem findings remained the basis of interpretation, less as such than in the form of its physiological derivatives.

Although Corvisart was accustomed to thinking in physiological terms, he saw no clinical value in the available chemical knowledge and opposed de Fourcroy's plan of installing a chemistry laboratory in every hospital. In his works he recorded the palpable thrill of mitral stenosis and enlargement of the heart's cavities and reported the autopsy finding of fatty infiltration of the heart. In his chapter on *La Maladie Bleu*, he clearly recognized the differences between arteriovenous mixture and venoarterial mixture, as well as the fact that blood could bypass the lungs entirely. His perceptive conclusion was that an auricular septal defect, a ventricular septal defect, an overriding aorta, and a patent ductus arteriosus were physiologically similar in that they all might cause cyanosis, its degree dependent on the size of the shunt and the amount of venous admixture. His treatise on heart disease never achieved maximal greatness because Corvisart was not able to include data on auscultation, which had yet to be discovered.   (When it was discovered, it was by his pupil Laennec.)

Corvisart's highly practical concept of clinical medicine was expounded best in his own words. Gates, the translator, not only mentions Corvisart's emphasis on the primary role of observation, but also adds a sentence on the secondary role of what the French always have called the "accessory" sciences (referred to in German and American as the "basic" sciences). The Preface states the following:

> The essay which I am publishing is a work purely practical, founded on irrefragable observation; hence clinical medicine rests solely upon the old and durable basis, *observation*. Doubtless, many works, to be commended, have been published in modern times on the healing art. All the accessory sciences seem to be intelligently united to enrich medicine with their new discoveries; yet the light which they have imparted, has reflected merely a glimmering ray on a path where many of those who are hastening have already been bewildered.

Also it is remarkable that Gates, translating Corvisart's own words, grouped the lesions in the heart by tissue classification, an approach allegedly peculiar to Bichat:

> The heart, like all the other organs, is formed by the assemblage of several different tissues. A cursory view of the lesions of this organ exhibits them always near the same in the analogous tissues, and evinces in the different tissues, particular modifications, which proceed partly from the different organization of the injured tissue. From this consideration, I conceived that I could assume, in the same tissue of the heart, the division of its lesions. This order is, indeed, more anatomical than medical; but if one reflect much on the nature of organic diseases, he will doubt

with me, whether any other be more conve-
nient.   Besides, I have adopted this order
mostly for the purpose of facilitating a satisfactory distribution of the materials which I
had to treat, and which will be arranged in
five classes.

1st.   The first will treat of the *membranous
envelopes of the heart.*

2d.   The second will comprise those of *its
muscular substance*

3d.   The third will explain the lesions of the
tendinous or fibrous tissue.

4th.   The fourth will embrace the affections
which involve the *different tissues,* and the
preternatural states which are considered as
diseases of this organ.

5th.   The fifth will give a brief account of
the aneurisms of the aorta.   In fine, the work
will be concluded by corollaries in which I
shall speak of the causes, signs, progress,
prognosis, treatment of the diseases of the
heart, and of the means of distinguishing them
from the affections with which they have
been confounded, &c.

Corvisart's successor as Physician to the Charité
was his pupil, Bayle, who had been born in Provence in
1774 and was the son of a lawyer.   Young Bayle showed
much interest in entymology, but chose to study theology
and law.   In 1793, at the age of 19, he entered politics as
a counterrevolutionary.   Like many other young people of
any era, he was against the existing system.   Perhaps as a
disguise, he became a medical student at Montpellier,
where he distinguished himself more by his poetry than by
his scholarly accomplishments.   Drafted into the army, he
worked in a hospital at Nice and then, in 1798, entered
the Ecole de Santé at Paris.   He was attracted by the

clinical teaching of Corvisart, especially its basis in pathology, and he, Laennec, and Dupuytren collaborated in studies.   Bayle became one of the founders of the so-called *Congregation*, a secret students' counterrevolutionary group headed by the Jesuit Father Delpris, and recruited Laennec into that group.   Both of them remained ardent royalists.   Bayle became not only Corvisart's student, but also his collaborator, and succeeded him on his retirement from the Charité.   Three years later, in 1802, Bayle received his M.D. degree.   Although he was a good clinical observer, he marred his work by forcing his data into idiosyncratic classifications (Rousseau, 1971).   He was an expert on tuberculosis and died of it in 1816, at the age of 40.   He was friend and teacher to Corvisart's more famous pupil, Laennec.

Laennec was born in 1781 in Quimper, in Brittany, and died there of tuberculosis in 1826.   He had a disordered childhood, his mother having died when he was five.   His father, a lawyer who wrote poetry, lived above his means and was always in debt.   He wanted the boy to swim, ride, play the flute, sing, dance, draw, and study only literature and politics.   Young Laennec was brought up by uncles, first by a priest and then by Guillaume, Chief Physician at the Hôtel Dieu in Nantes.   The latter complained about Laennec's persistent interest in music, dancing, and drawing (Fox, 1947; Kervan, 1960).   From his window in Nantes the boy witnessed the operation of the Terror: The house in which he lived faced the square that contained the guillotine.   The disparate influences in his early life created a curious mixture.   Outwardly humorless and conservative to the point of primness, he loved to return to Brittany, where he rebuilt his ancestral farm.   When he could, he enjoyed the seashore and the countryside and pursued his studies on the Breton language, literature, and music.   In 1821 he hired a housekeeper (in Paris), a widow older than he, whom he had met 16 years earlier.   After three years, apparently in response more to gossip than anything else, he married her (Miller, 1967).

Laennec's medical uncle, Guillaume, had had an excellent education at Montpellier and in Great Britain, and he guided the boy's career.   At 14 Laennec was a military surgeon, third class, in the army, and at 20 he was able to

go to Paris to complete his studies and also to join a secret counterrevolutionary group. He was influenced most
strongly by Corvisart, as was shown by his interest in
pathological anatomy post-mortem and percussion *in vivo*,
particularly with respect to the chest. Another of his favorite teachers was Bichat, whose writings about membranes had impressed him. One of Laennec's first studies
was published as a report on peritonitis in the *Journal de
Médicine* in 1802. In 1803 he received prizes in medicine
and surgery at the Ecole de Santé, after which, on the
basis of what he had learned from Corvisart, Dupuytren,
and Bayle (his co-conspirator), he began to give his own
course in pathology. In 1804 he went into practice for financial reasons, since he was denied a high academic position. He had as patients some of the most distinguished
persons in Napoleonic Paris; however, not until the
restoration of the Bourbons did he become head of a hospital, the Necker. In that year, 1816, he discovered auscultation. Never popular with his fellow physicians, most
of whom were liberals, he had to wait for Napoleon's fall
to make use of his Jesuit-Royalist connections to secure
advancement. It is interesting to note that after Laennec's death his positions were given to Recamier, so faith-
ful a royalist that he resigned in 1830 rather than serve
under Louis Philippe. Laennec's life previously had been
made particularly unhappy by the attacks of the followers
of Broussais, who were wild republicans.

Laennec published his treatise on auscultation in
1819, and its use spread in Paris and Great Britain
(Scudamore, 1826); however, it was treated with scorn in
Germany for a half-century. He retired to Brittany in
1819, when his tuberculosis began to trouble him severely.
On returning to Paris, he became Professor of Clinical
Medicine at the Charité, Professor at the Collège de
France, and Physician to the Crown Prince. In 1826,
shortly after completing the second edition of his book, he
died of tuberculosis at his Breton home. His influence on
medical practice is incalculable. Collin, an associate who
had helped Laennec with the second edition of his classic,
wrote a treatise of his own on auscultation in 1824, in
which he described the pleural friction rub and cor pulmonale, as well as other discoveries. The book was used

widely, and English, German, and American editions were published. In England the spread of stethoscopy was uneven and at times sluggish (King, 1959). In Ireland, Stokes in 1825 contributed a brilliant treatise on its place in clinical medicine. The use of auscultation-either directly or by means of a stethoscope-to hear fetal heart sounds occurred early (Trolle, 1975). Ultimately bowel sounds also came to be studied in this way.

Laennec's chief adversary-in fact almost everybody's chief adversary at the time-was another Breton and physician, Broussais. He was one of the great dogmatists of medicine and one of the most exuberantly vitriolic. The volume and viciousness of his denunciations equal those of Paracelsus in medicine and are in the same category in these respects as the oral and written productions in the 1840s and 1850s of Marx and Engels, on the one hand, and of materialists and socialists who disagreed with them on the other.

The fall of the Napoleonic Empire and the restoration of the Bourbon monarchy were bound to have effects on medicine. Leading physicians and teachers, such as Corvisart, withdrew from medicine entirely when the Jesuits were restored to their previous positions of influence and authority in educational matters. Some physicians were dismissed in the 1822 purge; others survived, and even prospered. Laennec prospered, despite his personal unpopularity and poor qualities as a teacher, because he was known for his lasting loyalty to the Bourbons.

Broussais prospered for quite another reason, and since that prosperity owed nothing to Bourbon politics, it lasted beyond the fall of their kingdom in 1830. Broussais was born in St. Malo in 1772, the son of a surgeon. Years later Chateaubriand wrote about their days at school together at Dinant: "The students were taken bathing every Thursday, like the clerks under Pope Adrian I, or every Sunday, like the prisoners under the Emperor Honorius. Once I was nearly drowned; on another occasion M. Broussais was bitten by ungrateful leeches, which failed to foresee the future." From 1792 to 1794 Broussais was an enthusiastic fighter in the Revolution, battling with the counterrevolutionaries in Western France. In 1795, on Christmas Eve, his "loving father" and "respectable mother" were killed by counterrevolutionaries. After a brief education as a surgeon, he served at sea, mostly on privateers, from 1795 to 1798. He then entered medical school in Paris, graduating in 1803 with a thesis written after the fashion of Pinel. Thereafter, until the fall of Napoleon, he served in his armies in the Netherlands, Germany, Austria, Italy, and Spain. His energy and exuberance attracted the attention of high-ranking military persons, both in the line and in the medical establishment.

In addition to his military duties, his time was occupied in collecting clinical and post-mortem data, the result of which was his treatise on chronic inflammatory disorders. He described these conditions, not simply as fevers, as Pinel would have done, but more in terms emphasized by Bichat, as inflammations located in tissues. However, he declared that all inflammations were situated in two tissues, the gut and the lung, and he failed to distinguish between tuberculosis and pneumonia. In general, he presented the post-mortem material unclearly and too briefly. Accordingly, his treatise did not give him the fame he craved.

After the Empire collapsed, Broussais was made second in rank at *Val-de-Grace*, the military medical school and hospital. This appointment was possible because the French army was solidly Bonapartist and had an almost independent status. The Napoleonic surgeon, Desgenettes, controlled the army medical service, and Broussais was one of his favorites. By 1820, when Broussais became chief at the hospital and Professor of Medicine at the University, he also became the self-appointed reformer of medicine. For one thing, as a devoted Bonapartist, anything from England, *perfide Albion*, was abhorrent to him. For another, he probably had been influenced to some degree by the Brownian system so popular in Italy, where he had served. (The Brownian system, in fact, was introduced into France by army surgeons returning from Italy.)

In 1816, Broussais published *Scrutiny of the Generally Adopted Medical Doctrine*, in which he thoroughly demolished Pinel's rigid and unrealistic *Nosographie Physiologique*. Broussais stated that all treatment must be antiphlogistic because he believed that all disease was an inflammation, most commonly of the gut. Antiphlogistic treatment consisted of starvation and repeated bleeding, chiefly by the use of leeches, a treatment in direct contrast to Brown's equally irrational treatment, mainly involving stimulation. Broussais is said to have been responsible for more blood-letting than anyone, except Tamerlane. He called his medicine "physiological" because it was a popular term, just as Pinel called his nosology "philosophic" because at that time that was the popular term.

Whatever Broussais' qualities as a thinker, there is no doubt about his skill as a sarcastic, scurrilous, *ad hominem* orator. He had enthusiastic followers on the Continent and in the United States, but his greatest admirers were the medical students in Paris (an example of the Pied Piper phenomenon affecting students during periods of social instability). Academically, students follow the noisy figures whose politics they find congenial and whose attacks on the current establishment they find exhilarating. (Of course, students were primarily republicans.)

With the passage of time, Broussais' fervor diminished, his novelty faded and, very importantly, his most significant statements were proved false. By the 1830s he was passé, an almost extinct volcano occasionally spewing up a cloud of dead cinders and smelly gas. He had few followers in his later years (Ackerknecht, 1953). Today he is regarded either as a ridiculous figure because of the manifest absurdities of his unrealistic dogma, or else as a menace because of his treatment. However, he deserves better than that.

Broussais' early admiration of Pinel was followed by a persistent interest in mental disease. His early work on mental disease, *De l'Irritation et la Folie* (1828) was deservedly successful; it was translated into English in 1831 by Thomas Cooper, M.D. Like some of his contemporaries, Broussais adopted some phrenologic ideas. (Many psychiatrists of the early 19th century were oriented phrenologically.) His ambitious book, *Cours de Phrenologie*, was written in 1836, but could not compete with the brilliant clinical writings of Esquirol, Guislain, and other French psychiatrists of that great era. On the other hand, his *Irritation and Insanity* went into an enlarged second edition in 1839. Its most interesting contents comprise a critique of some of Freud's ideas many years before Freud's birth. Broussais' book contained remarkable discussions of the concept of the Ego and of the values and drawbacks of the concept when introduced into clinical psychiatry. He warned emphatically against setting up a hypothetical abstract entity as the executive agent in a functional process. Regarding the use of free-association and the advice that we must "listen to ourselves alone and think," he wrote, "It will be impossible to assert, after this inspection of the interior, a single fact that will not require to be verified by the senses." This mild comment was followed by a much more vigorous attack on those who used introspection for studying the mind. Like almost all previous authors, he emphasized the importance of sexual factors in hysteria.

Broussais was one of the last outstanding dogmatists of internal medicine and one of the first of modern psychiatry. Because he was a dogmatist, he neglected to apply to his own ideas the standards by which he criticized the ideas of others. If he had been content merely to criticize the poorly founded ideas that pervaded the medicine of his time, he would have been known historically as a great reformer. Certainly his critique of psychoanalytic ideas a half-century before they were supposed to have been invented later would have evoked wonder at his mental abilities.

The period of medical repression, in which only the military had relative freedom, came to an end after the revolution in 1830. Louis Philippe became King and lived the life, outwardly at least, of the conventional conservative middle class. However, his 18-year reign was a time of considerable turmoil, with the old ideas of the great Revolution and the Empire continually asserting themselves. During that period French medicine-nourished both on bedside practice, including the use of percussion, and also on the findings of the post-mortem examination-came to maturity under the influence of auscultation, the influx of clinicopathological material from Great Britain and Ireland, and the growth of physiology.

In the reign of Louis Philippe, Paris was the intellectual center of Europe and, hence, of the world. The sciences, theoretical and practical, and the art, written, visual, and musical were in a state of lively growth. Medicine, in a state of revulsion against dogma and theory, likewise was growing actively, but it was hampered, and finally slowed, by a new kind of repression. The period was one in which a bourgeois society was developing for the first time in France, owing in large part to the advanced status of the industrial revolution, which kept pace with that in Great Britain, both outstripping by 50 years that in the German states. The political revolution of 1830 added to the power of the upper middle classes. In medicine this new society instituted a new kind of repression, one of family and political connections. The degree to which hospital and university posts in medicine depended on these connections far exceeded anything that Americans, however cynical, can appreciate (Ackerknecht, 1967). That situation had its inevitable effects in slowing the growth of medicine, and that became apparent in the latter part of Louis Philippe's reign.

Nevertheless, before the decay became pronounced, French medicine had produced a host of outstanding clinicians (Ackerknecht, 1967). Of that great number, two, Louis and Andral, will be considered, since they represent the high points of French medicine at the beginning and at the end of the period.

Louis had a remarkable career. Having graduated in Paris in 1813 at the age of 26, he practiced successfully in Russia for seven years and then, believing his knowledge to be inadequate, he returned to Paris to enlarge his experience. Broussais was then the leader of clinical teaching there, but Louis would have none of him. Louis turned to his friend Chomel at the Charité (he became head of it in 1827) and was given permission to study there alone. Through his own efforts, he accumulated thousands of clinical cases, many having post-mortem studies. He never held a university post, but had appointments at the Hôtel Dieu and the Pitié. He was very popular with American students, who found him painfully thorough in his work, modest in success, and fearless when facing false authority. Since his discussions required considerable maturity of knowledge, he was followed more by American than French students, for the Americans were almost without exception postgraduates. Louis relied heavily on accumulations of data: His researches on tuberculosis, typhoid fever, and blood-letting in pneumonia, many checked by post-mortem studies, involved almost 2,000 cases and hundreds of autopsies. He was not only a fine clinician but also, as was common among the French, an expert anatomist. Although statistics had been suggested as a guide to medical studies by several authors previously (Bariety, 1972), Louis had to work out for himself the detailed procedures for collecting and analyzing the data.

Although other French physicians who wrote soon after the Revolution continued to claim that they were disciples of Hippocrates, Louis did not. He opened his discussion of typhoid fever with a quotation from Rousseau, "I know that the truth is in the things and not in my mind which judges them. The less I put of my own into these judgments, the surer I am to approach the truth." In his work he emphasized the need to systematize clinical observations, post-mortem findings, and statistical analyses. The earlier accounts of disease were to him too imprecise to be of any value. He rejected the idea that such sciences as anatomy, physiology, and pathology, including animal experimentation, could help in making therapeutic decisions. One could learn to make these decisions, he maintained, only by observing sick people, much as Sydenham had stated. In 1825 he published his great book on tuberculosis; it had twice as much space devoted to clinical manifestations as to pathologic anatomy. Although he added little to what Laennec and Bayle had written, his "numerical method" gave the findings added authority. He wrote a similar book on typhoid fever in 1829, emphasizing its localization to Peyer's patches and other lymphoid structures. Three of his American pupils, Gerhard, Rennock, and Shattuck, showed the difference between typhus and typhoid fever in 1835. Several of Louis' papers on blood-letting appeared in the meantime and showed the inutility of that practice, thereby destroying Broussais' credibility.

Louis' teaching gave statistics a solid place in clinical medicine; however, making use of statistics did not originate with Louis. Statistics had been used in public health since the 17th century, although not necessarily by physicians (Rosen, 1955; Kargon, 1963). In the 18th century the writings of Condorcet had a decisive influence in this regard (Rosen, 1955; Baker, 1975).   As a mathematician and *encyclopédist*, he wrote extensively on the use of mathematical methods to study and reform human society. It is interesting to note that Diderot, who edited the *Encyclopédia*, was highly skeptical about whether mathematics could explain anything at all that concerned living things, and the then-ruling Jacobins opposed Condorcet's views because they believed that they would create an intellectual elite.   Nevertheless, Condorcet persisted in his notion that the mathematical approach would lead to the perfection of man and the triumph of preventive medicine.   Twelve years after the posthumous publication of Condorcet's work in 1795, his friend Pinel used probability statistics to try to prove that the psychotherapeutic treatment of the insane was effective.   To some it seemed that probability theory would answer questions about certainty in medicine which were raised during the Revolution.   A number of physicians and others in France and England in the early 19th century used the huge collection of data to buttress their conclusions.   Louis was one of these (Rosen, 1955), and his American students carried his emphasis on statistics home with them.

Andral represented the high-water mark of French clinical medicine before 1850.   Physicians as disparate as Holmes in America and Virchow and Wunderlich in Germany were among those who so characterized him.   Born in 1797, he was the son of physician Guillaume Andral, who showed his adaptability by being physician to Murat in Napoleon's time and after that to King Charles X, the last Bourbon monarch.   Young Andral graduated in 1821, receiving much of his training at the Charité under Corvisart's pupil, Lerminer.   During that time he was friendly with Louis.   Between 1823 and 1827, he published with Lerminer the first edition of *Clinique Médical* in parts. Between 1829 and 1833, Andral alone published the second edition.   This highly successful work was based on actual cases, each of which served as a text for part of the discussion.   Among other things, he edited the works of Laennec, and his case discussions were full of detailed physical findings, arranged to show the progression of the diseases.

Andral opposed all dogma and fanaticism in his writings. His rise was rapid, and the fact that he had married the daughter of a prominent political figure probably did not hurt his career. In 1826 he founded the *Journal Hébdomedaire* with Bouillaud, the pathologist, and Raynaud, famous for his temperature studies. His rise, begun under the Bourbons, continued under Louis Philippe. In 1829 he wrote *Précis d'Anatomie Pathologique*, in which he stated, "Where anatomy no longer finds changes, chemistry shows them to us, and I do not doubt that it will become more and more the foundation of pathogenesis...." It is to be noted that his collaborator in some of his laboratory studies, Gavarret, was a physicist by training, took his M.D. degree, and then gave up medicine to become Professor of Physics at the University of Paris.

Andral's brilliant combination of clinical history, physical findings based on percussion and auscultation, laboratory findings both hematological and chemical,and, whenever available, post-mortem findings made him one of the best clinical teachers of his era. The American students, particularly the Bostonians, linked him with Louis in the most laudable sense. Today, if he is mentioned at all, it is as the father of hematology, a characterization that still leaves him virtually unknown. To Holmes he was perfection.

The increasing interest in auscultation of the heart naturally led to studies on the origins of heart sounds and murmurs. Many physiologists, such as Magendie, participated in these studies, but the writings of two clinicians are of primary interest.

Savart, born in Mézière, France, in 1791, was one such clinician. His father worked at the artillery school at Metz, where the boy was educated. In addition, the father taught his young son precision in mechanical arts. Savart's grandfather had been assistant to Nollet, the physicist who incidentally had done some work on the medical uses of electricity. Young Savart had an uncle and a brother who were army engineers, but he decided on medicine as a career and began his training at the hospital at Metz in 1808. He served as Regimental Surgeon in an engineering unit from 1810 to 1814 and then, after his discharge, entered the medical school at Strasbourg. He received the M.D. degree in 1816 and began to practice medicine at Metz in 1817. Practice was slow, and he spent much time in the physics laboratory and in making instruments. In 1819 he went to Paris, where, among other things, he pursued his interest in acoustics. He worked in this field with Biot, the man who also had encouraged Pasteur. Savart taught physics and came to succeed Ampère as Professor at the Collège de France. His professional life included studies on the acoustics of stringed instruments and the siren. His importance lies in his work on eddies as the source of cardiovascular sounds and on the propagation of sound. In addition, he is an example of the physician-turned-physicist, a fairly common species in the 19th century.

Rouanet was even more interesting, not only because he actively practiced medicine, but also he was able to fill the gaps left by Laennec relating to cardiovascular sounds (McKusick, 1958). Born in 1797 in Southern France of illiterate peasant parents, young Rouanet was evidently precociously intelligent, thereby attracting the support of a local elderly rich woman, who had him educated for the priesthood. He learned Latin and Greek before entering a seminary in Paris around 1820, but he soon gave up the idea of becoming a priest in favor of becoming a tutor in those languages. He received a bachelor's degree in 1829, enjoyed the life of a student, including taking a walking tour through Normandy, and studied medicine probably from 1828 to 1832. Prior to that time he was Secretary to the Princess of Talmont and later became her physician. In 1832 he wrote his thesis for his M.D. degree in which the origin and mechanisms of the heart sounds were discussed. He started a private practice in Paris, but it did not prosper; however, he continued his interest in heart sounds. Apparently, some speculations in the stock market were unsuccessful, and he moved to America in 1847, later sending money back to France to pay his debts. That year he was licensed in New Orleans where he lived almost a monastic life as a "sober" bachelor. His reputation as a diagnostician grew rapidly. One day a young colleague brought him a goose's heart, representing it as that of a human infant. Another colleague wrote some doggerel verse about the episode. A duel with pistols followed. The first shots grazed the two duelists, and Rouanet wanted to fire again, but the referee declared that honor had been satisfied.

In his profession Rouanet's work on heart sounds was recognized as outstanding. Not only did he prove the origin of the sounds, using models, but he also defined the contribution of each valve to murmurs from the location and timing of the sounds. He was also a skillful surgeon, much in demand as a collaborator in operations. Although his work - presented in 1832 and extended in 1844 - became known, it was not accepted universally; however, subsequent observers proved the correctness of his ideas. It is interesting to note that Flint also was practicing in New Orleans at the time, but it is not known whether Rouanet had anything to do with Flint's discovery of the murmur named after him.

Thus far, two French physicians who did little or no pratice, but who chose careers in the accessory sciences, have been discussed: de Fourcroy in chemistry, and Savart in physics, chiefly acoustics. Another name should be mentioned in this connection, Poiseuille. Born in 1799, he was trained in mathematics and physics, but turned to medicine instead, receiving his M.D. degree in 1828. His doctoral thesis on the design and use of a device for measuring arterial blood pressure, was published in the *Journal de Physiologie et de Pathologie Expérimentale,* of which Magendie had been founder and still was editor. Poiseuille continued to study and write about fluid dynamics more in terms of physics than physiology, and today he is famous for his mathematical equation describing the behavior of liquids moving in capillary vessels. He summarized his work and formulated his law - Poiseuille' law - in the *Comptes Rendues de l' Académie des Sciences* in 1840.

The medicine of the Napoleonic era also was notable for some of its surgeons. One was Baron Larrey, born in the foothills of the Pyrenées in 1766. After studying medicine, he signed on as surgeon to a frigate stationed off Newfoundland to protect the French fishermen. On his return in 1789 he found himself in the midst of the Revolution. For a time he studied in Paris with Desault and then was sent to join the fighting on the Rhine when the war began. From that time his life was one campaign after another - 26 to be exact - and many battles. His administrative reforms, designed to improve service to the wounded, caught Napoleon's attention and ultimately led to his being given the post of Surgeon-in-Chief. He also became famous for innovative changes in treatment. Although devoted to Napoleon personally, Larrey recognized that Napoleon was destroying the Republic by making himself Emperor and that such an action would be his downfall. With the restoration of the Bourbons, Larrey was deprived of rank and pension, but remained Surgeon-in-Chief to the Guard's Hospital. After 1830 he was Surgeon-in-Chief to "les Invalides," the Veterans' Hospital. He practiced little but traveled abroad and there received many honors (Dible, 1959). So well had he organized the treatment of casualties in the French army that long afterward, in the Crimean War, the French treatment stood in marked contrast to the English (Lawson, 1968).

Some French surgeons of a later day were also famous. At a time when there was no anesthesia, the qualities of speed, precision, and confidence were essential, as was the most detailed knowledge of anatomy, including the normal variations. The abdomen was forbidden territory at that time, since antisepsis and asepsis had not yet been invented. When these and anesthesia were developed around midcentury, the character of surgery changed, although finesse was still essential. Dupuytren was so outstanding that he was called "the Napoleon of surgery," the greatest compliment that could be paid anyone at the time. He was scornful of theory and formalized knowledge: His idea of teaching was to show how to apply his knowledge and skill to the development of modified or even new surgical techniques that might be demanded by unusual situations. He was proud of his diagnostic ability and his speed in surgery. On occasion he might appropriate another man's ideas or techniques with no reference to their source. With patients he exhibited extreme brutality, sometimes berating or even striking one who gave too slow an answer, or a wrong one. He was cruelly sarcastic to students, and his boisterous quarrels with some of his colleagues were famous. (His comments about Lisfranc, one of his rivals, and the latter's responses, became especially famous [da Costa, 1922].) Nevertheless, his outstanding skill, deftness, and ability to improvise caused him to be followed by large numbers of students, including Americans.

Quite unlike Dupuytren in behavior was Roux, a senior surgeon at the Charité He was extremely careful and considerate to patients, particularly in the dressing of their wounds, and his gentleness was especially apparent in his plastic surgery. Roux's remarkable dexterity attracted large numbers of students, but his lectures, which he initiated in 1812, were boring. In 1815 he published his extended, detailed observations on surgical practice in London, declaring it to be the only rival to the French. He succeeded Dupuytren as Chief at l'Hôtel Dieu in 1835.

Velpeau was another surgeon who was highly regarded by the American students. A poor peasant who had taught himself to read and write (da Costa, 1922), he had no resources except for his intellect and his character. He went first to Tours to study medicine, becoming an assistant to Bretonneau, and then he made his way to Paris. Eventually he rose to the highest levels of Paris medicine, becoming Professor of Clinical Surgery and Anatomy, Surgeon-in-Chief at the Charité and Surgeon at La Pitié. He was an enormously hard worker and never seemed to tire. Like other leading French surgeons, he was an expert anatomist, but he was unusual because of his broad reading and the utilization of information from many sources, including American writings. His books on operative surgery and obstetrics were used widely in Europe and America.

In an era in which every superior physician and surgeon was also a superior pathologist, choosing one who was outstanding is difficult, unless he had some unusual feature. Cruveilhier was that one. He was born in Limoges in 1791, the son of a military surgeon. He hoped to enter the church, but his father ordered him to study medicine, which he did in Paris beginning in 1810. He received the M.D. degree in 1816 after having caught the attention of Dupuytren. Although he had returned to Limoges to practice after graduation, he was appointed Professor of Surgery at Montpellier in 1823, through the influence of his old master. Again through Dupuytren's influence, Cruveilhier was appointed Professor of Descriptive Anatomy at Paris in 1825, where he helped Dupuytren establish his museum of morbid anatomy. When Dupuytren died he left a sum of money to establish a professorship of pathological anatomy, and in 1836 Cruveilhier was given the post, which he held for 30 years. He did his post-mortem work at the Charité and at the Salpetrière and had a busy private medical practice. In addition to his discoveries in general pathology, he made notable ones in neuropathology (Flamm, 1972). He had to work very hard, because he and his family had no private means. Cruveilhier was not only a great pathologist, but he was also the most important creator of illustrations of morbid anatomy until that time. His great *Anatomie Pathologique* (1829-1843) sold for 450 gold francs (Goldschind, 1952). It employed the newly developed and expensive process of making lithographs colored by hand. Only 409 copies were distributed. The work was clearly a labor of love and nobody, least of all Cruveilhier, made much money from it. The work, published in two parts, represented the height of medical illustration; its 233 lithograph plates were works of art as well as of information. Among the diseases Cruveilhier first described were multiple sclerosis, hypertrophic pyloric stenosis, and gastric ulcer. He was regarded highly as a teacher and was well known for his five-volume text written for more general use, *Treatise on General Pathological Anatomy*. The example of his appointment to a separate chair of pathology in Paris stimulated similar appointments in America.

Discussion of the period ending in 1848 should include the name of one person who, though never taking the M.D. degree (it offended his egalitarian principles), was important to medical history. Raspail, born in 1794, remained dedicated to the most extreme radical tenets of the Revolution and its terror, although they had for the most part become passé by the time he was old enough to know what they had been. His early training in a seminary at Avignon ended abruptly when he found that he had lost his faith. He then turned to scientific studies, involving both the biological and the physical sciences, but continued to be active in radical politics. By the time he reached the age of 26 in 1830, he had already published 50 papers, anticipating not only the cell theory of Schleiden and Schwann, but also by a quarter of a century the cellular pathology of Virchow. Also, by his work on microincineration and microanalysis, he anticipated modern approaches to histochemistry by many decades.   When the Revolution of 1830 forced out the Bourbons and put Louis Philippe on the throne, Raspail, always the ardent republican, took part in an uprising against the new King.   He spent two years in prison as a result, and had the leisure to write extensively on many subjects, including organic chemistry and plant physiology.   Although well qualified by his studies to take the M.D. degree, he refused to do so out of principle.   Nevertheless, in 1840 he began to practice medicine and pharmacy, taking no fees from the poor whom he treated.   This unauthorized practice occasioned more trouble with the authorities (Wiener, 1968).   The Revolution of 1848 engaged his full activities, and he was chosen to read from the Paris City Hall the proclamation establishing the Republic.   Elected to the Chamber of Deputies, he ran for the presidency, but was defeated by Louis Napoleon.   When a few years later Napoleon made himself Emperor, Raspail went into exile, and during the next nine years he edited a radical newspaper, agitated for free medical care for all, and created a line of valueless pharmaceutical remedies, in which he firmly believed.   He saw himself as a reformer not only of the administrative aspects of medicine but of medical practice itself.   When the Empire of Napoleon III collapsed after Sedan, Raspail took part in the revolt that established the Commune in Paris, and he survived its bloody defeat.   He died in 1878, probably never having experienced a boring minute after leaving the seminary.   His erratic life, and particularly his radical politics, overshadowed his important studies in the medical sciences.   He was, however, not a clinician.   If he had lived a century after he did, he undoubtedly would have been a radical activist during and after the years of the Vietnam conflict.   He should be remembered, however (although he is not), for his *Nouveau Synthèse de Chimie Organique*, which proposes his intelligent reasoning about the role of cells in physiology and that living matter merely represents a higher level of organization of the same things found in nonliving matter.

After the Revolution of 1848 and the dictatorial seizure of the government by its elected president, Napoleon III, a few years later, French medicine began to lose much of its impetus.   In 1848 economic conditions, the smoldering republican spirit of earlier times, and the furor created by the gathering in Paris of most of the malcontents of Europe combined to produce revolutions, successful in France and unsuccessful in the German states.   The enfranchisement of the peasants in France had the inevitable effect of making Louis Napoleon President of the Republic, a trust he violated a few years later by making himself Emperor Napoleon III.   He had none of the imagination, administrative ability, or leadership qualities of the first Napoleon, and his reign was characterized by a new repression.   For example, Chomel, who had succeeded Laennec at the Charité in 1827 and had helped Louis become an outstanding clinician, resigned in 1852 rather than take the oath of loyalty to Napoleon III. Moreover, although he sought popularity through military victories, this Napoleon's military adventures did not turn out well-Italy, the Crimea, Mexico, and finally the disaster at Sedan.   The sorry events did not finish with him, for the end of his reign saw the battle with the Commune in Paris, in which many thousands were killed.   French clinical medicine, a creature of the central government, demoralized by political and financial disorder, lost its preeminence except, for reasons unknown, in clinical neurology and psychiatry.   Here superiority was maintained throughout the rest of the century.   The so-called ancillary sciences - physiology, chemistry, and bacteriology - also prospered, as well as or better than might be expected during times of financial stringency.   However, they took directions that often led them away from the everyday aspects of clinical medicine and into areas more basic than clinical.

To summarize, the accomplishments of French clinical medicine to around 1850, perfected physical diagnosis, supported by post-mortem studies and also by the beginnings of laboratory studies in disease, created concepts and procedures that were bound to stimulate the development of clinical medicine for decades to come.   There were, however, two negative aspects: Students did not often participate in the new medicine except as observers, and many practicing physicians outside the Paris hospitals did not accept the new physical diagnosis.   In fact it was physicians across the Channel, at first chiefly in Ireland, whose actions led to a widespread use of percussion and auscultation and the involvement of students in their use. Moreover, the development of French medicine centered in large hospitals impaired the development of the doctor-patient relationship that is the basis of the best clinical medicine.

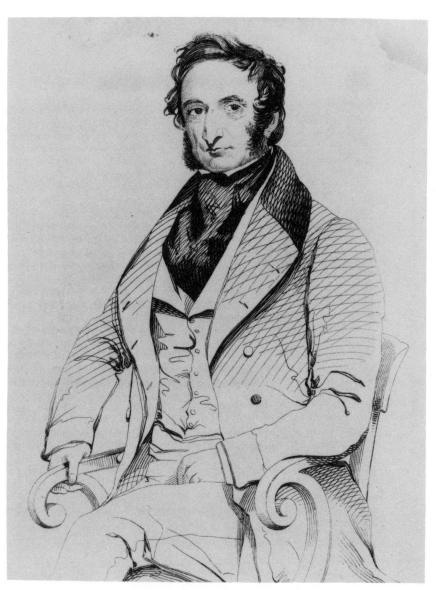

Robert J. Graves, 1796–1853

THE SCOTTISH RENAISSANCE IN EDINBURGH and other cities had a smaller counterpart in Dublin. Even before Dublin gained its great medical renown it already had established one tradition that was to spread and become important in British and American medicine. What was to become a tradition was the new idea of the voluntary hospital, in contrast to the religious or government hospital. Thus, in the 18th century - years before Guy's, the first voluntary hospital in London, was established - Dublin eventually had a number of them: the Jervis Street, the Meath, Sir Patrick Dun's, the Stevens, and later Mosse's, the last better known as the Rotunda.

Overpopulation and poverty had been endemic in Ireland - almost 1,000,000 Irishmen had gone to America *before* the great famine sent great numbers of them overseas in the 1840s. Such poverty and misery cannot be imagined today. (A visitor to Dublin commented that at last he knew what happened to the clothes discarded by London's beggars [Cummins, 1957; Fleetwood, 1951].) On the other hand, there was considerable concentrated wealth, much of it in the hands of the descendants of Cromwell's colonels who had seized extensive lands but usually lived in England. Dublin, the capital in Georgian times, had a large wealthy and cultivated class; however, the poor in the slums lived in unimaginable misery, a misery made darker by William and Mary's tax on windows. Misery and injustice precipitated the rebellion of 1798, and after it was quieted, the Act of Union in 1801 deprived Dublin of its status as the seat of government, although it was still second city of the Empire. After Waterloo there was fivefold inflation, and recurrent typhus and cholera epidemics occurred over the next decades.

Nevertheless, the Irish intellectual renaissance developed and, medically, it was far out of proportion to the number of physicians involved.   A small group of Irish physicians carried forward the advances in clinical medicine which had made Edinburgh and Paris great, not only accelerating these advances, but also helping to make them acceptable to the English-speaking world.   Accordingly, during the first half of the 19th century Dublin became an important site of medical education for the Atlantic community.   During the early part of this era medical education was carried on largely in unregulated, private medical schools, much like those in London; however, none was as famous as London's Great Windmill Street School.   In addition, the College of Physicians in Dublin gave courses; but, there were no clinical facilities until 1810, when Dun's Hospital became the clinical facility for the University of Dublin.   For some time men who had received part or much of their training in Ireland had to go elsewhere for a few years of clinical experience.   Nevertheless, Dublin's medical growth, like London's, began with the establishment of private medical schools and voluntary hospitals.

Many of Ireland's physicians were Scottish-trained, for Edinburgh provided more medical practitioners to Ireland than it did to Scotland itself.   One of Edinburgh's famous Irish alumni was Colles, born in 1773 near Kilkenny of an English family long established there.   As a schoolboy he found a textbook of anatomy that had washed up from a local doctor's house during a flood.   From then on he was committed to medicine, although Burke, a family friend, wanted him to develop his already evident skills in political satire.   Colles entered Dublin University in 1790 and simultaneously was apprenticed to the resident surgeon of Stevens' Hospital.   He obtained the diploma of the Irish College of Surgeons five years later and then entered the medical school at Edinburgh.   Having obtained the M.D. degree, he went to London, where he assisted Cooper in dissection and studied at London hospitals.   Colles returned to Dublin in 1797 and began a general practice, having been appointed Visiting Physician to the Meath Hospital, another voluntary hospital.   He gave up medicine for surgery two years later and was appointed Resident Surgeon to Stevens' Hospital, a post he held until 1813 when he than became Visiting Surgeon to that hospital.   In

1804 he became Professor of Anatomy and Surgery in the Irish College of Surgeons and held that post until 1836.

Colles became known as a cool, dexterous operator, exhibiting a great deal of ingenuity in difficult and complicated situations. For years he continued to practice dissection for several hours daily, and his knowledge of anatomy grew. Although he was accomplished in many areas of surgery, he is best remembered for Colles' fracture of the radius. His abilities as a lecturer enhanced Dublin's reputation as a center for medical education and attracted many students. He disdained preformed notions and avoided speculation, and his lectures, published in 1844 in two volumes, are models of clarity and concentration on salient points. He was described as cheerful, generous, and modest, and a liberal in politics. He despised fanatics and charlatans equally, and he was frank when acknowledging errors in his own judgment.

A son, William Colles, gained fame in the medicine of Great Britain and Ireland for his surgical skills and fresh and lucid comments on an old disease - gout - in his treatise in 1857. His reputation in Ireland as a surgeon and as an anatomist, especially abnormal anatomy of disease, led to his election three times as President of the Royal College of Surgeons in Ireland, to his appointment as Surgeon to the Queen in Ireland, and finally in 1861, to his being made Regius Professor of Surgery at Dublin.

One of the first of Edinburgh's alumni in Ireland to achieve international recognition was Cheyne, born in Leith, Scotland, the son of a general practitioner. After completing his primary education at Leith, he was sent to a secondary school in Edinburgh, where he evidently had a generally unpleasant time. He started his medical education at the age of 13, when he began to assist his father. He entered Edinburgh, and in 1795, with a superficial knowledge of medicine but with the help of a famous coach, he obtained his M.D. degree. Subsequently, he entered the army, serving with an artillery regiment for four years and spending his time, according to his own account, in "frivolous pursuits." After retiring from the army, he joined his father in practice and also ran the ordinance hospital in Leith. That was the real beginning of his medical career, and he wrote clinical treatises based on his observations of diphtheria, pulmonary diseases, and hydrocephalus, among other things.   (Some of these works contained beautiful illustrations by Bell.)   At the age of 32 he moved to Dublin, where he practiced for more than 20 years.   In 1811 he was appointed Physician at the Meath Hospital and later Professor of Physic at the College of Surgeons.   His experience during the epidemics of 1817 to 1819 led to his fine treatise on febrile illnesses, but he achieved immortality as the Cheyne of Cheyne-Stokes breathing.   Outwardly he seemed indifferent to suffering, but as his health began to fail - he ultimately developed gangrene of the legs - he devoted all of his time and great clinical abilities to the medical care of the poor who lived near his estate in Buckinghamshire.   A devout Christian, he considered it his duty to make his personal and professional behavior serve as models to his younger colleagues.   Although a competent and devoted physician and a good clinical observer, he at no time gave any evidence, or himself believed, that he was, in fact, ushering in the Dublin revival.   It is interesting that his writing late in life included several treatises on the impossibility of curing insanity by psychotherapeutic means.

Another pioneer in the Dublin revival was Adams, whose accomplishments were noteworthy but not among the greatest.   Adams, like Cheyne, achieved immortality by having his name linked with that of Stokes in the description of a clinical syndrome, the Stokes-Adams syndrome. Little is known about Adams' early life except that he was born in Ireland in 1791.   He attended Trinity College in Dublin, where he was granted the Bachelor's degree in 1814, a Master's degree in 1832 and, finally, the M.D. degree 10 years later at the age of 51.   Actually he had begun to study medicine years before, when he was apprenticed to a practitioner, and he was licensed after taking the examinations given by the Royal College of Surgeons of Ireland shortly after receiving his Bachelor's degree. He spent some years on the Continent in further medical education and then opened his practice in Dublin, where he was regarded highly and was soon elected Surgeon to the Jervis Street hospital and later to the Richmond Hospital. At the latter institution he helped to organize a hospital medical school, in much the same manner as the early medical schools of London. His career emphasized clinical observation, and in 1826 his description of the manifestations of heart-block in the *Dublin Hospital Reports* was recognized immediately as a classic. Although Adams was eventually Regius Professor of Surgery at Dublin, his predecessor in that post - Abraham Colles - was by far the more famous in that field.

The Dublin medical renaissance clearly became recognizable in the work and career of Robert Graves. Without him and his student, colleague, and friend Stokes, it would be impossible to establish without disagreement that there was the great era of Dublin medicine that we now recognize (Riesman, 1922; Doolin, 1947). Graves was born in 1796, the son of the Professor of Divinity at Dublin University and Dean of Armagh. The family was descended from one of Cromwell's army officers, who had established the family fortune as a result of that service, "acquiring considerable property in the county of Limerick." Graves studied at the University of Dublin, taking both liberal arts and medical courses, and his performance was such that he won every available prize. He then had three years of study with outstanding teachers in London, Germany, Austria, Copenhagen, and Edinburgh. In his travels he exercised his great abilities with languages (resulting in his being arrested as a spy) and with oil paint (traveling with Turner in the Alps). On his return to Dublin in 1821 he was elected Physician at the Meath Hospital, where he startled both students and staff by blaming many deaths on the staff's not teaching the students adequately. Graves also became a founder of the Pack Street School of Medicine. In his teaching he insisted that the students work up cases themselves. He also was appointed Professor of the Institutes of Medicine at the Irish College of Physicians and lectured there on physiology for many years. His physiologic competence was not limited to lectures, for he published original essays in this field in the *Dublin Journal of Medical Science*, a periodical he helped to found and edit. His *Clinical Lectures* (1834-1837) and *System of Clinical Medicine* (1843) were translated later into French, and led Trousseau, himself one of the greatest clinicians of the century, to declare that they had inspired him. Graves also wrote many articles on clinical subjects in which he insisted that the treatment of fevers should be based on nutrition. He wanted his epitaph to be "He fed fevers." Like other Dubliners, his name is attached to a disease, Graves' disease. (The Germans prefer to call it "Basedow's.") Not the least of his writings was his answer, as co-author with Stokes, to Clutterbuck's criticism of auscultation and percussion in medicine. Graves also showed his appreciation of emotional factors in disease, using the then-current writings of Hall in London on visceral reflexes. He was warm-hearted and appreciative in his relationships with colleagues and former students in every country. His one serious error was his insistence that all fevers were the same, although he quickly admitted the mistakes when Gerhard in Philadelphia separated typhus and typhoid fevers by their clinical and post-mortem features.

Graves' status is impossible to separate from that of his pupil, Stokes, because Stokes built upon Graves' work and carried it forward, often in conjunction with Graves. The Stokes clan was another English family that had immigrated to Ireland. They arrived in 1735, when the first of them, Gabriel, was a scholar and clergyman, a fellow of Trinity College, and the holder of a number of ecclesiastical posts. This Gabriel had a son, Whitley, who took a Bachelor of Medicine degree at Dublin and a few years later the M.D. degree. he was connected for a time with the revolutionary movement in Ireland and accordingly was suspended from his academic duties. He remained a patriotic Irishman throughout his life, not only founding the Irish Society, but translating the New Testament into Gaelic. He later was reappointed and continued to gain prominence until he became Regius Professor of Medicine in 1830, holding that post for 12 years. Whitley Stokes was Physician to the Meath Hospital when the young Graves was appointed to the staff in 1821, and he immediately instituted the latter's innovative ideas. Stokes' opinions of Graves' ideas are not recorded specifically, but he encouraged the close ties that developed between Graves and his own son William.

William Stokes was born in Dublin in 1804 and was tutored in classics and mathematics by a fellow of Trinity College, and in the sciences by his own father. He went to Edinburgh to study medicine and graduated in 1825. On his return to Dublin, he was licensed by the College of Physicians there and immediately elected Physician to the Meath Hospital. Also in 1825 he published his treatise, *An Introduction to the Use of the Stethoscope*, dedicated to Cullen of Edinburgh. Two years later he published his work on the use of the stethoscope in chest diseases. From the very first he worked closely with Graves in the reform of practice and teaching in Dublin. He was a more brilliant lecturer than Graves and an indefatigable observer and recorder of clinical phenomena. The year 1837 saw the publication of his great work on the diagnosis and treatment of chest disease, a critical analysis of the works of Laennec modified and fortified by his own extensive case material. In 1838 he founded the Dublin Pathological Society, antedating the founding of the London society. He had an amateur interest in art and antiquities, and he traveled in Europe not only to enrich his medical knowledge, but also to pursue his other interests. At home he reserved every Saturday evening for a gathering of the young men in every branch of science and art, helping some of them individually. In 1854 he published his greatest work, *Diseases of the Heart and Aorta*, followed in 1863 by *Studies in Physiology and Medicine*. He was Regius Professor of Medicine at Dublin from the time of his father's retirement from that post in 1843. In addition to his treatises on medical subjects, he wrote about the life and work of archaeologist Petrie, his friend. He encouraged studies of Irish archaeology, art, architecture, and music, participating himself. One of his sons became a surgeon, and another a well-known Celtic scholar. During his lifetime he received many of the highest honors in Ireland, Great Britain, and on the Continent.

Modern clinical teaching owes its existence to the efforts of Graves and Stokes, who in large part were responsible, together with Hope in England, for making use of auscultation and standardizing percussion in medicine; moreover, they made the students learn these methods. Stokes' clinical contributions included the creation of much of today's cardiology as well as a good portion of our understanding of chest diseases. The fame of the pair was worldwide; for example, their influence on the development of clinical medicine in Philadelphia in the 19th century helped to make that city outstanding (Riesman, 1942). Graves and Stokes incorporated the innovations of the greatest medicine of their era - French - with their own, thereby propelling medical education, particularly with respect to diagnosis, along the road that was to carry it forward during the rest of the century in Europe, and to some extent in America.   Their assimilation of the use of the stethoscope into clinical medicine would have been enough to make them great, but it was not unopposed. Clutterbuck, a leading Irish practitioner, strongly was opposed to the use of percussion and auscultation in the 1830s.   (The opposition of German physicians in the 1840s through 1860s will be noted later.)   Clutterbuck filled many pages in journals with his criticisms.   One of his papers, published in the *London Medical Gazette* for July 28, 1838, particularly was spirited; Graves and Stokes replied in the *Dublin Journal of Medical Sciences* (1839, page 138), of which they were editors.   They enumerated in detail the diagnoses that could be made only by percussion and auscultation, and closed with the warning that the diagnosis of heart diseases was not yet founded securely. Despite Clutterbuck's excellent reputation, Graves and Stokes fortunately prevailed.

The greatness of those two men should not overshadow completely the somewhat lesser figures working in Ireland during that time, one of whom was Wallace of Dublin, who introduced the use of iodides for the treatment of syphilis.   Using his own funds he established a clinic for the poor suffering from venereal diseases and founded his own medical school adjacent to it (Merton, 1966).   He died at an early age from typhus contracted from a patient; thus, what might have been a fine teaching career ended.   Today he rarely is remembered.

Corrigan suffered no such fate.   He lived to achieve fame, although some historians disparage his accomplishments because he did not refer to the works of all of his predecessors.   For example, his biographer in *Dictionary of National Biography* states that "He had received little general education, and had no knowledge of the writings of his predecessors, but he was the first prominent physician of the race and religion of the majority in Ireland, and the populace were pleased with his success, and spread his fame through the country, so that no physician in Ireland had before received so many fees as he did." This insulting comment seems to be dictated by prejudice, since it is not inconsistent with established facts. It is true that Corrigan was born at the edge of a slum and was of Gaelic origin and Catholic religion, unlike the other leaders of Irish medicine discussed in this section, all of whom were of Anglo-Saxon origin, Protestant in religion, and mostly of distinguished families. Corrigan's family were hardworking and intelligent people, and they did everything possible to give him a good education. He entered the medical school at Edinburgh after some informal study with a local doctor and received the M.D. degree in 1825 at the age of 23. (Among his fellow students were William Stokes of Dublin and Hope of London.) He returned to Dublin and began to practice. In 1832 his paper, "On permanent patency of the mouth of the aorta, or inadequacy of the aortic valves," was published in the *Edinburgh Medical and Surgical Journal* and immediately was recognized as an excellent description of the clinical syndrome. It was praised by Graves and Stokes, and Trousseau in France called the disease "la maladie de Corrigan." (Later, while traveling in France, Corrigan had the interesting experience of being asked whether he was descended from the famous Dr. Corrigan of Dublin. Some historians, however, have criticized Corrigan for not noting that Cowper as well as Vieussens had described the disease years before that time, and that Hodgkin had discussed it in two letters a year or two earlier. Actually, any dispute that might arise about whether Corrigan was the first to describe the manifestations of aortic regurgitation, or whether it was Hodgkin, is superfluous.) In 1833 he was appointed Lecturer in Medicine at the private Carmichael (formerly Richmond) School.

An earlier description of the major clinical manifestations of that syndrome was made by another Irishman, Cumming. Born in Ulster in 1798, he was destined for the church but preferred medicine, taking the M.D. degree at Edinburgh in 1818 and then settling in Dublin, where he participated actively in medical affairs. He became Physician at the Dublin General Dispensary and several other institutions, and he lectured at the Richmond School of medicine.   Later in life he returned to Armagh where he practiced for some time, becoming known for his treatment of fevers.   The third volume of the *Dublin Hospital Reports* contained Cumming's observations on aortic regurgitation, which were made in 1822.   First seen in 1820, his patient exhibited anginal pain, exaggerated arterial pusations, and pulmonary congestion, which Cumming correlated with the post-mortem finding of aortic valve disease.   The case report (published by Cumming under the title, "A Case of Diseased Heart") indicates that the patient had the paroxysmal disorder described by Thomas Lewis a century later as occurring in aortic regurgitation.   Cumming emphasized the notable arterial pulsations of the disorder seven years before Hodgkin and two before Corrigan.   He commented accurately on the different pulse forms of aortic regurgitation and aortic stenosis.   Cumming's report was unusual also in that he ascribed the pulmonary congestion to back-pressure, a concept that Hope proffered a decade later.   Cumming treated the patient with digitalis.   At post-mortem examination the coronary arteries were found to be normal, showing that coronary atherosclerosis was not essential for cardiac pain.   His report is remarkably accurate, except regarding the etiology of the disorder, which he believed was due to excessive playing of the flute.

Corrigan's other major academic contribution was in the field of pulmonary fibrosis.   He maintained the opinion, now regarded as correct, that pulmonary fibrosis caused bronchial dilation, whereas others, such as Hope, held that bronchiectasis caused fibrosis.   Corrigan was criticized severely at the time for that viewpoint, but history has vindicated him.

From 1840 to 1866 Corrigan was Physician to the House of Industry Hospitals and also managed a huge practice.   In 1841 he was appointed a Member of the Board of the new Queen's College and in 1871 became Vice Chancellor.   It is interesting to note that in 1846 he pointed out that starvation led to epidemics of fevers, a concept preceding Virchow's more widely applauded similar idea. Corrigan was elected President of the Royal College of Physicians and served for five terms.   In addition to his very busy practice, he was very interested in politics and was elected to the Parliament in Westminster from Dublin as a Liberal, but opposed Home Rule. He also opposed the opening of pubs on Sunday. As a member of the General Medical Council, he made every effort to involve the ordinary general practitioners in medical politics; however, he was unsuccessful. His large practice and his very active public life did not interfere with his becoming a force for excellence in medical practice.

This group of Irishmen quickly recognized the importance not only of clinical observation along the lines initiated by Sydenham and Locke, but also of new methods for enhancing and broadening the value of clinical observation, which increased doctor-patient contact and further improved clinical practice.

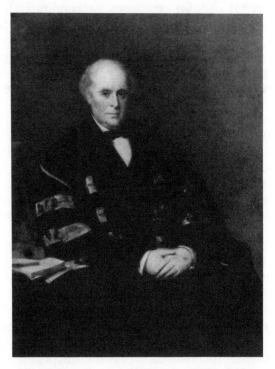

Sir Dominic Corrigan, 1802–1880

As previously noted, medical education in 18th-century london was carried on in private medical schools and in hospital medical schools, often with overlapping staffs. Although what were called the "collateral" sciences - mal anatomy, comparative anatomy, and the rather primitive physiology and chemistry - were not neglected, the main orientation was clinical, or disease related.

The great social changes attending the industrial revolution of the late 18th century increased in the early 19th century. The cities grew, and a prosperous middle class developed; but the number of poor increased. The social change that characterized 19th-century England began to accelerate rapidly after 1830. That year the death of George IV and the accession of William IV made Parliamentary elections mandatory. It was a time of poor trade and economic distress in the land, with incendiarism on large agricultural estates and disorder in industrial towns. The year 1830 was also one of economic depression and political revolution on the Continent, where the general misery was increased by the widespread severe cholera epidemic, which crossed into England the next year. The Parliamentary election in England was won by the Liberals, and after political maneuvering, the House of Lords was forced to agree to the Reform Bill passed by the House of Commons. The political power of the middle class was established and that, together with its growing wealth and determined pursuit of education, characterized subsequent decades in England. A need for increased numbers of well-trained doctors was evident. Medical education in hospitals increased. (These hospitals usually were called "infirmaries" in order to distinguish them from religious foundations.) In addition to those hospitals of London that had instituted organized teaching in the mid- to late 18th century, a half-dozen others were established in the 19th century.

Two of the older hospitals of London, St. Bartholomew's and St. Thomas', presented organized teaching in medicine in 1731 and 1740, respectively. Three others, founded in the 18th century as outgrowths of humanitarian movements, instituted medical teaching in that century, Guy's in 1740, St. George's in 1752, and the London in 1785. The 18th-century growth of cities accelerated the establishment of the new criteria of medical education derived from Leyden *via* Edinburgh.

The Middlesex instituted teaching in 1822, and the Westminster in 1841, although both had been founded as hospitals in the preceding century. Two other hospitals, founded in the 19th century, had been organized with a view toward medical teaching, the Charing Cross in 1821 and St. Mary's in 1846. Appointments to the staffs of these and other hospitals in London were not always based on merit; rather, favoritism and even bribery seemed to have been factors (Singer and Holloway, 1960). In addition to the hospitals, free "dispensaries" also became involved in clinical teaching (Cope, 1969). The dispensary movement, initiated for the relief of the poor, began with the founding of the Dispensary for Sick Children in London in 1769 (Poynter, 1957) and spread throughout Great Britain and to America. These dispensaries had not only out-patients, but in-patients and home-patients in varying numbers.

Changes in licensing also came to the fore around that time (Newman, 1957), creating a need for more formal training not only in clinical subjects, but also in the clinically related, or so-called collateral, sciences. By the middle of the century there were six new medical schools in London, but only two of them were university connected (Singer and Holloway, 1960).

There was no university presence in London medical education until 1828, when London University was founded. It soon had its own hospital, the University College Hospital, which had been the North London Hospital. King's College, founded in 1836, began organized medical teaching in 1839. Nevertheless, for a long time most medical training was carried on mainly in the famous independent London teaching hospitals.

The founding of universities in London was regarded as an affront to the hitherto ruling Tory class (Singer and Holloway, 1960), which considered only the ancient universities of Oxford and Cambridge capable of serving the country's intellectual and professional needs. However, the various reform movements of the early century pushed the Tories into the background and, despite their voiced opposition, the University of London was founded. But the old universities still were regarded highly.

London medicine in the early 19th century was responsible for great clinical accomplishments. Many men and a number of institutions were involved. In this period the accumulation of observational data which was to create modern clinical medicine grew out of the contributions of numerous physicians. Although the interest in those developments overshadows that in the individual men who created them, special attention will be given to some men's lives and works. Some of these men were members of that remarkable group working at Guy's Hospital (Ober, 1973; Handler, 1976). This is not intended to belittle the outstanding contributions of men at other hospitals, most notably the surgeons at St. Bartholomew's (Medvie and Thornton, 1974); nor is it necessary to dwell on the temporary decline of teaching at St. Thomas' after its separation from Guy's (Foster and Pinniger, 1963). Indeed, not all of the great events occurred in London, for the York Medical School gave us Hutchinson and Jackson, among others, around this time (Wetherill, 1961). York was but one of the nine provincial medical schools founded in England between 1824 and 1834, and provincial medicine of the period had some practitioners as good as any in London. For example, Carson, an Edinburgh M.D. of 1799, opened a practice in Liverpool and made important contributions. Whereas others discussed only the pumping action of the heart as the mechanism of circulation, he emphasized the elasticity of arteries and the effects of negative intrathoracic pressure in sucking blood from the periphery back to the heart (Cohen of Birkenhead, 1972). He also invented artificial pneumothorax for the treatment of tuberculosis 70 years before the date that historians apply to its discovery in Italy.

Special attention should be given to the London Hospital, for the first of the specifically designated medical schools derived from hospitals in London originated there. The name of Blizard is associated with that event. Born in 1743 and the son of an auctioneer, Blizard received his early medical training as apprentice to a surgeon. Later he studied with John Hunter, under Pott at St. Bartholomew's, and finally on the wards of the London Hospital, a charity hospital. With Lettsom he was one of the founders of the Medical Society of London in 1773. For a time he taught surgery at a private medical school, and he was appointed Surgeon to the London Hospital in 1780, petitioning its governing board the following year to be allowed to teach there. Permission was granted, on condition that he use none of its patients in his demonstrations (McConaghy, 1958). That was probably a hardship, for Blizard was said to have been a poor lecturer but a brilliant teacher. In 1783 the staff petitioned the governors to build "a proper building" for the teaching of the various branches of physic and surgery by means of lectures at the Hospital. Blizard himself made a large contribution toward the cost of the new school and also circulated a fund-raising pamphlet called, "An Address to the Friends of the London Hospital and of Medical Learning." The London Hospital School of Medicine was founded in 1785. Blizard lectured there and elsewhere but was not popular with students, who referred to him as a snarler.

Blizard was extremely formal in manner and dress, sometimes to the point of being ludicrous, but by nature he was high-spirited, irascible, and daring. (On one occasion he leaped from his carriage to seize an armed highwayman by the throat; on another, he challenged a man to a duel which, fortunately, never was held.) Although students disliked him, mature physicians such as Abernathy and Lettsom praised his qualities as both practitioner and teacher. Except for his role in establishing the first of London's great teaching hospitals, his place in the history of medicine is not noteworthy. He did gain some note as a poet (whose works were collected). His poems were written in the flowery, pompous style of that time, but whatever their technical qualities, their content was not outstanding. One critic suggested that Blizard might have been included in Pope's *Dunciad*. If there is any interest in his poems today, it is because they presented the medical ideas of his times. Nevertheless, he remains immortal as a leader in the development of hospital medical schools.

The philosophy that had become established in London emphasized that clinical observation had to be confirmed by post-mortem findings. However, since there was much to be learned, and sick people could not wait for research to solve the problems, physicians had to be tolerant regarding the use of unestablished or incomplete concepts. Farre, founder of the London Dispensary for Curing Diseases of the Eye, described the situation well in 1819:

> The wants of man, and his impatience to remove them, have always engrossed man's attention and he is instinctively led to regard, in the first place, those (wants) which he feels to be most urgent. Therefore, we do not despise popular medicine, although we cannot commend it....The science of medicine does indeed rest on the basis of observation but that observation is of two kinds - clinical and anatomical. Anatomical observation preceded by clinical observation, affords the only means of distinguishing between diseases of function and diseases of structure. It is (also) capable of introducing great simplicity in methodical arrangement of diseases. For in tracing by dissection the morbid changes of internal organs, it is impossible not to perceive that numerous diseases are, in truth, but varieties in the stage, or in the seat, of one and the same disease.

Nevertheless, for the most part the advances were based on clinical findings plus those of morbid anatomy, supplemented by some chemical data.

In the first half of the 19th century London clearly had numerous physicians who were notable as practitioners and contributors of data to clinical medicine. They were also noteworthy because of the diversity of their specific interests, both in medicine and elsewhere. The reason for that diversity is not evident, but it is interesting that few of London's outstanding physicians were interested in experimental science before their medical training; their scientific interest (if any) was in botany, natural history, and geology. Clearly, they did not go into medicine in order to pursue careers in science. Most of the medical educators of the period stressed the need for a broad cultural education, which usually meant an education in the classics (Peterson, 1978). However, few men could afford the arts degree before medicine, the implication being that not having it was no hindrance: Then, as now, there was no evidence that any one type of premedical education leads to production of better doctors than any other. What happened in the hospital or hospital medical school - granting individual differences in intelligence, interest, and human understanding - was crucial. There is perhaps a lesson here.

Another point is less clear. At that time there was a good deal of tension between the hospitals' lay governing boards and the clinical staffs regarding teaching. The laymen believed that the main role of the charitable hospital was to treat the poor, or at least "the deserving" poor, while many of the professional staff believed that the role of the hospital patient was simply to be teaching material - an audiovisual aid to teaching, as Peterson (1978) put it.

Another conflict that arose in London a century ago seems familiar today. When the governors of St. Thomas' Hospital allowed Florence Nightingale to set up a nurses' training school in their hospital, they did not consult the medical staff. Some physicians objected because they believed that the nurses would take over the hospital, a belief presumably based on the ancient masculine conviction that unmarried women with a mission who are given any encouragement cannot be stopped.

All London teaching hospitals had staff members who made notable contributions to clinical medicine. In the case of Guy's Hospital, several such men were there at about the same time, and the hospital accordingly had a remarkable reputation. Originally Guy's and St. Thomas' together became the United Borough Hospitals but, when they separated, they agreed that the teaching in medicine and surgery should take place at Guy's and St. Thomas', respectively. The men of Guy's were a remarkable group, some of whom shaped the course of clinical medicine in the Western World. Three men at Guy's - all contemporaries - were perhaps the most famous, the name of each becoming the basis of an eponym.

Bright, the first (temporally) among them, was born in Bristol in 1789 and brought up in a home of wealth and culture. As a youth he showed great interest in geology, an interest that was encouraged by Babington, a physician at Guy's Hospital. At the age of 20 Bright began medical studies at Edinburgh but, after a few months, left for London. He applied for a position with Sir George MacKenzie, a well-known explorer, who was planning a trip to Iceland. Until that time Iceland, although not far from England, for the most part was unknown to the English; however, after it was captured by them during the Napoleonic wars, it became open to them. Accompanied by his friend and schoolmate, Holland, Bright joined the expedition that set sail for Iceland, via the Orkneys, in April of 1810. MacKenzie wrote a book about Iceland which contained important contributions by Bright, some of which were the engravings illustrating the work. The return trip was like the trip out, a long and stormy one; the group had returned from Iceland after an absence of five months.

Bright immediately went to London where he resumed his medical studies at Guy's. Initially interested in morbid anatomy, he studied it with Cooper, and the drawings he made at the time were marvelously accurate. However, he did not abandon his interest in geology, and Babington of Guy's continued to encourage him in that work. Ultimately, his association with Babington grew closer, and Bright married his daughter a few years later. In 1811 Bright read a paper before the Geological Society and then returned to Edinburgh to study geology and natural history. Nevertheless, he did not neglect medicine and received his M.D. degree in 1812. After a brief period at Cambridge, which he disliked he returned to London to resume his medical work. He again became restless and went to the Continent, mostly for the sake of traveling, but also to study wherever there were opportunities. Bright visited Holland, Belgium, and Germany, and although the social life of Vienna during the Congress of Vienna intrigued him, he found time to study at the Allgemaine Krankenhaus. At that time his writings were much like illustrated travelogues (Chance, 1940). From Vienna he went on to Hungary, visiting the university and the museums of Budapest. His *Travels from Vienna to Lower Hungary* came to be regarded as an authoritative handbook because of its accuracy and thoroughness. In fact, his description of the land around Lake Balaton became recognized *in Hungary* as an authoritative work (Boksay, 1970).

Between trips Bright was licensed in medicine and was appointed to the staff of the London Fever Hospital in 1816. In 1820 he was back in practice. He pursued his teaching at Guy's from 1824 to 1843, after which he retired and limited his practice to consultations. His daily work at Guy's consisted of six hours of lectures and postmortem studies. His *Reports of Medical Cases* (1827) was notable for the discussion of the difference between cardiac and nephritic edema; and, his writings on the finding of albumin in the urine in nephritis and its association with contracted kidneys and oliguria led others to name the disease "Bright's disease." For his studies he was given two wards, with attached consulting rooms and laboratories, at Guy's Hospital.

In his teaching, Bright refused to theorize, insisting on presenting only his observations. He made notable contributions to the clinicopathological findings in diabetes mellitus, pancreatic steatorrhea, acute yellow atrophy of the liver, Jacksonian epilepsy (not yet given that name, of course), otitic brain abscess, hemiplegia, and various other conditions. His illustrations were works of art. He had adopted the clinicopathological approach of the Paris school and carried it forward, both by his own studies and by example.

Bright's slightly younger contemporary Addison was also his friend and close associate. Born in Newcastle in 1895, Addison went to Edinburgh to study medicine, graduating in 1815, and then went to London to work in dermatology. (Bright also had worked there for a time with Bateman, the most famous dermatologist in England.) Addison's interest in skin changes in disease continued for the rest of his life. He began to study at Guy's in 1820, at which time his friend Bright was Assistant Physician there. Whereas Bright habitually used pathological data to support his clinical findings, which he considered the most important, Addison emphasized the pathological at the expense of the clinical. His papers on pulmonary diseases, including tuberculosis, helped distinguish one from the other. Addison realized that the role of pathologic studies was to aid in defining conditions but not to explain them. Also, he was also greatly influenced by Laennec's publications, and his papers included detailed comments on auscultatory findings and the frequent difficulties in explaining them. In 1849 he gave his famous lecture on anemia, which he claimed was due to destruction of the adrenal cortex. At first he confused clinically observed primary anemia with the condition caused by bilateral adrenal disease seen at post-mortem examination (Keele, 1969); however, by 1855 his pioneering work on disease of the adrenal glands clarified the confusion. (Today we recognize Addison's disease [of the adrenal glands] and Addisonian anemia, a condition later defined by Biermer in Germany.) Addison's meticulous accounts of the clinical manifestations and post-mortem findings in that adrenal disease led Trousseau in Paris in 1856 to name adrenal insufficiency, "Addison's Disease." His studies in other aspects of medicine also were noteworthy but did not attract as much attention. Addison was extremely shy and sensitive, and consequently lacking in the personal qualities of a good practitioner. In manner he was cold and haughty to the point of being repellant. He lived entirely for his hospital work and was admired and respected, but not loved, by his students and colleagues, who recognized how much his teaching contributed to Guy's great reputation at the time.

The third of the great Guy's triumvirate of that era was Hodgkin, who, even more than Addison and totally unlike the outgoing Bright, was a less-than-outstanding practitioner. He was born into a Quaker family in Tottenham in 1798, and after early local education entered the medical school at Edinburgh, graduating in 1823. Although he became a member of the College of Physicians in London in 1825, he refused to accept the title of Fellow because it offended his egalitarian principles. He had been doing clinical work at Guy's when he introduced the use of the stethoscope there in 1822, three years after Laennec's first publication on the subject (Liebowitz, 1967). After travel in Italy and studies in Paris with Laennec, he returned to London, where he was appointed Curator of the Pathological Museum and Demonstrator in Pathology at Guy's Hospital. However, his duties were primarily clinical and, after a decade, he tried for an appointment as Assistant Physician at the Hospital but was rejected because of his idiosyncratic independence of spirit and his republican political views. He left Guy's Hospital and for a time was associated with St. Thomas'.

Hodgkin's writings included a discussion of appendicitis long before it was recognized by others, and he wrote about aortic regurgitation several years before Corrigan's paper on the same subject. However, these reports were presented obscurely as letters and, therefore, they did not receive much attention at the time. In 1832 his famous paper on diseases of the spleen and lymph nodes was published, but that also received little attention then.

He had a great interest in philanthropy and in the rights of the oppressed, and this led to his close friendship with Montefiore, with whom he traveled and whom he served as Personal Physician. Hodgkin's accounts of his travels contained drawings and lithographs that reveal him to be an accomplished artist. Hodgkin died in Jaffa while accompanying Montefiore on philanthropic enterprises designed to aid the Jewish people; his grave and its monument are in Jaffa. Montefiore was a most humane man, and the two worked hard and traveled far in the interests of social justice (Stern, 1967). Montefiore's nephew, Nathaniel, qualified at Guy's Hospital in 1858. He married Emma, the daughter of Sir Isaac Lyon Goldsmid, one of the founders of London University. It is interesting that Hodgkin also was involved in the founding of London University and was one of the first members of its senate.

The extensive bibliography of Hodgkin's writings shows the breadth of his knowledge (Kass and Bartlett, 1969), which is much greater than that indicated by those who limit his fame to the discovery of the disease that bears his name. For example, his concept of the nature of metastasis in cancer is the one we hold today, rather than the mystical notions of Virchow and others that metastases developed from new cells formed at a distance in the imaginary *blastema* (Onuigbo, 1967). Hodgkin formulated these views around 1830, before the introduction of the microscope into routine medical studies. He maintained that parts of a cancer migrated to other areas, often selectively, and most commonly *via* lymphatics, although the bloodstream also might be the avenue. Moreover, he stated that a cancer might remain localized for years and then begin to spread, maintaining that a healthy system had barriers that normally limited spread. His careful observing and clear reasoning added to the reputation of Guy's Hospital during his short affiliation with it. Although his departure from Guy's was not a happy one, today he is claimed by the men of Guy's as one of the Hospital's greatest.

It is possible that the justifiable emphasis on the work of Bright, Addison, and Hodgkin at Guy's Hospital regrettably has overshadowed the work of others, who became distinguished for approaches other than the clinicopathological. One such man was Marcet. Although he was a physician on the staff of Guy's Hospital, little is known about his apparently successful clinical practice; however, a great deal is known about his largely unsuccessful attempts to advance the science of animal chemistry to a point where it would be useful to practitioners in their daily work. Marcet was born in Geneva, Switzerland, in 1770, the son of a merchant of Huguenot descent. Although his father wanted him to remain in the family business, young Marcet preferred the profession of law. When he and his young friend de la Rive became involved in the disturbances that accompanied the French Revolution, both were sent to prison. After Robespierre's downfall in 1794, they were set free, but banished from Switzerland.

Marcet and de la Rive went to Edinburgh, where in 1797 they graduated in medicine and started practice. De la Rive returned to Geneva two years later and joined the faculty of the university there, but Marcet went to London, where he secured positions on hospital staffs, made a good marriage to the daughter of a wealthy Swiss merchant, and became naturalized in 1800 (Colby, 1968). He was appointed Physician to Guy's Hospital in 1804 and held that post until 1819. During that period he served for a time in a temporary military hospital in Portsmouth and caught a fever, probably typhus, from his patients, and recovered narrowly.

In London at that time there was a growing interest in the possible applications of chemistry to medicine. The students at Guy's were hungry for chemical knowledge that might bear on medicine, but there was little to tell them. Animal chemistry consisted of analyses of kidney stones, urine, blood, and body fluids. The information available about them was fragmentary and either inaccurate or downright wrong. Inorganic, rather than organic, analyses were more likely to be correct, and Marcet's book on kidney stones was a good one. Together with Bright's mentor, Babington, and others, Marcet gave lectures to the students, mainly in general chemistry, with few clinical applications. Nevertheless, Marcet's interest in animal chemistry led to a friendship with the famous Swedish chemist, Berzelius, who visited London and saw Marcet actually demonstrate chemical reactions during his lectures, a procedure that was novel at that time. Berzelius adopted that method. The unsatisfactory state of animal chemistry then is illustrated by the fact that Marcet's observation - that sodium was the main alkaline element in body fluids - started a fierce controversy that lasted for years.

During all of that time Marcet also pursued the private practice of medicine. It was probably Marcet's reputation as a chemist that led the authorities at Guy's Hospital to accept his recommendations about improving the patients' diets. Although dignified and somewhat unbending, he was nevertheless friendly and sympathetic; patients, students, and colleagues held him in great affection. In 1819 Marcet's father-in-law died, leaving a huge fortune. Marcet lost interest in the practice of medicine and resigned as Physician at Guy's Hospital, but continued to lecture in chemistry there. He visited Geneva and was welcomed happily by his old friend, de la Rive, who had become a Professor of Chemistry at the University. The city received Marcet with honor and offered him a professorship in chemistry. He returned to England to prepare for his move to Geneva but died after a brief illness. Marcet's career of medical practice cannot be evaluated. However, he made contributions, chiefly methodological, to the science of chemistry, but failed in his serious effort to make it a usable branch of medicine. (Several decades later another physician-chemist, Bence-Jones, used advances made by that time to accomplish this end.)

Prout, another physician-scientist whose work failed to influence medicine (Brock, 1965), is known today not by his medical works, but by his hypothesis that the atomic weights of the elements are always multiples of the atomic weight of hydrogen. Nevertheless, he should be remembered as a physician and a man with an inquiring mind. He was remarkable for his firm conviction, stated in 1817, that chemistry would become the basis of medicine, with the reservation that since chemical remedies caused many side effects, chemistry would not be useful in treatment, only in prevention. He was never able to advance any data to support those views, but that did not keep him from reiterating them emphatically and frequently. They were for him a matter of faith.

Prout exhibited an interesting personality early in life. Born in 1785 into a family of Gloucestershire farmers, he learned reading and writing at local schools, but his early education ceased when he was 13. At the age of 17, determined to improve his education, he attended a private academy to learn Greek and Latin. Dissatisfied with his progress he took the unusual step of placing an advertisement in a local newspaper, asking for advice on how to proceed. A clergyman in Bristol invited him to enter his academy, which Prout did, paying for it by tutoring the younger students in chemistry. In 1808, at the age of 23, he entered Edinburgh and, after three totally undistinguished years there, took his M.D. degree. His schoolmates included such great physicians as Hall, Holland, and Elliotson, who became his close friend. In London he walked the wards at Guy's and St. Thomas' Hospitals, coming under the influence of Cooper and Marcet. Although active in his practice, he began to pursue his chemical interests, giving private chemistry lectures to a select audience that included Cooper. Prout's first paper was on the production of carbon dioxide in himself, which he measured almost hourly for three weeks. Although well executed technically, these studies were conceived so poorly that their net result was nil except for arousing his curious notions regarding the processes involved in respiration. He studied the composition of the air and concluded that one change in it which he had observed was probably the cause of a cholera epidemic. Like Marcet he analyzed kidney stones and wrote a treatise on the subject. His practice increased greatly, but a large source of his income was the analyses of numerous stones sent to him. On the other hand, he did discover the hydrochloric acid of gastric juice, thereby starting a controversy with others who held that such acid was lactic or butyric. That positive contribution was offset by his refusal to acknowledge the existence of pepsin in the stomach, reminiscent of his discovery that all atomic weights were multiples of that of hydrogen, which was offset by his refusal to accept Dalton's atomic theory. His theory of how food was changed into blood was sheer nonsense, but he did divide the nutrients into water, sugar, fat, and protein. That perceptive concept was counteracted by his insistence that carbon, oxygen, nitrogen, and hydrogen alone were the basic elements of life. In short, he was a curious mixture of observer, mystic, and dogmatist. When the eighth Earl of Bridgewater died and left 8,000 pounds to the Royal Society as a prize for "a work on the Power, Wisdom and Goodness of God, as manifested in the Creation," Prout was invited to submit a treatise on this subject, which he did. And when Tyndall, the physicist, was asked to edit the treatise for publication, he wrote,

> I should have thought more highly of Dr. Prout had I not read his book. Certainly if no better Deity than this can be purchased for the eight thousand pounds of the Earl of Bridgewater, it is a dear bargain. It is very evident that Dr. Prout would never have written such a book through the spontaneous promptings of his own spirit; it was written for money, and lack even common scientific depth, not to speak of religious inspiration.

In short, Prout had done what was usual for him; namely, producing a mixture of hard observation and abundant fanciful interpretation, while ignoring the works of others. There remains a composite of a good observer so opinionated that he could not profit from either his own observations or those of others, thereby straying from the mainstream of biochemistry. However, it should not be forgotten that it was he who suggested to Elliotson that iodine should be used to treat thyroid disorders. Prout was a curious mixture of a man.

Elliotson was not one of the men of Guy's, but he was important in the medical life of London. Although trained in the tradition of clinicopathological correlations, including percussion and auscultation of the chest, he took a different road. Born in London in 1791, the son of a chemist-pharmacist, he studied at Edinburgh and Cambridge. His medical training consisted of three years at Guy's and St. Thomas' Hospitals, after which he received the M.D. degree in 1821 and was then elected Assistant at Guy's. A decided individualist, by 1826 he was known already for eccentricities in dress and for having a beard when most others did not. An early defender of Laennec's auscultation, he nevertheless tempered enthusiasm with sound comments, writing that

> Auscultation, however, can never justify us in the least neglect of the general symptoms and history of the disease. This would indeed by unphilosophical; for the symptoms of auscultation are but one set among a host of others. But if to neglect the general symptoms were unphilosophical, it would be equally so to despise those which present themselves to the ear. If the functions of the heart and lungs are naturally performed with peculiar sounds, and in diseases the sounds are altered, these deviations demand equal attention with those discernible by the other senses....

Such a simple, clear, and forceful statement on the multifactorial nature of the diagnostic process applies equally well today; in fact, neglect of this concept has had highly destructive effects on medical practice.

Elliotson gave the Lumleian Lectures before the Royal College of Physicians in 1829, discussing the most modern ways then available to diagnose diseases of the heart. Illustrated with remarkable lithographs showing the morbid anatomy of the cardiac diseases, those lectures were published in 1830. A year later Elliotson was appointed Professor of the Practice of Medicine at the University of London, and he spent the next few years organizing the University College Hospital. He also alarmed many London physicians by giving accepted remedies in doses very much larger than those generally used. Probably particularly disconcerting was that neither good nor bad resulted. Despite this idiosyncrasy, by the late 1830s Elliotson had the reputation of being one of England's ablest physicians and teachers and, as was then the custom regarding outstanding lectures, his were regularly reported in *The Lancet*.

Elliotson was recurrently idiosyncratic in medical practice. The leaders of London's, as well as Dublin's, medicine had shown themselves eager to adopt the French innovation of medicine: physical examination by palpation, auscultation, and percussion, supported by pathologic anatomy. Elliotson chose to adopt other Continental innovations as well, for he was interested in phrenology and mesmerism, both Viennese superstitions that had become established in France and then crossed the Channel. He founded the Phrenological Society of London and subsequently became a mesmerist, attempting to experiment in mesmerism at his hospitals, which the governors forbade. He held seances in his own house, offending his colleagues. The ensuing controversies led to his resignation in 1838 from his professorship, but in no other way was his individuality impaired. He continued to practice mesmerism and, indeed, published a paper in 1843 in which he described surgical operations conducted with the subject in a trance, rather than anesthetized. In 1849 he established a hospital for mesmeric treatment and gave public demonstrations of mesmeric healing. It should be noted that Elliotson was not alone in these endeavors. Braid, a Scot who had settled in Manchester, at one time stated that mesmerism was based on "collusion and illusion"; but, he later got the faith and became a hypnotist. Even more noteworthy was the work of Esdaille, also a Scot, who performed hundreds of surgical operations in India on patients mesmerized only.

Whatever Elliotson's views, superstitious or sound, he was clearly a fine medical practitioner. His reputation was that of kindliness, sympathy, and interest in the patient and in all manifestations of disease. One of his patients was Thackeray, who dedicated his novel *Pendennis* to Elliotson, commenting on the physician's life-saving watchfulness and skill, and his goodness and kindness, "when kindness and friendship were most needed and welcome." Dickens was Elliotson's close friend.

Today it is impossible to know how much, if any, harm or good, Elliotson's belief in the superstitions of phrenology and mesmerism may have done. At the time, the effective medications, barring a considerable number of emetics and cathartics, could be counted easily on the finger of one hand. Therefore, under these circumstances the factors responsible for a physician's success or failure are difficult to establish.

One of Elliotson's students was Peacock, another unusual London physician, born in 1812 into a middle-class Quaker family in York. After seven years at school in Scarborough he wanted to go to sea, but his father persuaded him to study medicine. As a Quaker, young Peacock was excluded by religion from Oxford and Cambridge and from the Church, and by pacifism from the Army and Navy. He went to London to serve for five years as apprentice to a fellow Quaker, Fothergill, and received his formal training at the University College Hospital, where he studied with Elliotson. Having fulfilled the requirements, he was licensed in 1835. He experienced two voyages to Ceylon as ship's surgeon in 1835 and 1836, and on his way home studied in Paris for a few months. From 1836 to 1841 he served as House Surgeon to the Infirmary in Chester, where his family lived. He then went to Edinburgh, where he served as House Physician and Pathologist at the Edinburgh Royal Infirmary and later was awarded the M.D. degree there. His service at the Infirmary was notable for his copious case notes and exact records of post-mortem findings. In 1844 he went to London, opened an office for the practice of medicine, and was appointed to the staffs of several hospitals. Peacock maintained a major interest in morbid anatomy, founding the Pathological Society of London in 1846 with Bence-Jones and others. Over 100 physicians in every branch of medicine were members. Proceedings, which contained the clinical and pathologic findings of numerous patients, were bound in volumes with the portrait of Baillie stamped in gold on the cover. The Society maintained an independent existence until 1908, when it became the Pathological Section of the Royal Society of Medicine and had in its remarkable collection of medical data approximately 160 reports delivered by Peacock. He founded a dispensary on Liverpool Street which became the Victoria Park Hospital for Diseases of the Chest. In addition to his flow of case reports, Peacock in 1847 published his invaluable table on normal organ weights and his writings on the great influenza epidemic of that year. In 1849 he became Assistant Physician at St. Thomas' Hospital and taught clinical medicine at the bedside. To those who knew him well he was kind and generous, while to others he seemed a reserved, serious, austere, and cold person who showed quiet persistence and steadfast reliance on detail in history and physical findings. His reputation presented him as a man of stubborn honesty and integrity, with a capacity for sustained work, but without brilliance or sparkle in work or private life. In the 1850s he published his famous *On the Weights and Dimensions of the Heart in Health and Disease* and *On Malformations of the Human Heart*. He rose in rank at St. Thomas' Hospital, becoming Dean of its medical school in 1871. Although he retired in 1877 for reasons of health, he continued his private practice and his activities in medical societies.

The career of Hope of St. George's is an example of independence combined with intellectual brilliance. Born in Cheshire in 1801, the tenth of twelve children of a very wealthy retired merchant and manufacturer, he revealed his high intelligence before the age of nine by creating a large chart summarizing the history of England. Although he already was reading Milton, he also showed himself to be skilled in all boyhood sports. When he was about 18 years old, he wanted to become a lawyer, but his father preferred that he go into business. Young Hope did nothing for about a year, at which time the Manchester riots were occurring and he joined the Yeomanry as a lancer, again distinguishing himself. His father then proposed medicine as a career and Hope agreed only on condition that he be allowed to practice in London. He was at Oxford briefly and then entered the medical school at Edinburgh in 1820. He found dissection very distasteful and, as a result, wore gloves and used forceps; however, his diffidence vanished when he learned that Baillie, then a recognized leader of London medicine, had become famous through his studies of morbid anatomy. In fact, Hope devoted almost all of his efforts for a time to the study of anatomy. The next year he was induced to join the Royal Medical Society of Edinburgh, which required each member to prepare a paper on a subject to be debated at one of the meetings. Hope's paper on the heart was so well received that he was determined to work in that specialty; later he published a monograph on it. While he was a student he also pursued flute-playing, painting, and drawing as avocations, giving special effort to his anatomical drawings. In 1824 Hope was chosen House Physician at the Royal Edinburgh Infirmary and ten months later he also was made House Surgeon. He took his M.D. degree in 1825 and went to London for training in surgery at St. Bartholomew's Hospital. In the Spring of 1826 he passed his licensing examination in London and then went to Paris for a year, quickly learning to speak the language fluently. After spending two or three weeks at each of several hospitals - starting each day at 5:00 A.M. - he decided on the Charité with Chomel. Hope was appointed Clinical Clerk and Chomel had him make three or four drawings of specimens each week, which he did very well. After a year, he toured Switzerland and Italy, learning the languages and visiting the hospitals. On his return to London in 1828 he opened an office for the practice of medicine and, without friends or other connections, did poorly, surviving only with his father's financial aid. His father had a low opinion of doctors, pointing out that he had reached the age of 80 without ever having seen one, whereas four of his children had died younger than 25 after, of course, having been treated by physicians. Nevertheless he kept his commitment to his son.

Young Hope opened a private dispensary and became very popular among the poor of the neighborhood. He persuaded St. George's Hospital to establish clinical clerkships and became the first to hold that position there. He chose St. George's Hospital as the best site for the development of his ambitions and walked its wards with the visiting physicians, introducing the systematic recording of clinical notes there. His treatise *Diseases of the Heart and Great Vessels* (1831) had an enormous positive effect on his reputation and greatly enlarged his practice. Although his *Morbid Anatomy* (1835) was also a fine work filled with remarkable lithographs, the cardiology treatise is one of the great works in that specialty. In it the various diseases of the heart are described in terms of their symptoms, physical signs, and pathological findings, with many illustrations enhancing the descriptions. The work went through several editions in England, was published in America, and was translated into German and Italian.

At the young age of 31 Hope often was consulted as an outstanding clinician, and in 1834 he was made Assistant Physician to St. George's. He had always had strong personal ambitions in his medical career, and he was determined to become the leader in the introduction of auscultation into English medicine (Blieth, 1970). However, the next ten years were not easy for him. He worked hard to accumulate clinical material, and he did experimental work on the genesis of heart sounds in animals. Although his publications gave him standing as an expert on diseases of the heart, his status still was insecure because many physicians distrusted his reliance on the stethoscope (King, 1959). He conducted public demonstrations on the use of the instrument, a procedure that, if anything, turned more physicians against him. Years of public controversy followed, but his beliefs at last began to be accepted by London physicians, having been accepted already by the Irish group. Hope attained one of his ambitions when he was chosen Chief Physician at St. George's in 1839, but he died of tuberculosis only two years later, barely able to enjoy his personal advancement and probably not fully aware of his role in promoting the practice in England of one of clinical medicine's greatest advances.

Actually, the men of Guy's Hospital showed interest early in Laennec's methods, but that work did not attract widespread notice.   In 1822 Hodgkin presented a paper on the subject at the Hospital, even before he was appointed to the staff (Leibowitz, 1967), and Addison likewise studied and used these methods in his student days at Guy's in the early 1820s.

One case was presented and its study using the stethoscope was described at a meeting of the University of London Medical Society in 1834 (Newman, 1958).   A few years later other cases were inscribed in the records of the University College Hospital, but the use of the stethoscope remained limited.   After publishing five papers on the physical examination of the chest after 1837, Addison concluded in 1846 with a thorough and temperate discussion of the errors and fallacies of the methods (Keele, 1969), all in marked contrast to the emotional and often ill-tempered criticisms of Hope's writings on the subject.

The account of the stethoscope's introduction into English cardiology includes error, competition, and the bitter falling out of friends.   The two English physicians involved were Hope and C.J.B. Williams, who was trained in Paris in 1825 under Laennec at the Charité and who also studied experimental physiology with Magendie and clinicopathological correlations with Andral.   He was early interested in the use of the stethoscope and wrote his first work, *Rational Exposition of the Physical Signs of the Diseases of the Lungs and Pleura*, in 1828.   In it he attempted to define stethoscopic findings in lung disease, not merely in terms of what was audible, but on the basis of the physics of acoustics - a regrettable approach since acoustics was not yet highly developed.   A few years later, because of his friendship with Hope, he turned his attention to heart sounds and improved the stethoscope, changing its shape and adding the diaphragm to cover the mouth of the bowl.

Hope also had gone to Paris to study at the Charité, in 1827, when Chomel had succeeded Laennec.   On his return to England he began his studies of heart sounds in frogs, rabbits, and donkeys.   He had little but speculation, which yielded nothing certain, but he discussed the subject in 1831 in his *Diseases of the Heart and Great Vessels*. A fine clinical treatise, it was marred by Hope's attempts to explain what he had observed without anything approaching satisfactory knowledge of fluid dynamics or cardiac physiology.

For a decade (1828-1838) Hope and Williams worked together in animal experiments designed to elucidate the origin and mechanism of cardiovascular sounds. In his book written in 1835, Williams concluded that the first sound was due to the contraction of the ventricles, while the second was caused by the snapping shut of the aortic and pulmonary valves as the ventricles ceased contracting. Williams claimed these ideas as his own, but Hope dissented bitterly, stating that he had planned the crucial experiments; he wrote in this vein in his works of 1835 and 1838. The decade-long friendship of the two men soon vanished. Each independently wrote his ideas on the genesis of murmurs, ending up similarly after many revisions. Hope's few remaining years before his death in 1841 were embittered by his lost friendship with Williams and other disappointments. Williams still was claiming the ideas as his own in 1884 (Keele, 1973). It is interesting that in 1839 Skoda in Vienna published his famous work on percussion and auscultation, concluding that it was impossible to describe the findings on the basis of the then-known science of acoustics.

Later in the century acoustics began to catch up to other sciences. Reynolds, an engineer of Manchester, advanced the applications of Poiseuille's law, developing descriptions of the behavior of blood during both streamlined and turbulent flow (McKusick and Wiskind, 1959). He demonstrated that the formation of cavities was a result of turbulence in a flowing stream, a concept that is highly important in the genesis of sounds in the heart chambers and blood vessels. In the 20th century other acoustical physicists made additional contributions, and now there is some understanding of the matter. Nevertheless, the history of percussion and auscultation exemplifies how phenomena of clinical medicine fully become recognized, despite the absence of an adequate basis of knowledge in physical science. In fact, as is often the case in medicine, the clinical findings uncover a previously unknown phenomenon or at least lead to a better-founded study of it than was previously possible.

Remembered today chiefly because of his name was Bence-Jones, a practicing London physician who exemplified the early beginning of a new trend, a trend toward chemical studies after the Leibig mode.   However, he was a good physician, having been trained at St. George's Hospital.   He was born in 1814, a son of Lt. Col. William Jones of the Dragoon Guards, and grandson of Bence Bence, a clergyman of Thorrington Hall, Suffolk.   At age 12 young Bence-Jones entered Harrow and at 18 began his studies at Trinity College, Cambridge.   His degrees, in succession, were B.A., 1836; M.A., 1842; M.B., 1845; and M.D., 1849. Before winning his first medical degree, he studied at St. George's Hospital in London as well as in the chemistry laboratories of University College in 1841.   Later that year he went to Giessen to study with Leibig.   He was licensed in medicine in 1842, became a fellow, and then was appointed Senior Censor of the Royal College of Physicians. In 1846 he became Fellow of the Royal Society, and from 1860 onward was its Secretary.   He was elected Assistant Physician to St. George's Hospital in 1845, and Physician in 1846.

Bence-Jones obviously was an important person in the academic medical establishment, and his large and highly remunerative practice, mental activity, genial nature and, of course, his wealth and connections, made him a social success.   His closest friends, however, were English and foreign scientists, who were not necessarily physicians. He worked diligently in his chosen field of chemical research as related to medicine and also was interested especially in making scientific studies in all fields.   His own papers and longer works were all on chemical subjects, chiefly analysis of urine constituents, and as was true of many medical chemists of that era (and every other), he attempted to explain too much on the basis of fragmentary and often erroneous chemical information then available. Nevertheless, the discovery by Bence-Jones of a special protein in the urine was an important one, and his career illustrates the beginning of the turning away from French medicine and morbid anatomy to German chemistry-based medicine.

One of the most remarkable physicians of the early Victorian era in London was Hall. He had the largest clinical practice in London, made momentous contributions to physiology, and played a highly important role in medical education, especially in America (Green, 1958). Hall was born in 1790 near Nottingham, the sixth of the eight children of a prosperous cotton manufacturer who had introduced chemical and mechanical innovations into the manufacturing process. One of Hall's brothers was a chemical inventor also. Perhaps these factors had something to do with Hall's early interest in chemistry, leading to his reading of Lavoissier's and others' works. In addition to his ordinary schooling, he spent some time with a nearby chemist. In 1809 Hall went to Edinburgh to study medicine. His favorite subject was chemistry, until a Dr. Belcombe of York said, "I never knew a great chemist make a good physician." His contemporaries included Holland, Prout, and Elliotson. Hall worked very hard and soon was elected to the students' medical society, the Royal Medical Society of Edinburgh. He decided to make himself expert in diagnosis. In 1812 he graduated and was appointed Clinical Clerk (equivalent to our resident house physicians). In the following year he gave a series of lectures on "Principles of Diagnosis," which was expanded into a book a few years later. In 1814 and 1815 he visited Paris, Berlin, and Göttingen, covering 600 miles of the trip on foot, and then returned to Nottingham to practice, becoming Physician to the General Hospital there in 1825. The next year Hall moved to London where his practice grew, principally among the aristocracy. He never held a regular academic or clinical appointment in London; he applied for the Professorship of Medicine at the University of London but was advised to withdraw. He did some lecturing at a number of non-affiliated medical schools and for a time at St. Thomas'; however, trouble with his voice caused him to stop lecturing in 1839, and increasing trouble with his throat forced him to retire in 1852. He and his wife had developed the custom of traveling in Western Europe every year "about the end of the London season" starting in 1830. After his retirement he toured America for 15 months, lecturing in Washington, Baltimore, Philadelphia, and Chicago; in several Canadian cities; and in Havana (in French). He also traveled in the back country and visited Indian tribes. Returning home in 1854, he remained active (taking time to learn Hebrew) until his death in 1857.

Hall's writings were remarkably extensive in terms of quantity and diversity of subjects. His earliest papers were on subjects in chemistry, and he published occasional papers along these lines for many years after that time. His many medical publications included a great number of case reports, but it was his book, *The Diagnosis of Diseases*, that began his fame. Published in 1817, it was written literally at the bedside of patients. A second edition was published in 1834, and the book then became part of *Principles of the Theory and Practice of Medicine* (1837). Hall wrote special works on the diseases of women and functional disorders (which he called "mimoses") and more general discussions on almost every aspect of medicine. Interspersed among these were articles on the physiology of vision, speech, and vomiting. His studies on the capillary circulation in frogs and fish were rejected by the Royal Society, although Müller in Germany declared them to be extraordinarily interesting. He also wrote learnedly on hibernation, and his home was said to contain a menagerie of animals accumulated for his studies.

Hall's work on the reflex arc, however, has led some historians to refer to him as a great physiologist rather than a great clinician. It was Whytt in Edinburgh who had put studies of reflex phenomena on sound bases, and others after him, notably Legallois and Flourens in France, had increased knowledge of the phenomenon. Hall's research established the central role of the spinal cord in reflex arcs, although, as he pointed out in his meticulous reports, earlier observers had commented, albeit inaccurately, on these matters. His reports were rejected by the Philosophical Transactions of the Royal Society but were presented before and published by the Zoological Society. He received some praise in England, but much more on the Continent. A committee of the Royal Society recommended him for the Copley Medal, but the Society rejected the recommendation, and he was not considered for any other award; however, in 1850, he was elected to the Council of the Royal Society, an occurrence for which *The Lancet* claimed credit!

In addition, Hall wrote on mathematical topics, Greek grammar, sewage disposal, slavery in America, resuscitation in drowning, and the establishment of a group to study public health. All of this miscellaneous writing was done while he was busy with other work: his physiological studies (in his home); the most remunerative practice in London; and clinical writings that were to have great influence on medical practice and education. Perhaps he was able to accomplish so much because he had neither academic or hospital ranks nor administrative duties. At any rate, his avoidance of these hindrances to accomplishments made him unusual, and perhaps his failure to become part of the academic medical establishment was the cause of the failure of English medicine to accept his remarkable accomplishments. (Hall had one other distinction: He never was called a Renaissance man.)

Another practicing physician who became famous, despite the fact that he did not belong to any London academic establishment, was Birkbeck. He was born in Yorkshire in 1776, son of a Quaker banker and merchant, but little is known of his early life. Birkbeck studied medicine at Edinburgh, receiving the M.D. degree there in 1799, and for a time studied medicine in London. At the early age of 23 he became Professor of Natural Philosophy at Andersonian University in Glasgow. Having observed that some laborers in the factories wanted to learn science but had difficulty doing so, he inaugurated in 1800 an inexpensive series of lectures at the University for them. (In 1823 that series of lectures became the independent Glasgow Mechanics Institution.) Birkbeck started his medical practice in London in 1804, and it prospered. Later he was active in the founding of University College in London. In 1824 a mechanics institute was established largely because Birkbeck loaned it 3,700 pounds and had himself elected president. It survived the ridicule of its enemies and the quarrels of its promoters, for a time bearing the name "The Birkbeck Institution," and served as an example to many institutes being founded in other cities. (Birkbeck lectured at most of these institutes at one time or another [Kelly, 1959].)

A man of enormous altruism and energy - always a dangerous combination - he was described as arrogant, vain, dictatorial, and humorless, attributes that tradition-ally have been found in reformers. However, despite the demands of his busy practice he found time to pursue his other interest, adult education. Little is known about the quality of medicine he practiced; however, he must have had a reputation of some eminence, for he acted as con-sultant, with Clutterbuck, in the notorious case of John Tilly Matthews, a true paranoid who convinced the Com-mittee of Public Safety in Paris during the Revolution that he was receiving airborne messages from the King of Eng-land promising peace. After a time Matthews was impris-oned and deported, eventually ending up in the Bethlehem Hospital in London. Examined in court at the behest of relatives, he was declared sane by Birkbeck and Clutter-buck, until Haslam, the Physician in Charge at Bethlehem, skillfully turned the discussion to the subject of Russian spies and murderers, airborne messages, and sexual assaults. To the chagrin of the consultant physicians, Matthews then revealed himself to be crazy (Altschule, 1977). Birkbeck's zeal for human rights was not dimmed by this humiliation, however, and in other respects he may well have been a good doctor.

Another interesting London physician of the era was Wells, who was born in 1757 in Charleston, South Carolina, but received his preliminary and medical education in Edin-burgh. Refusing to be disloyal to the King, he gave up his American connections and remained in London, where he practiced medicine until his death in 1817 (Keil, 1936). He lived an isolated life; his high standards of duty and his hypersensitivity, introspection, and humorless cold man-ner alienated people. Although his practice was not finan-cially successful, his accomplishments evoked the admira-tion of physicians such as Pitcairne, Holland, Elliotson, and Budd, and his elegant literary style made him widely read. Such accomplishments included studies on nephritis, which actually served as the basis of Bright's work, and an ex-cellent account of the relation between rheumatic fever and heart disease (Keil, 1936). He was equally productive in another area, being responsible for reforms in medical education, including the removal of the restrictive practices of the Royal College of Physicians. Altogether he seemed an uprooted, lonesome man, but one of great talent who preferred to be himself rather than a pretentious person. His contributions to the development of the concept of rheumatic heart disease are most noteworthy.

Budd was perhaps one of the most original of London physicians. Born in Devon in 1808, the son of a surgeon, he took his bachelor's degree at Cambridge in 1831 and studied medicine in Paris and at London's Middlesex Hospital. In 1837 he wrote a popular article on the stethoscope and that same year was appointed Physician to the Seamen's Hospital at Greenwich, where he conducted studies on scurvy, among other subjects. In 1840 Cambridge granted him the M.D. degree, and the next year he was appointed Professor of Medicine at King's College in London, while at the same time maintaining a large practice. He held the chair until 1863.

Today Budd's reputation rests on two excellent books, *On Diseases of the Liver* (1842) and *On the Organic and Functional Diseases of the Stomach* (1855). As was characteristic of the period, his books were based on both clinical and pathological data. His book on the liver is especially noteworthy in that his classification of liver diseases is remarkably modern. (Frerich's famous book on the liver, published in Germany later, resembled Budd's in many respects.) However well conceived and executed, Budd's two books were not his only contributions. Another even greater contribution, which regrettably received little attention at the time, consisted of five articles (based on his lectures) published in the 1842 *London Medical Gazette*. In that series, entitled "Disorders Resulting from Defective Nutriment," he clearly stated his conviction that there were essential accessory food factors, the absence of which caused clearly definable deficiency diseases. He included scurvy and two others to which no name was given, but which today easily are recognizable as Vitamin A deficiency and Vitamin D deficiency. Thus, his work preceded the development of the concept of vitamins by more than 50 years. The modern ideas on this subject finally grew out of the error that Voit and other German nutritionists made when they assumed that man's needs for food could be grouped under five categories: protein, carbohydrate, fat, water, and minerals.   Only when they and their followers tried to maintain animals on synthetic diets did they recognize their error, leading to a search for the accessory factors - many decades after Budd.   Budd deserves to be considered one of the greatest men in an era of great clinicians in London.   In his position as Professor of Medicine at King's College and by his popular writings, he greatly influenced medical practice.

Another of London's highly original thinkers was Snow.   Born at York in 1813, a son of a farmer, he was educated at a private school until the age of 14 and then apprenticed to a surgeon in Newcastle-on-Tyne, during which time he swore to abstain forever from alcohol and meat.   He served for a short time as a colliery surgeon during the cholera epidemic of 1831 to 1832, although still not licensed.   He studied at the Great Windmill Street Medical School and the Westminster Hospital, beginning in 1836.   Licensed in 1838 and awarded the M.D. degree at the University of London in 1844, he lectured for a short time at a private medical school, the Aldersgate School of Medicine, until its closing in 1849.   He became interested in asphyxia and resuscitation early in his career and wrote about them in 1841.   In 1846 he began the technique of its administration.   Snow became the principal etherizer in London, but he also appreciated the value of chloroform as an anesthetic and wrote about that substance.   In fact, he administered chloroform to Queen Victoria in 1853 and 1857 during the birth of two of her children.

Although appreciated as a pioneer in anesthesiology, Snow is more famous today as a pioneer in epidemiology (Barrett, 1946).   In 1854 he mapped the distribution of the cases of cholera in one area of London and showed their clustering around a single pump that provided water for the neighborhood.   That pump was found to receive the overflow from a nearby sewer.   After he persuaded the authorities to remove the pump handle, the epidemic subsided in that area.   The Institute of France offered a prize for the discovery of the cause of cholera, and Snow applied for it, but did not win (Edwards, 1959).   Thirty years later Koch isolated the bacterium that caused cholera, having found it in some water tanks in Hamburg. It was Snow, however, who showed that the disease was spread not by contact, as occurred in contagious diseases, but by contamination of a water supply. Although his contemporaries regarded him highly - and justifiably - as an outstanding anesthetist, Snow's contribution to the study of cholera is his claim to fame today.

Snow, quite properly praised for his epidemiologic studies, was not alone in these pursuits. There was a great deal of interest in what was called "the numerical method," which was, in fact, nothing but an aspect of epidemiology. In an era preceding the acceptance of bacterial infection, nutritional deficiency, chemical intoxication, or genetic biochemical dysfunction as etiologic factors, the definition of specific diseases depended not only on the observable manifestations of the acute stage, but also on the course and outcome. Information on these two aspects of disease was furnished by the so-called *sanitary physicians*, who specifically studied and reported on these matters. Although the statistical approach to clinical phenomena had been used systematically by Pinel, and more thoroughly by Pierre Louis, the development of epidemiology as a governmental function was a London phenomenon (Lilienfeld, 1979).

The examples cited in this chapter - and the number easily could have been made larger - show clearly that the medical scene in early 19th-century London was much more varied than that in Edinburgh or Dublin. London contained men as distinguished as any in the other two cities, but who had a greater diversity of interests and careers. Prominent London physicians were receptive to ideas from the Continent. Whereas the Dubliners developed mainly along the lines of Parisian medicine, with its physical diagnosis backed up by morbid anatomy, and some London physicians followed that path, others followed the lead of Gall and Mesmer, on the one hand, and of Leibig on the other. Was this diversity mainly due to the numbers involved? It is possible. However, the fact that medical education was centered in a number of different hospitals in London rather than in a monolithic university organization, emphasized clinical medicine, and that kind of medicine must allow for the diverse natures of physicians and their patients. Moreover, by the mid-19th century exact clinical observation had become the rule. The growth and expansion of clinical medicine, based on the application of clinical thinking in new areas, was inevitable. It was stimulated by meticulous clinicopathologic studies performed by the men of Guy's and others, like Peacock, plus the more liberal thinking of such universal clinical geniuses as Hall and Budd.

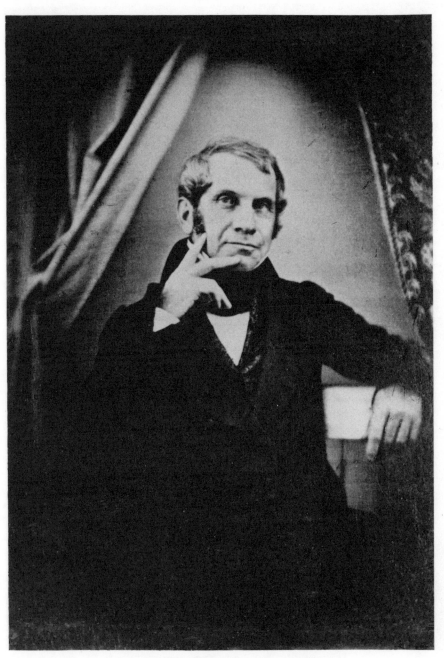

Jacob Bigelow, 1787–1879

Chapter 11: *European Influences on American Medicine to the Mid-Nineteenth Century*

THE DEVELOPMENT OF MEDICINE IN BRITISH AMERICA followed patterns that were not the same everywhere. In some places, local factors determined local differences in ways easily recognized; whereas in other cases the reasons for local differences are not evident. When the colonists came to what is now this country in the 17th century, some medical personnel were among them, including physicians, barber-surgeons, and midwives, the last two outnumbering the first. In some areas and at some periods, however, most of the medical care was given by the clergy. Accordingly, the number of persons holding the M.D. degree or equivalent training at a medical school in Europe was small. Regional differences in this respect are apparent. The first physician in New Amsterdam, for example, was a Leyden graduate of French Huguenot extraction (Snapper, 1966; Heaton, 1941). In that period one quarter of the immigrants to that town were either refugee Protestants or descendants of refugee Protestants who had gone to the Netherlands from other countries to escape persecution (Snapper, 1966). By the end of the 17th century, however, the numbers of Edinburgh and Leyden men in New Amsterdam were approximately equal (Snapper, 1966). New Orleans was different in that there was a considerable French medical presence, and the holders of Parisian medical degrees there were considered by everyone, including themselves, to be superior, which, under the circumstances, they probably were.

Circumstances were different in the English Atlantic colonies where university-trained men were uncommon. By the mid-18th century the English Colonies increased the number of physicians by permitting physicians already there to train apprentices, some of whom went to Europe for formal medical education, after beginning as apprentices and perhaps having attended private anatomy lectures.

Starting in 1749, and before 1775, there were 41 Colonials registered at Edinburgh to study medicine, 14 of them from Virginia.   Between 1776 and 1800, 76 more registered at Edinburgh, 30 of them from Virginia.   Shippen, Rush, and Morgan came from Philadelphia.   Morgan had a brilliant record at Edinburgh, studied in Paris, again with brilliant results, and finally went to Italy (Kieffer, 1942; Pace, 1945).   Bond, Colden, Nicoll, and James Jay, all from New York, received the M.D. degree at Edinburgh.   John Jones of New York studied at Edinburgh, London, Paris, and finally took his degree at Rheims (Hume, 1943).   His training was remarkable, and he showed himself to be a remarkable physician.   He was a Revolutionary Army surgeon, a distinguished practitioner, and the author of America's first medical book.   There were well-known men who studied in London during the colonial period, including the aforementioned Shippen and Physick of Philadelphia, and a number of others from New York (Heaton, 1945) and Boston (Cash, 1981).

Edinburgh men created the University of Pennsylvania Medical School and were instrumental in establishing the one in New York.   Through his emphatic comments, Bond of Philadelphia gave patient-oriented medicine a prominent place in that city (Bridenbaugh, 1947).   Morgan and Shippen not only were influential in medical education in Philadelphia; during the Revolution they rose to high positions, and their fierce quarrels that started as a purely local matter about education, came to be of national importance (Kieffer, 1942).   The situation in Boston was different from that elsewhere in the country.   New England men preferred to go to London to attend the informal private and hospital schools rather than to the Scottish university schools.   Of the 45 physicians who practiced in Boston from 1760 through 1798, 15 studied abroad; of these, only two took their foreign training at Edinburgh; 10 studied in London; and 2 studied in London plus either Edinburgh, Aberdeen, or Paris.   The reason for the subordinate role of Edinburgh, and its replacement by London, in Boston medicine is not evident, but it is possible that the Bostonians preferred practical to theoretical training.

Books and other publications were another source of European influence on American medicine.   English works were sold to Americans here or abroad, or they were reprinted in American editions. A considerable number of non-English works were translated and republished here during the early years (Gaskell, 1970). In contrast, American materials such as pamphlets, letters, and journal notes generally were well received in Great Britain and on the Continent because they were considered to represent experiences that Europeans could not have. However, there was one exception to this rule, probably trivial at first, but given great significance. In 1818 Seybert, a graduate of the University of Pennsylvania Medical School, published a paper on the nonmedical subject of vital statistics, which was reviewed by Sydney Smith, one of the founders of the *Edinburgh Review* (who falsely claimed to have been its editor). Smith had audited medical lectures at Oxford and at Edinburgh. His review criticized taxes in America, a perennial subject usually raised by Americans and not foreigners. In the course of his review Smith wrote, "What does the world yet owe to American physicians or surgeons?" Those words of a non-physician, in a review of a nonmedical subject, seemed purposeless at the time; however, they were given purpose by Chapman, who in 1820 was inaugurating *The Philadelphia Journal of the Medical and Physical Sciences* (which became *The American Journal of Medical Sciences*, the name it bears to this day). Chapman printed Smith's words in a prominent place on the first page of his journal (Eckman, 1941), thereby establishing himself as a founding father of publishing-related advertising. Whether Chapman's action caused increased sales of that journal never will be known; but, the quotation did keep alive a feeling of some Americans that they were the victims of arrogant British animosity. Such animosity did not seem to affect the frequency with which American physicians went to London for postgraduate training, although after the American Revolution, the numbers going to Edinburgh declined as the quality of medical education there declined. Thus 145 Americans earned the M.D. degree at Edinburgh in that 50-year period (1769-1819), while about 24 did so the the next half-century. (These figures are misleading in that almost twice as many Americans took courses as took the degree.)

Actually, the popularity or unpopularity of a given culture or political system seemed to have little to do with whether American physicians went to a given country for their training.   Thus, while the enthusiasm for Edinburgh medicine was declining slowly, that of French medicine was increasing rapidly, with French medicine becoming the world's leader until the time of Louis Phillipe's reign, at which point it was recognized everywhere.   That medicine was patient-oriented and from the first based on pathological-anatomical findings, and once physical diagnosis (as performed by palpation) and auscultation were added to it, French medicine became supreme.

After the Revolutionary War hundreds of American physicians who wanted European training went mainly to Paris for postgraduate education, and this number increased after the War of 1812.   In almost all cases a visit to Dublin or London schools, or a short stay at them, might precede the period of Paris study; in fact, medical books written by Dublin or London physicians were used in America, largely because by then Dublin and London were clearly the daughters of Paris.   The men who returned from Paris study to practice in their own cities naturally brought back different impressions of the information; however, nearly all of them became convinced, or had their convictions reinforced, that pathological anatomy and bedside medicine had to go hand in hand.   Others came back impressed by the new methods of physical examination, while a few returned with little more than some ideas relative to surgical techniques.   Oddly enough, and for no evident reason, Boston tried to bring back most of French medicine.   James Jackson of Harvard and the Massachusetts General Hospital sent his son to London for a year and then to Paris for two; Holmes went to Paris and came back with extensive notes of Andral's lectures.   Accordingly, although Paris medicine entered into medical practice and teaching in many parts of this country to varying degrees, it preponderated in Boston, at least in some of its aspects.

All of that change occurred despite the fact that for decades French culture was considered decadent: The high moral hopes of the French Revolution had been superseded by the brutality of the Terror, the militarism of the

Napoleonic empire, and the absolutism of the Bourbon restoration. Then toward midcentury, when Paris became the great artistic, literary, and musical center, its culture was considered shallow, frivolous, and even immoral. In contrast, German philosophic, ethical, and theologic ideas were popular in at least the Northeastern United States. Nevertheless, American physicians flocked to Paris, sometimes after a short stay in London. A total of 616 Americans went to Paris for medical studies in the 40 years starting in 1820, most of them actually from 1830 to 1850. However, only 24 of them took the M.D. degree, 20 of whom were from New Orleans. Most of the Americans in Paris had taken the M.D. degree in America previously or, in a few cases, were to take it later on their return there. Of the identifiable men who did not take degrees, 198 were from the two Philadelphia schools, 60 from Harvard, 51 from South Carolina, and only 16 from New York's College of Physicians and Surgeons. A total of 202 held or, more commonly, came to hold American academic posts, including the surprising number of 16 at the Medical College of Ohio. Not all went for clinical studies: S. Wier Mitchell expressly went to study with Glaude Bernard (Middleton, 1966).

Accordingly, early in the 18th century American physicians, long dependent on English medicine for information and training, came to recognize the need to keep up with French medicine. Leading professors such as Gross and Stillé of Philadelphia, and many who were less famous, translated French works into English. In the 1820s and 1830s American medical journals discussed the advances in French medicine, and among them were Chapman's journals: *Journal of Foreign Medical Science, North American Medical and Surgical Journal*, and *American Journal of Medical Sciences* (Blick, 1957). *The New Orleans Journal of Medicine*, as might be expected, emphasized French findings, since practitioners in that city included émigrés from France, who proudly added the letter "P." after "M.D." to indicate its source in Paris. In 1836 Jackson wrote, "For 30 years I have been satisfied that the physicians of Paris were laying the firmest foundation for the science of therapeutics by studying the natural history of diseases; and by this giving us rules for diagnoses and prognoses."

Pierre Louis was especially popular with Americans, having as pupils the Boston teachers Bowditch, Holmes, James Jackson, Jr., Shattuck, John Collins Warren, and John Mason Warren. From New York came Metcalf, Charles L. Mitchell, and Mott. The notable Philadelphia teachers who had studied with Louis were Gerhard, Pennock, Pepper, Stillé, and S. Wier Mitchell.

Paris served as a model to American medical educators. Stillé compared French and American education, much to the detriment of the latter; on the other hand, the Paris hospital system of practice did not emphasize the doctor-patient bond. Many American doctors criticized their French surgical teachers because they seemed to be more interested in the performance of beautiful operations that tested their diagnoses, technical abilities, and prognoses, than in the patients' welfare.

The political upheaval of 1830 evidently had little effect on the popularity of French medicine. However, following the republican revolution of 1848 - when Louis Napoleon had himself elected President - Napoleon waited only a few years before making himself Emperor. He forced the retirement of popular medical teachers, thereby offending some of the foreign physicians. By the 1850s the French, like the English, were unpopular in America, unlike the Russian-American friendship, which was very good. At the outbreak of the Crimean War about 30 American physicians then studying in Paris volunteered for the Russian Army, serving at Sebastopol. The first two were King from South Carolina and Draper from Massachusetts, both of whom died of typhus, along with many others. When Pirogov, Surgeon-General of the Czar's Army, arrived in 1854, he found that the foreign physicians were instructed poorly in surgery and subsequently wrote his own book on the subject (Dvoichenko-Markov, 1954).

Although members of the faculties of a number of medical schools studied in Paris, they were affected in different ways. Some were influenced mainly by the technical proficiency of French surgeons. Others, like Metcalf of Philadelphia, praised the length and format of the French medical curriculum. The men from Boston, most notably Holmes, wanted to bring back both the format and content of French medicine to their own universities (Beecher and Altschule, 1977).

By the middle of the 19th century many leading physicians of the important American cities had been trained to be competent clinicians in Edinburgh, London, Paris, and Dublin. When back in America, they presumably practiced clinical medicine as ably as did physicians in those western European cities where they had received their training. For some time medical education in America could not advance to a comparable degree, because the American universities had no facilities for clinical teaching; however, two exceptions were the dispensaries associated with Jefferson Medical College in Philadelphia and the University of Vermont Medical School in Burlington. The other dispensaries located in Philadelphia, New York, and Boston were not sites of clinical teaching under the auspices of university-connected medical schools in those cities. Most bedside teaching, if it existed at all in America, was not conducted within the framework of a university medical school. In Boston, therefore, non-university clinical teaching was conducted at the Boston Dispensary (founded in 1795) and at the Boston Marine Hospital (which later became the Chelsea Naval Hospital). Some of the men who did that teaching were members of the university-connected medical school faculty, others were not. Similarly, some of the students being taught in these unofficial courses might have been registered at the university-connected medical school, whereas others were not so registered but were apprentices to some licensed physician. Today few historians appreciate the part played by these unofficial teachers and the private medical schools they founded, particularly in Boston, in order to pursue the kind of teaching they favored (and to collect the fees). Some of the private medical schools were founded by members of the Harvard faculty who were able, as a result, to teach the clinical medicine that the university-connected school was neither willing nor able to teach. Those private medical schools of Boston, Philadelphia, and New York were created after the precedent of the private medical schools of London. For decades they carried on clinical teaching at a time when university-connected schools were doing little, if any, and when hospital-connected medical schools like those dominating the London scene were not functioning in America (Smith, 1979). The Boylston Medical School, which was one of the Boston private schools, actually was given a charter by the State.

The teaching of physical diagnosis based on percussion and auscultation developed in America largely due to the activities of the private schools. Instruction in those procedures was first given in America at Boston's Tremont Medical School in 1838 under Holmes, who had learned such procedures in Paris. The diaries of Harvard medical students indicate that in 1841 the teaching was introduced in a fragmentary way at their medical school, but that approach was not emphasized. The second institution to make this instruction a formal part of the curriculum was the private medical school at Woodstock, Vermont, where Clark was a professor. Clark had learned physical diagnosis in Paris through an interesting series of events. He had become Physician to Jerome Bonaparte who, after graduating from Harvard College, married an American woman and remained in America. Bonaparte took a trip to Paris in the late 1830s and invited Clark along as his personal physician. Clark studied in Paris for the next three years and after his return taught percussion and auscultation, beginning in 1842. The words "physical diagnosis" were used first by Worcester, a graduate of Harvard College and Dartmouth Medical School, when he taught at the private Ohio Medical College starting in 1842. It will be recalled that the migration of New Englanders to the Midwest between 1820 and 1850 chiefly involved the rural residents and included many graduates of New England's private medical schools (Waite, 1945). At that time New England had only 17% of the country's population but contained more than 40% of its medical educational facilities, largely at private medical schools. In fact, a graduate of one of these rural medical schools at Castleton, Vermont, became a regent at the University of Michigan, and he persuaded that university to open a medical school in 1851, with graduates of Castleton making up half the faculty, including the dean. This is only one example of the respect accorded physicians trained at New England's rural medical schools.

When the American Medical Association held its first meeting in 1847, it voted to recommend that all medical schools have university connections. Certainly such a connection would minimize the administrative instability and the financial insecurity hampering the activities of the private schools, ultimately forcing them to close. Boston's private schools closed in the late 1850s, but their contributions should not be forgotten. In addition to their progressive views on clinical training and their reluctance to adopt medical superstitions, these schools produced a number of leaders in education at university-controlled medical schools.

Connection with a private medical school in no way was degrading, because their faculties contained many men who taught simultaneously or subsequently at university medical schools. The career of John C. Dalton, Jr., affords a noteworthy example. One of the group of Harvard men who founded the private Boylston Medical School in Boston in 1847, he went to France in 1850 to study with Bernard and later became Professor of Physiology at Buffalo, New York. He held the same post at the College of Physicians and Surgeons in New York from 1855 to 1875, becoming one of America's leading physiologists.

It is clear that the need for bedside training officially came to be recognized everywhere in the country only after having been recognized unofficially in the activities of some of the private medical schools. Although clearly successful when judged by the quality of some of its products, the prevailing training-by-apprenticeship of the earlier years was not acceptable in the modern era of the early 19th century, in which collateral or accessory science became important in clinical medicine. Even more crucial, however, was the inefficiency, variability, and unpredictability of clinical teaching by apprenticeship. The private medical schools early recognized the inadequacies of apprenticeships and helped start the development in America of clinical medicine after the models of Paris, London, and Dublin.

Holmes and Bigelow were important not only as pioneers in the introduction of physical diagnosis in clinical teaching, but also as the medical writers who gave America it first modern textbook of medicine in 1839, the revised and enlarged Hall's *Principles of The Theory and Practice of Physic.* Bigelow and Holmes wrote that they had selected Hall's work as the textbook on *The Theory and Practice of Medicine* in their private medical school, adding

> [it] has been found necessary to condense some of these subjects....Some controversial parts have been omitted, also a few other portions, which appeared to have only a personal or local interest. Large additions have been made, consisting of subjects not contained, or imperfectly treated, in the original volume. In certain cases, where the science has advanced, the chapters and sections have been rewritten....The whole of the first four chapters, also the seventh, the last, and the larger part of several intermediate chapters are furnished by the editors, which with the other interpolations, amount to about one-third of the entire volume.

In describing the elements of clinical medicine they wrote the following:

> Disease when made the subject of study, presents itself to our contemplation under several points of view, so that some ambiguity exists in the application of the term. In its most common or vulgar acceptation, the word disease means the symptoms which are present during illness, and which interfere with the ease and welfare of the patient. Thus dysentery is considered as consisting of pain and soreness in the abdomen, with tenesmus, and mucous or bloody discharges. Phthisis or consumption is said to consist of cough, pain in the chest, dyspnoea, hectic and emaciation. And when common patients are interrogated in regard to the nature of their own disease, the only satisfaction they can give us, is by enumerating the symptoms of

which they are conscious. Upon these collections of symptoms are founded many of the older nosologies which have been introduced for the purpose of defining and classifying the morbid affections of the body.

But disease, more rigidly and scientifically considered, consists not in the symptoms, but in the morbid changes, or pathological condition, of the organs, in which it is seated, and of which the symptoms are merely consequences. Thus dysentery consists in a certain inflammation in the intestines, and phthisis in a tubercular affection of the lungs. Colic, in which there may be no structural change, consists not in the congnizable symptom of pain, but in the irregular, and supposed spasmodic performance, of an internal function. Disease moreover is not in most cases a simple alteration of structure or function. It consists more commonly in a series of consecutive changes, commencing with a slight deviation from the healthy condition, and increasing till it involves extensive tissues, and deranges many functions of the body.

For our knowledge of the morbid changes which constitute disease, we are dependent, during life, upon our observation of the symptoms. This evidence, although indirect, is the only one which we are able to command, when vital organs are concerned, for no one can obtain ocular evidence of the condition of the brain, lungs or heart. The science of pathology has been built up by a careful observation of symptoms, and a comparison of these with the anatomical appearances exhibited in those who die. In this way we have become able to infer the existence of internal and hidden changes, by external and cognizable phenomena.

Symptoms are divided into what are called rational and the physical signs. The rational signs, strictly speaking, are those which we derive from the testimony of the patient himself, and which we are obliged to receive from him upon trust, because we have no better means of obtaining satisfaction. Thus pain is a rational sign, of which we should be ignorant, but for the assurances of the patient. In like manner dizziness, noise in the ears, various defects of the senses, thirst, anorexia, nausea, &c. are all rational signs, the knowledge of which we obtain not from our own senses, but from those of the patient.

The physical signs on the contrary, are those which we learn from our own personal inspection, as we should learn the qualities and phenomena of inert matter. Some of the physical signs are obvious at sight, others are appreciable only by circuitous exploration. The color and aspect of the face, and the temperature of the skin, are physical signs. The state of the pulse is a strictly physical sign, about which the patient knows little or nothing from his own sensations, and in regard to which we should not trust him if he did. The condition of the surface of the tongue, the appearance of the sputa, the alvine and urinary discharges, the phenomena of tumor and depression, hardness and softness, distortion of shape and irregularity of motion, are among the physical signs. Lastly, the results of the modern modes of exploring the chest, and other cavities, by auscultation and percussion are called physical signs by way of eminence, and these are often intended alone, when the term is used...

Judiciously blending history, physical findings and laboratory data, the book continued by discussing the diseases, organ by organ. For example, in reference to the kidney, it stated in part:

When the urine has an albuminous character, so that it is coagulated by heat, or by the action of strong acids, &c. there is usually though not always, a granular disorganization of the kidney. Dropsy is a frequent concomitant of this symptom.

When the urine is excessive in quantity, with a sweet taste and smell, and afford sugar by evaporation, the disease is diabetes mellitus.

When there is pain and tenderness in the lumbar region, shooting downward toward the thighs, with nausea or vomiting, frequent micturition, numbness of the thigh and retraction of the testicle, we infer that there is inflammation of the kidney.

When in conjunction with some of the foregoing symptoms, the urine deposits a sabulous or sand-like sediment, there is renal calculus, or gravel in the kidneys.

When there is acute pain and a sense of weight in one lumbar and iliac region, without most of the symptoms which have been previously mentioned, and without disturbance of the pulse, we may suspect obstruction of the ureter by the passage of a calculus.

Pain felt in the glans penis, and unattended by disease in the part itself, is indicative of calculous affection in some part of the urinary organs.

> When there is pain in the glans penis,
> with frequent desire to pass urine, attended
> by a sudden stoppage of the stream, there is
> probably calculus in the bladder, the existence
> of which can be certain by striking it with a
> sound.

In addition to condensing Hall's work, they added much from Andral.   Except for the elegance and precision of the language, the Bigelow-Holmes volume resembles modern works on the subject.

Holmes is written about more often as a literary figure than as a physician, being well known as a poet and essayist before he became physician.   Born in Cambridge, Massachusetts, the son of a Calvinist minister, he spent his early years in a home full of books and people who pursued intellectual interests.   He was educated first at Andover and then Harvard College, from which he received the A.B. degree in 1829.   Unwilling to follow his father's wish that he enter the clergy, he tried but soon abandoned the legal profession; however, he became well known for his writing.   He decided to become a physician and, after a few years at a private medical school in Boston, he entered the Harvard Medical School.   Holmes traveled in Europe and came under the influence of Louis and Andral in Paris.   Returning in 1835, he received the M.D. degree from Harvard, but was more interested in writing than in medical practice; however, he was appointed Professor of Anatomy at Dartmouth, a post he held until 1840.   In 1847 he became Dean of the Faculty and Parkman Professor of Anatomy and Physiology at Harvard, holding the former post until 1853 and the latter until 1882.   In addition, he continued to write, helped Lowell organize the *Atlantic Monthly*, and was associated closely with the great writers and poets of America.   Holmes did not himself produce much of medical note except for his lecture on puerperal fever, which he declared was derivative.   He was very interested in microscopy and was a great collector of medical books and prints, which he bequeathed to the Boston Medical Library.

A man of tremendous ego, Holmes was the most photographed subject of his time.   While he was Chairman of the Committee on Medical Literature of the American Medical Association, his frankness and witty sarcasm immediately involved him in a furious controversy. In commenting on Dowler's paper in the *New Orleans Medical and Surgical Journal*, he wrote, "Obviously an acute thinker and original observer, this gentlemen allows himself to mingle so many acid, astringent, effervescent and overheating elements in the large libations he pours on the altar of science that all but the very thirsty are likely to sip rather than drink of the strange composition." He also commented on the poor quality of the Southern and Western (Chicago) medical literature, and *The Southern Medical and Surgical Journal* responded in furious and minute detail, stating, "We deny that a Diploma from Pennsylvania or Harvard conveys any distinction whatever upon its possessor....It may be that if we of the South and West contribute less to the medical literature of our country, that little is more original." Holmes' reply was moderate and relatively short, but the *Journal* went on furiously and at length. Some years later, Holmes wrote on "the hydrostatic paradox of controversy....If you had a bent tube, one arm of which was the size of a pipe stem and the other big enough to hold the ocean, the water would stand at the same height in one as in the other" (Marshall, 1948).

Historians have looked for hidden greatness, or even significance, in Holmes' medical works. One of them called Holmes a great psychologist, an actual precursor of Freud (Oberndorf, 1943). This seems to me to be quite unjustified. Holmes is an example of an outstanding medical editor who wrote little about medicine *per se*; but, what he wrote about medical education itself reveals him to be a fine medical educator. His views expressed in his "Introductory Lecture to the Medical Class of Harvard University" were delivered on November 6, 1867, a significant date, since it was 30 years after the Bigelow-Holmes "Preface" and shows that Holmes at least still adhered to what Flexner, decades later, sarcastically referred to as "clinicism." A few medical educators in other cities made similar comments, although in far fewer words and with less eloquence:

The most essential part of a student's instruction is obtained as I believe, not in the lecture-room, but at the bedside. Nothing seen there is lost; the rhythms of disease are learned by frequent repetition; its unforeseen occurrences stamp themselves indelibly in the memory. Before the student is aware of what he has acquired, he has learned the aspects and course and probable issue of the diseases he has seen with his teacher, and the proper mode of dealing with them, so far as his master knows it. On the other hand, our ex cathedra prelections have a strong tendency to run into details which, however interesting they may be to ourselves and a few of our more curious listeners, have nothing in them which will ever be of use to the student as a practitioner. It is a perfectly fair question whether I and some other American Professors do not teach quite enough that is useless already. Is it not well to remind the student from time to time that a physician's business is to avert disease, to heal the sick, to prolong life, and to diminish suffering? Is it not true that the young man of average ability will find it as much as he can do to fit himself for these simple duties? Is it not best to begin, at any rate, by making sure of such knowledge as he will require in his daily walk, by no means discouraging him from any study for which his genius fits him when he once feels that he has become master of his chosen art?

Bigelow was not only Holmes' co-author of the first outstanding American medical text, albeit a derived one. He was Visiting Physician at the Massachusetts General Hospital and the author of the outstanding, illustrated *Medical Botany* (1817-1820). Today he is best known for his article "Self-Limited Disease" (1855), which pointed out the uselessness of much of the medical treatment then widely used. Bigelow also should be remembered for his oblique but perceptive comment on statistics, which appeared in his address, in 1860, at the banquet of the Fourth National Quarantine and Sanitary Commission:

> It is vain that the unhappy inquirer resorts to his statistical tables to inform himself whether there is most danger in a steamboat or on a railroad, - he unfortunately learns that the most dangerous thing a man can do is to go to bed, for more people die in bed than anywhere else.

Harvard also followed Paris in the matter of faculty chairs. Like Paris, Harvard early established a separate Chair of Pathological Anatomy and had Professors of Medicine come up through pathology. Fitz at Harvard was one of these, the last being Henry Christian in 1912. Like Paris, Harvard considered pathological anatomy highly important, evident in Isaac Ray's thesis at Bowdoin. Ray was at Harvard Medical School in 1825 and then went to Bowdoin, taking his M.D. degree there in 1827. Without forgetting his Harvard lessons and using very forceful language, he declared that a personal experience with pathological anatomy was absolutely essential to the study of medicine, and that post-mortem examinations were done to learn about disease, not merely to prove diagnoses. He showed great familiarity with the French writings in pathological anatomy. What is remarkable is not that a young physician should think the French example important, but rather that he should become a world-famous psychiatrist, known chiefly for his writings on the medicolegal aspects of insanity. His *A Treatise in the Medical Jurisprudence of Insanity* was considered so authoritative everywhere that it became the basis of the McNaughton Rule laid down in England in 1843; moreover, he was also the founder of what is today called the American Psychiatric Society.

The school of Bigelow and Holmes had a commitment to the patient care derived from bedside medicine which lasted for decades. It manifested itself in different ways from time to time, as when, in the early 20th century it led to the creation of the first hospital social service department in the country (Beecher and Altschule, 1977).

Another New Englander who was an outstanding medical thinker was Bartlett, who, after attending medical lectures in Boston and Rhode Island, took the M.D. degree at Brown University in 1826. He then spent a year in Paris, never forgetting its lessons. After his return he was given, in 1832, the Chair of Pathological Anatomy and Materia Medica at the Berkshire Medical Institution in Pittsfield, Massachusetts.   (At that time the Berkshire generally was considered superior to Harvard.) In 1839 he moved from the Chair of Pathological Anatomy at Pittsfield to that of Practice of Medicine at Dartmouth. Thereafter, sometimes simultaneously, he held chairs at Vermont, Transylvania (Lexington, Kentucky), Louisville (1850-1852), New York University (1850-1852), and the College of Physicians and Surgeons, New York, in Medical Jurisprudence and Materia Medica (1852-1855).   Except for the years in New York, he also practiced in Lowell, Massachusetts, where he was twice mayor and once state legislator (de Bauer, 1945; Ackerknecht, 1950).   His book on fevers, written in 1842, received worldwide recognition.   However, his most important work was *An Essay on the Philosophy of Medical Science* (1844), a precise, clear, logical exposition of the nature of medicine according to his own ideas, including a considerable amount of French thinking on the subject. Among other things he pointed out the ease with which we fall into error, the fallacies of speculation, and the fact that physiology is not deducible from anatomy and *vice versa*. He had many other interesting ideas, such as the possibility of disease classification by response to therapeutic agents. Although Bigelow often is listed as early America's main, or perhaps only, medical philosopher, it is clear that Bartlett, with his breadth and wisdom, should rank first.

A final note should be made about the Americans educated in Great Britain who preferred that country to their own during the War of the Revolution. For example, Wells of Charleston, South Carolina, graduated at Edinburgh and refused to return to America. He practiced in London until the end of his life.

Another American, Jeffries, had a more varied career. Having graduated in arts at Harvard in 1745, he was an apprentice to Lloyd of Boston, the man who trained many of Boston's outstanding physicians before the Revolution. Jeffries went abroad for further study, receiving the M.D. degree at Aberdeen in 1769, and then studied in London with Hunter and others. In 1771, back in America, he was appointed surgeon to a British ship of the line, with a hospital on shore, a position he held until 1774. Thereafter he remained loyal to the Crown, and when the British Army evacuated Boston, he left for Halifax, where he was appointed Surgeon-Major to the British forces in America. When the war ended, he settled in England, where he not only pursued his medical career, with emphasis on midwifery, but also carried on detailed studies in meteorology. The latter interest led him to make a balloon flight over London, during the course of which he dropped greeting cards addressed to his friends and admirers. He reached an elevation of more than 6,500 feet, collecting samples of air in bottles at different levels. Five weeks later he flew with a companion across the English Channel from Dover to the forest of Guienne in Artois. He was America's first aeronaut. Returning to Boston in 1790 he practiced surgery, medicine, and midwifery, leaving detailed reports on all of his cases upon his death. Although Jeffries was a good doctor, his main contribution was to aerial travel.

By the beginning of the Civil War the Eastern States and Louisiana had many physicians trained in European schools. Newport, New York, Philadelphia, and Charleston, South Carolina, in the earlier years mainly favored Edinburgh, with some changeover to Paris later. Boston favored London in the early years of that period, subsequently giving Paris training a preponderant status in its medical education. Apparently, Boston wanted more practical and less theoretical training than did the other cities; that is, more patient-oriented practice than theory-oriented medicine. Grafting the Paris medicine of that period onto the London-Dublin medicine that it favored was easy. However, several *caveats* must be offered. For one thing, Paris medicine was hospital-centered and as such did not permit the development of the doctor-patient interactions that form the basis of medicine; English and Irish medicine were more satisfactory in that regard.   Moreover, universities were slow to accept the new medicine officially and when they finally did, a new element for making change appeared, the scientific medicine of Germany. Thus, at that time the development of sound patient-doctor interactions was impaired by a partial return to the hospital medicine of 19th-century Paris and by the injudicious imposition of new viewpoints that arose in Germany after 1848.

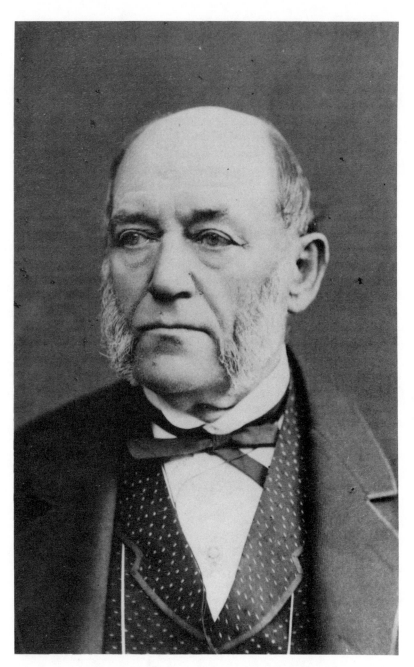

Carl Rokitansky, 1804–1878

Part II: Austrian and German Influences in Nineteenth-Century Medicine

Chapter 12: Vienna, The Great Medical Center: 1848-1918

IN THE 18TH CENTURY VIENNA WAS UNABLE to become an heir to Leyden, a feat accomplished by Edinburgh and, to some extent, Paris. There were two impediments: The rigid, dictatorial organization of medical education and practice, in which the wrong kind of man in the dictator's seat could retard, or even reverse, progress; and, the boring, time-wasting, and generally destructive German propensity toward theorizing on the basis of inadequate or nonexistent data. The former occurred during the tenure of Baron von Stifft, Physician to the King, head of Austria's medical profession, and Director of Teaching at the Univerity. The latter came into play after von Stifft's death at which time Vienna favored theory, unlike other cities, despite the fact that Vienna originally had followed the lead of Paris medicine and then that of London and Dublin.

The history of the involved doctrinal disputes occurring before and during the von Stifft period were presented with brilliant clarity - a most difficult task - by Lesky (1976). Those emotion-laden conflicts, made even more senseless by the professional inadequacies of many of the protagonists, create a sorry picture of Viennese medicine at the time. In a more positive sense von Stifft dismissed or forced the resignation of phrenologists and Brunonians because their ideas were not traditional, rather than because they adhered to error. However, he did not prevent the prevailing German superstition of "Natur-Philosophie" from contaminating Viennese medicine. Moreover, for reasons not clear now, he decided that pathological anatomy was the jurisdiction only of the anatomists, thus attenuating its role as a basis of clinical medicine.

Whatever von Stifft's ambiguous rationale may have been regarding medical theory (or perhaps dogma), no uncertainties were apparent in his rule over the faculty and students. The atmosphere of repression - the insistence of returning to old ways and old ideas and the exclusion of all that came from the West (at least as far west as France) - was maintained, although it did not represent necessarily his own convictions. As a high official serving a strong-willed reactionary monarch, von Stifft may have believed that any inclination of his to independent thought or action was best controlled. However, at the time he was becoming a villain because of his repressive acts, a hero was working quietly for the regeneration of Viennese medicine. That man was von Turkheim, the man to whom Skoda, otherwise a consistently unsentimental man, referred to as "a second van Swieten, who worked for many years on a reform of medical studies in Austria, which would not limp behind progress but would stimulate progress, and who was prevented from implementing it by death alone." (Since von Turkheim died in 1846, we can only surmise how it was possible for him to accomplish that under the circumstances.)

Von Stifft's early life prepared him for a conservative career. Born in Lower Austria in 1760 of a middle-class family, he practiced largely among the nobility in Vienna, after graduation from the Medical School. One of his patients was the Emperor's physician, von Lagusius, who died in 1795 and presumably had recommended von Stifft to Emperor Franz II. Although accepted procedure required that Storck, van Swieten's successor, serve as the Emperor's physician, Franz preferred von Stifft and in 1798 appointed him Acting Personal Physician. When Stork died in 1803, von Stifft was given those posts once held by van Swieten - Physician to the Imperial Family, Head of Medical Education, Director of Public Health and State Medicine - all of which he maintained until his death in 1836.

His successor as executive, von Turkheim, studied in Vienna and graduated in 1800. While at school he had been a member of the circle of Frank's Brunonian's, at that time out of favor because they followed the foreign erratic guru, Brown of Edinburgh, rather than local leaders. Nevertheless, von Turkheim received an important appointment in the health department of the court chancellery and, hence, became a close collaborator with von Stifft. He also held several other titles, including that of Vice-Director of the Faculty. The fact that this young man of somewhat heretical opinion was acceptable to the ostensibly archconservative von Stifft is puzzling. Was von Stifft really less conservative than his position required, or was he unwilling to complain of the appointment because von Turkheim's father was a state councilor and a man of power in the inner circles of the government? These questions cannot be answered using the available information. Comparatively speaking, the intricacies of academic life in Vienna at that time made the activities of the medieval Byzantine court seem to be the height of integrity, candor, and generosity. Suffice it to say that von Turkheim early showed his sound qualities as well as his influence. In 1811 von Stifft wanted to make pathological anatomy an appendage of the surgical assistant's post, whereas von Turkheim wanted it to be a separate position; the latter prevailed.

Later von Turkheim became more active in his reform efforts. In 1836, after von Stifft died, his son-in-law Raimann succeeded him. However, Raimann was a man of neither energy nor enterprise, and von Turkheim openly took charge. Beginning in 1837 he made it possible for students and young physicians to meet and present papers, which then were published. In 1840 he created a special thoracic service for Skoda at the Allgemeine Krankenhaus. Two years later he arranged for von Hebra to give clinical courses on skin diseases, and he sent Rokitansky and Skoda to Paris to study. In 1844 he created a full professorship of pathological anatomy, giving the chair to Rokitansky. The next year Hyrtl, a fine lecturer, was brought in to teach anatomy, and he insisted on the need to emphasize regional anatomy, thus making the material maximally useful to clinicians. Von Turkheim either created new departments or strengthened old ones in pathological chemistry, microscopic anatomy, pediatrics, surgery, gynecology, otology, psychiatry, and other areas of medicine. He wrote a draft of his administrative master plan for the reform and rejuvenation of Viennese medicine and held many discussions with members of the faculty to persuade them to adopt his plan rather than impose it as an order. Regrettably, he died in 1846 before the plan could be completed formally. Today von Feunchtersleben usually is credited with the plan, for he was dean during the revolution of 1848, when students and faculty presented their revolutionary demands. Von Feunchtersleben then announced (without attribution) the administrative changes on which von Turkheim had been working. (Those wanting an account of the administrative changes should read Lesky's meticulous description of them and how they came to pass. For our purposes, changes in the faculty and in what and how they taught are the salient features.)

The revived medical school eventually was called the Second Vienna Medical School and initially was centered around Rokitansky's autopsy teaching. Rokitansky's personality and training were noteworthy. He was born in 1804 in Moravia, the son of a clerk in a local government office. His mother was partially of Irish descent. When his father died in 1812, the family was put in a difficult situation; nevertheless, Rokitansky was determined to pursue a medical career, and he entered the University at Prague where he was required to take a three-year course in philosophy. Throughout his life he maintained an interest in philosophy, particularly the works of Kant and Schopenhauer, the latter's pessimistic outlook suitable to Rokitansky's tendency to brood. Although he was required to memorize the books used, he tried to understand the meanings behind the words; essentially, therefore, he was self-taught. Such an habitual philosophizing tendency played an important role in his studies at Prague from 1822 to 1824. The generation of hypotheses that comprised a large part of his first major work all but destroyed the book's medical usefulness.

From 1824 to 1828 he attended the Medical School in Vienna, becoming an unpaid prosector in pathological anatomy in 1827 and a paid assistant in 1830. His chief, Wagner, was a competent pathologist, but was content merely to describe any abnormalities that were discovered, without relating them to causative disease states. Rokitansky was well read in the French and English literature of the period and learned that in those countries the post-mortem examinations were performed by a patient's own physician, who then used the findings not only to check the diagnosis and effects, if any, of treatment, but more importantly to create a complete picture of the disease process as it manifested itself clinically. When Rokitansky became Associate Professor in 1834, he was in the position to see a vast amount of pathologic material at the Allgemeine Krankenhaus, where most of the sick of Vienna were concentrated. This extensive and concentrated experience was the basis of his creation, from static data, of a dynamic composite of the development of different diseases from their onset to their terminations.

The lesson he learned from the writings of French and English clinicians of that era was reinforced by his period of study in Paris, where post-mortem data was correlated with clinical data, thus having the obvious effect of sharpening the clinician's diagnostic faculties. For the teacher of medicine, it clarified the life histories of diseases. Whereas most earlier collections of pathologic anatomical material dealt only with those diseases seen in general medicine and surgery, Rokitansky's vast collections of data eventually included significant amounts of information in the fields of dermatology, ophthalmology, otology, obstetrics, and gynecology. It was this accumulation of sound anatomical data that, some decades later, led to the development of Vienna as a leading center of medical specialization. In addition, Rokitansky's data led to the formulation of the idea that there are specific disease processes in all branches of medicine. Such concepts often were incomplete because the role of microorganisms causing infections was still unknown; moreover, the specific nature of the pathologic changes caused by certain infectious agents was not recognized. It was only with the interpretive participation of Skoda and other clinicians that Rokitansky's massive amounts of data could achieve clinical significance.

Rokitansky's post-mortem conferences were so remarkable that all physicians who attended them, whether enthusiastic supporters or his most determined critics (like Virchow), stated that he had no equal in this endeavor; his careful dissections and accurate observations being made more vivid by his clear thinking and evocative language.

His publications on various single subjects were preludes to his greatest work, *Handbuch der Pathologischen Anatomie*, published over a period of years from 1842.   In many conditions, however, the symptoms were so diffuse and generalized that no local anatomic findings could explain them effectively.   For such situations, and for some others in which the anatomical findings themselves seemed adequate, Rokitansky formulated an etiologic theory that seriously marred his otherwise great contributions.   That theory, termed "crasis," held that diseases originated in changes or abnormalities in blood proteins, about which very little was known then.   However, that lack of information seemed to encourage rather than deter Rokitansky, since he had a need to explain what was not yet explained, a propensity common among medical academicians and one that unjustifiably weakens their credibility as observers.   Although this hypothesis-spinning occurs everywhere, it most generally is accepted - even praised - in German medical writings.   It is easy to see how Rokitansky fell into this morass, since as a student at the University in Prague, he was very interested in philosophy, particularly German.   German philosophies popular at the time were noted for their exquisitely logical formulations built on false, unprovable, or nonexistent data.   The "crasis" hypothesis fell into this pattern, and parts of Rokitansky's general comment were too speculative for his English translators and, therefore, were omitted (Ruther and Rohl, 1973).   Virchow reviewed Rokitansky's *Handbook* in 1846 and his comments about "crasis" were so harshly critical that Rokitansky deleted those sections from subsequent editions (Rather, 1969). (Of course, Virchow was not above creating some unsupported hypotheses of his own later.)

Rokitansky became dean of the school, was elected to high posts in professional societies and educational organizations, and also held government posts.   His great energy, combined with his usual geniality, made him an effective leader; his good sense, together with his strong devotion to freedom and progress, made him a popular one. Despite his many administrative and educational duties he continued to report his pathological observations; however, with the passage of time his youthful preoccupation with pessimistic ideas recurred, and the attraction of gloomy philosophy distracted him from his clinical work. *The Solidarity of All Animal Life,* published when he was 65 years old, was one of a number of his writings in this vein, in which he stated how the inborn "hunger of protoplasm" made all animals victimize each other. According to Rokitansky, humans because of their moral and compassionate impulses, could be different, but usually were not. He wrote that the fight for progress and freedom engaged in by many around 1848 largely was forgotten, and that liberal individualism was degenerating into ruthless egotism. Nevertheless, he continued to pursue his own ideals. As a member of the Upper House of the State Council, he worked for the removal of schools from church dominance. His influence in pathology itself continued to grow as his students and assistants came to occupy important posts. For some reason Rokitansky never became a leader in microscopic pathology, an unusual fact since the very first edition of his *Handbook* contained many microscopic findings. Several of his students, such as Engel, Wedl, and Stellwag, were making histologic studies and lecturing on them in the early 1840s. It was through Rokitansky's influence at that period that in 1853 the first Chair in Histology in a German-speaking city was established; however, Rokitansky chose to remain a macroscopic pathologist and was the most significant contributor to that field.

Skoda was Rokitansky's partner in starting the great period of 19th-century Viennese medicine and, like Rokitansky, he was a Czech. Whereas Rokitansky was genial and sociable, Skoda was a reserved and serious bachelor. Fearful of hurting the feelings of his tailor, a personal friend, he is said to have worn clothes he disliked for years. His remoteness and his unpredictability made him an object of respect rather than affection. Born in Pilsen in 1805, the son of a locksmith, he was too poor to buy oil or candles and had to study by firelight while in high school. Sent to the University by a wealthy manufacturer, he made his living by tutoring other students. While at the medical school in Vienna, he studied physics and mathematics, subjects which helped him clarify his ideas in percussion and auscultation. Disregarding the content of the lectures then being given at the medical school because they were more philosophical than medical, he trained himself to become an expert in the physical examination of the chest.   Skoda graduated in 1831 and the next year was made an unpaid assistant at the Allgemeine Krankenhaus.   He spent much time at percussion and auscultation, for which he was much ridiculed and criticized.   When on one occasion he did a lifesaving tracheotomy without having the permission of his superiors, he was taken off the medical wards and punished by being made to work in the psychiatric division.   Nevertheless he continued his studies, comparing the findings on auscultation and percussion with the findings at autopsy in men and animals and on artificial models.   His work clarified the clinical findings then accepted and the descriptive criteria he developed still is used today.

In his work on the heart, Skoda established the distinctions between heart sounds and murmurs.   In 1839 he felt ready to present his findings and conclusions formally. *His Treatise on Percussion and Auscultation* was published in that year, at a time when Skoda, discouraged by his treatment at the Krankenhaus, had given up work there and was practicing medicine in a poor suburb of Vienna. In 1840 von Turkheim removed him from this pedestrian occupation and had him put in charge of the newly created thoracic service at the Krankenhaus, which had treated him so poorly.   A year later von Turkheim had him promoted to the rank of Chief Physician.   Given that opportunity, Skoda quickly showed his diagnostic wizardry; however, his teachings got a mixed reception.   Some younger physicians were enthusiastic, while some of the older ones berated them.   A few, such as Piorry in Paris, claimed that Skoda had stolen ideas from him.

The combined activities of Rokitansky and Skoda produced an enormous expansion in the data of bedside medicine.   Physical diagnosis became a meticulously detailed subject dependent on careful and well-informed examination.   The pupils of Rokitansky and Skoda gradually came to fill the chairs in medicine at chief cities of the Austro-Hungarian empire - Prague, Pavia, Cracow, Lemberg, Budapest - and many physicians came from other countries, particularly America, to learn their methods. Nevertheless, despite the fact that Skoda made some treatments such as chest paracentesis more accurate and

effective, he and his pupils became fervid therapeutic ni-
hilists. That is not surprising because, as the autopsy was
an important part of their patient study, the patients at
that point hardly could be called therapeutic successes.
Their therapeutic skepticism aroused much criticism; nevertheless, Skoda actually was much broader in his therapeutic outlook than physicians who were merely content to
prescribe drugs whose value had never been demonstrated.
When Skoda's ideas about the municipal water supply were
carried out, for example, cholera all but disappeared. He
was never made head of the medical service, however,
since his mentor, von Turkheim, became ill and soon afterward died.

Although, in general, individual medical specialties
will not be considered in this work, mention must be made
here of the dermatologist, von Hebra, also a Czech, and
born in Moravia in 1816, the illegitimate son of an army
officer. Baptized Schwarzmann, his mother's name, he
later was legitimized and given that of his father. After
his early schooling he entered the medical school at Vienna. For reasons now unclear, the skin patients were attended to by Skoda's thoracic service in 1840. When von
Hebra graduated in 1841, he was put in charge of these
patients and rapidly rose in rank. Applying the new techniques of microscopic study to the investigation of skin
diseases (as the French and the English had just begun to
do), he soon became the leader in the creation of that
new discipline. His various treatises and atlases published
over the next decades became standard texts all over the
world. He was a popular lecturer, not only because he
was expert in pointing out the distinguishing features of
rashes, but also because he was good-humored, sarcastically
witty, and anything but stuffy in manner.

As has been noted, the most effective teachers at
the medical school in Vienna in the 1840s were three
Czechs - Rokitansky, Skoda, and von Hebra - and a Hungarian, Hyrtl. The generally accepted originator of Vienna's medical rebirth, von Turkheim, had picked them out
of the crowd and had given them prominent places in the
hospital and university. Although von Turkheim died in
1846, his actions started the process that before the end
of the century made Vienna a great medical center. It

should be noted also that Viennese medicine could draw from not only Austrians but also Hungarians, Czechs, Silesians, and even persons from Austrian Poland (Cracow) and Austrian Italy (Pavia).

In Vienna, at midcentury, diagnostic bedside medicine reached its highest level. Those diagnostic methods used required close and, in fact, intimate contact with the patient. However, such medicine had several flaws. The patients on whom all of the advances had been made were far along in their diseases, most of them close to death; hence, the early stages of disease frequently were not taught. Also, the far-advanced diseases, in most cases, were beyond cure and, therefore, the prevailing attitude was one of therapeutic nihilism. And unfortunately, since most of the patients were patients of the hospital rather than of a physician, there was little chance for a doctor-patient relationship to develop. Whatever the doctors and their patients developed in their relationship they did in private practice. Only one of these three problems was remedied easily. That one - therapeutic nihilism - attacked in Vienna, and the man most responsible for that attack was von Oppolzer (also a Czech).

Born in Bohemia, von Oppolzer studied at Prague and graduated from its medical school in 1835. He was an assistant in the clinic there and, in 1841, became head of it. (It is worth noting that the other person considered for the post was Skoda; however, it is doubtful that Skoda was disappointed by not becoming Chief at Prague, because by then his future at Vienna seemed secure.) He developed his teaching along the lines being made famous by Skoda and Rokitansky; that is, clinical medicine based on the developments in physical examination and knowledge of morbid anatomy. His commitment to this kind of medicine was clear, but he added something of his own. His vast experience with people made it evident to him that therapeutic nihilism - almost a religion at Vienna - was not only wrong, but simply was not workable in the daily practice of medicine. That fact was well expressed by Kussmaul after attending one of von Oppolzer's lectures. Kussmaul had just come from Vienna, and to him the contrast between von Oppolzer and Skoda was striking:

> Von Oppolzer's talents could in no way
> match the genius of Skoda, but in his quality
> as a practical teacher we physicians placed
> him above the great critic and reformer. He
> possessed a vast and solid experience, was
> imbued with the humane spirit of his medical
> mission....Quietly and wisely he chose to
> forego mathematical certainty and with simple
> means obtained the best possible results,
> which is the hallmark of medical ability.

It is evident that a genius like Skoda could have been a somewhat better diagnostician than von Oppolzer, but there is little doubt that Skoda, unlike von Oppolzer, was lacking in some of the qualities of a good physician.

Von Oppolzer was invited to the Chair of Medicine at Leipzig and, hence, was instrumental in spreading the concepts of Viennese medicine (with the exception of therapeutic nihilism) in Germany. At that time there was a strong move in Germany to make medicine exist solely on the basis of physiologic information. Since such information was fragmentary, inaccurate and, in some areas, totally lacking, the proponents of that school of thought could do no more than utter insistent, unsupported statements about the validity of their ideas and further add, with equal certainty, that all of the weaknesses would vanish when more research data became available (the last a familiar refrain today). Von Oppolzer did not accept this view; however, he did recognize that pathological anatomy, a static discipline, could never be the sole basis of clinical practice. To him a functional approach clearly was essential, and he recognized that the physiology that was still in its infancy held promise of a solution. His tenure at Leipzig was brief, for in 1850 he was called to Vienna to rank with Skoda. His appointment there was not popular with the faculty; in particular, the other Czechs - Rokitansky, Skoda, and von Hebra - treated him coldly. However, his enthusiasm for teaching, sympathy for the sick, and his persistence and ingenuity in working out ways to make the patients feel better quickly made him popular with both students and patients. In addition, his foresight in encouraging young physicians such as

Breuer and Politzer to pursue studies in medical physiology gave Vienna the additional dimension it needed. Through the influence of von Oppolzer's activities, Vienna was stimulated further to become a great medical center, not only in clinical medicine, but also in surgery, the specialties, and the sciences collateral or accessory to clinical medicine. As is perhaps typical of a clinician like von Oppolzer, his writings were sparse and uninspired.

Some who read Lesky's deservedly praised book, either in its original language or in translation, may be fascinated - or revolted - by the jealousies and intrigues that seemed to motivate much of activities of Viennese medicine. Others may note with astonishment the assiduity, if not the ingenuity, with which the German mind created systems of ideas from nothing or next to nothing. Such fairy tales have had the dubious effect of providing some historians with a *raison d'etre*. Medical practitioners, however, will find Lesky's book an astonishing compilation, not only of important events, but of names outstanding in clinical medicine. The proportion of the listed names known to us today as eponyms with respect to a sign or symptom, syndrome, test, or diagnostic or therapeutic procedure is the mark of Vienna's greatness in the development of bedside medicine from 1840 to World War I and beyond. The dismemberment of the Austro-Hungarian empire after World War I was not only a political and social change, but it also signaled the separation of the Czechs, Hungarians, Silesians, Poles, Italians, and others who had come from the periphery of the empire and had contributed greatly to Viennese medicine of the past.

Viennese medicine has given us a host of great practitioners and some remarkable administrators, as well as providing its share of noble figures. One of the more interesting of the unusual men of Vienna was Gruby, born in 1810 in Hungary, the son of an impoverished Jewish farmer. He was a serious child, always interested in medicine; but there was no money to educate him. When he was 15, his father gave him a large loaf of bread and sent him on his way. Working his way from village to village, he ultimately reached Budapest; however, it seemed as if all was in vain, for he was refused admission to school because of his religion. Nevertheless, he stood in

the doorway of the schoolhouse listening to the lessons until the priest who conducted the school, evidently impressed by him, permitted him inside.   Gruby managed to
finish the required work and entered the medical school at
Vienna.   Too poor to buy a microscope, he made one himself and became expert in its use.   Rokitansky noticed the
young man and in 1835 encouraged him to publish his microscopic observations.   Gruby was awarded the M.D. degree in 1839, subsequently teaching anatomy and physiology
at the medical school.   He wrote a treatise on gross and
microscopic pathology which won him the offer of a professorship at Vienna.   Since the position was contingent on
his having himself baptized, he refused it.   In 1840, Roux,
Dupuytren's successor, invited him to Paris, and he worked
in several hospitals for the next eight years.   In 1841 he
proved that favus was fungal skin disease, unaware that
Schönlein had suggested that two years earlier.   Administrative obstacles finally defeated him, and in 1854 he gave
up research and entered private practice.   His patients
were the cultural leaders of the community, and he
achieved an extraordinary reputation as a practitioner.   He
is noteworthy not only for his remarkable life experience,
but also because he developed and retained the qualities of
a fine practitioner while pursuing his hobby of scientific
research.   There must have been many more like him, for
medicine otherwise could not have reached its present
level of development.

The case of psychiatry requires special comment.
The course of events in the rejuvenated medical school in
Vienna reveals differences in approach to psychiatry which
have occurred in this specialty for generations.   On the
one hand there were proponents of the so-called *mentalism*
that developed in Germany early in the 19th century.   In
Vienna the chief proponent of this view was von Feunchtersleben, Dean of the Medical School and Councilor
to the Emperor.   He was born in 1806, the son of a state
official of high rank.   His mother died when he was young,
and he spent 12 years at boarding school.   He proved to
be susceptible to brooding, depression, and hypochondriasis.
He studied oriental and other philosophies, and sought the
company of poets and artists.   His expressed wish to study
medicine was in large measure based upon a desire to

study mind-body relations, with emphasis on the role of the mind. His father finally consented, and the young von Feunchtersleben became a doctor at the age of 28. However, when the father committed suicide a short time later, the son had to go into practice. Four years later he published his *Dietetics of the Soul*, in praise of the healing power of one's own soul. He greatly admired Kant's writings in *The Power of the Mind to Control Morbid Feelings* and believed that physical symptoms were nothing but symbolic expressions of the Ego's thoughts. Von Feunchtersleben prospered, and his writings of the 1840s and 1850s went through repeated editions for nearly 50 years.

The opposing concept of psychiatry was exemplified by the views of Meynert, who also was raised in an artistic environment, the son of a writer and a singer in the Court Opera. Born in 1833 he acquired a reputation as a romantic poet as a young man. His other distinction during his youth was persistent loafing; however, after his graduation from medical school, which occurred late, he married a woman who gave direction to his life. In addition, one of his brothers-in-law happened to be an assistant to Rokitansky. After a period of, at most, nine months of clinical experience and a fairly extensive experience in the field of brain pathology, he applied for, and was given, permission to lecture in psychiatry, ultimately becoming Professor (Marx, 1971). Meynert conducted extensive studies on the pathology of the brain, and on the normal brain in humans and other mammals at different ages. He attempted to explain normal and pathological psychological phenomena on the basis of this information and, of course, was unsuccessful. On the other hand, his explanation of how a child develops consciousness of himself is, in my estimation, the only convincing one ever offered by anyone (Altschule, 1976).

Meynert's successor was von Krafft-Ebing, the finest clinician of his era in the field of psychiatry. He was sufficiently indiscreet to write a book then considered pornographic, *Psychopathia Sexualis*, and he lost much of his practice and reputation as a result. At about the time von Krafft-Ebing's career was approaching its close, Freud, a man of enormous ego, was beginning to formulate his views of mental function from fragments of the ideas of others. Although not given much attention at the time in Vienna, his dogma gained great prominence in America and wherever there was American influence after World War II, including Europe. Accordingly, whereas Vienna's contributions to nearly all branches of clinical medicine were highly beneficial, some were of mixed significance.

Thus Vienna, which should have been Leyden's heir, or at least should have followed the line taken by Paris, London, and Dublin, suffered a period of medical regression - superstition - in the early 19th century. Subsequently it was guided by von Turkheim, who recruited and furthered the careers of a group of remarkable physicians so that Vienna not only rejoined the mainstream of developments in clinical medicine, but became outstanding in it.

Chapter 13: Beginnings of the Definition of Syndromes and Concepts

WHEN SYDENHAM AND HIS FOLLOWERS BEGAN TO ISOLATE from the unformed mass of humorally defined conditions the syndromes that appeared distinct to them, the criteria they used were the clinical symptoms and their courses, plus some superficially evident physical findings. This approach, although valid, lacked precision and, hence, advanced clinical medicine little. The addition of the findings of pathological anatomy revealed at post-mortem became an effective means for the separation of syndromes that could not have been defined previously. Before this approach was developed to its fullest, percussion and auscultation were included as methods of characterizing specific disease states. Such new approaches, although developed in France, were not always well-received in that country, as was the case in Dublin and London; likewise, Germany criticized rather than praised. At about that time a few simple chemical tests were introduced, but it would be many decades before chemistry could be helpful to clinical practice. In addition, the antipathy that many French pathologists held toward the use of the microscope was not the situation elsewhere, and the use of this instrument later helped to distinguish syndromes. Although chemistry and microscopy were not ready to be used diagnostically early in the 19th century, collections of detailed information on the physical findings in life and anatomical findings post-mortem allowed for the distinction among syndromes. That happened with increasing rapidity through the middle of the century, subsequently slowing its pace but becoming more refined. (An exception to that statement was neurology, in which the most rapid advances occurred late in the century.) Most of the advances were made by practitioners.

Cardiology

In France Corvisart had made a good start toward distinguishing the various cardiac diseases early in the 19th century (Herrick, 1941; Luisada, 1944).   The next decades saw continued development with respect to valvular heart disease and congenital cardiac malformations (Luisada, 1944; East, 1957).   Most of those new definitions of cardiac diseases were originated by French, Irish, and English physicians.   Especially noteworthy were the contributions of the Dublin Group and Hope in london, with German authors entering the field later (Herrick, 1941).

Ideas about some other cardiac conditions had less than smooth developments (East, 1957).   Although Jenner and Heberden had emphasized that angina pectoris often accompanied coronary atherosclerosis, that connection was not acknowledged universally, because some persons with coronary atherosclerosis never had chest pain (Morgan, 1968).   The concept of such a relationship to coronary atherosclerosis received a further setback when Laennec declared that angina pectoris was merely an affection of the cardiac nerves rather than of the heart itself.   The idea that occlusion of a coronary artery could cause muscle necrosis, although demonstrated by Hammer in America, was rejected by Rokitansky and Virchow, who considered the necrosis merely a manifestation of chronic inflammation of some other origin.   Not until the clinical studies of Herrick and Levine were published in America in the early 20th century did the modern concept of coronary artery disease begin to take definitive form (Leibowitz, 1970).   The later clinicopathological work of Schlesinger and Blumgart greatly clarified some of the ambiguities.

The development of the concept that rheumatic fever was a cause of heart disease was also erratic. Around 1798 Pitcairne showed that acute rheumatism often preceded heart disease, a fact subsequently noted by a number of authors, including Jenner and Wells (Keil, 1936); therefore, the relationship between rheumatic fever and valvular heart disease was noted early.   Perhaps the earliest clinical account of the significance of rheumatic rashes and nodules in relation to rheumatic heart disease was in the work of Joseph Brown, a provincial doctor who practiced in towns near York and who was probably one of the first English physicians to use a stethoscope routinely. How that country doctor came to make his discoveries is worth analyzing.

Born a Quaker in Northumberland in 1784, Brown studied medicine in Edinburgh and London.   Despite his Quaker heritage, he joined the army in 1808 as an assistant surgeon and served with Wellington during the Peninsular Campaign, being present at a half-dozen battles, for which he was decorated six times.   After the Battle of Waterloo, he remained in France with the army of occupation until 1819, whereupon he retired on a pension.   He returned to Edinburgh to take his M.D. degree, married the widow of an officer killed at Waterloo, and started his practice in Sunderland.   Brown developed a large practice, became Chief of the Infirmary in that town, and also served as Mayor and Magistrate.   As mayor he worked actively to improve the housing of the poor.   His records suggest that he acquired a stethosocpe during his service in France and used it regularly on his return to England. Through his use of the stethoscope he acquired more accurate knowledge of heart disease than did others, estimating that in 50% of his patients with heart disease, rheumatic fever was the cause (Bedford *et al.*, 1976).   Of course, at that time the histopathology of rheumatic fever was not even imagined and, in fact, its development did not occur until a half-century after the use of the microscope was accepted in pathology.   Nevertheless, Brown's bedside studies yielded much significant information.

The subject of cardiac arrhythmias, today of major interest in medicine, could not be studied effectively in an era of pathological anatomy; rather, its growth had to be preceded by the polygraph and then the electrocardiograph. Nevertheless, for some time observant clinicians recognized the occurrence of very slow pulse or heart rates and their associated symptoms.   Although the names of Stokes and Adams quite properly are associated with the clinical syndrome of heart block, that striking disorder was noted by practitioners long before them (Flaxman, 1937).   Of greater interest is the possibility that Vesalius recorded a case of atrial fibrillation with pulse deficit, perhaps with peripheral embolization, due to cardiac mural thrombus (Leibowitz, 1963).

An important part of today's examination of the cardiovascular system is the measurement arterial blood pressure. As noted previously, the method of occlusion on which today's technique is based was described four centuries ago. However, as then proposed it was cumbersome and relatively inaccurate and, hence, was used little until Rivi-Rocca in the late 19th century developed the familiar cuff. The measurement of arterial blood pressure for clinical purposes was facilitated by the discoveries of Korotkov, a Russian military surgeon, about whom we know very little. (In fact, it is uncertain whether his photograph exists.) However, he made an outstanding contribution while stationed at a remote Siberian post during the Russo-Japanese War: He studied arterial wounds and described the arterial sounds we now use routinely in blood pressure measurements, evidently in order to alleviate boredom. There is nothing to indicate that this seemingly ordinary practitioner made any other discoveries.

Respiratory Disorders

The initial growth of the field of pulmonary and related diseases consisted mainly in scattered case reports from different parts of Europe. One notable exception was the discussion of asthma by Floyer around 1700, whose clinical writings added little to the subject. A century later Hutchinson described his invention of the water spirometer, a device still used today and with which he made approximately 4,000 measurements on patients. Hutchinson was more than a gadget inventor, for he made important clinical observations, including the familial tendency to tuberculosis and the occurrence of lung diseases in miners (Spriggs, 1971). He gained his clinical experience after graduating from London's University College, at which time he joined the staffs of the Brompton Hospital for Consumption, the Britannia Life Assurance Company, and other organizations. In addition to his clinical observations he made studies on the physiology of the lung and its subdivisions; however, his interests extended far beyond medicine and physiology. He had a fine ear for music and played the violin beautifully. In addition, he was an excellent draughtsman, painted in oils, cut silhouettes, and did creditable work in sculpture. When he went to the South Pacific in 1852, his career as an outstanding pulmonary physician rapidly came to an end. In Australia and Fiji he seems to have changed from a sensitive but precise and industrious person to an aggressive irresponsible one. The reasons for his migration and subsequent personality change are not known and, although there have been many conjectures, to this day they remain only conjectures. Hutchinson's concepts regarding lung function and the forces involved in breathing were used later by another practitioner, Salter, in his discussion of asthma (Neale, 1963). Salter's writings around midcentury not only described asthma in physiologic terms, but also emphasized the role of bronchospasm and recommended bronchodilatory drugs for treating the condition, a practice still pursued more than 100 years later. In addition, a good deal of clinical interest in artificial respiration (Baker, 1971) also occurred in the early 19th century. (Of course, mouth-to-mouth respiration had been described many centuries earlier in Kings II, 4, 34-35.)

The growth of understanding about pulmonary emphysema is an interesting story (Rosenblatt, 1969). The amount of information on this subject increased greatly during the 19th century, at first with contributions made mainly by French and English physicians, including Laennec, and then more and more by others. Similarly, the clinical picture of tuberculosis of the lungs was developed early by Laennec, then Stokes and others in England, and then Skoda in Vienna; but many other practitioners also made contributions. In contrast to that development was the story of the growth of knowledge about pleural effusion. After Emperor Leopold's death from pleural effusion, the Academy bearing his name put together a scholarly work in 1706 discussing the various features of that disorder and described its treatment - removal of the fluid through a trocar (Jarcho, 1971). The next contribution was the diagnostic discussion of Auenbrugger, who discovered percussion; but this was forgotten. A half-century later Corvisart republished Auenbrugger's discovery and emphatically called attention to the physical findings of fluid in the chest, after which the great stethoscopists of the era, notably Skoda, enlarged upon that topic.

Although the idea of pneumothorax for the treatment of tuberculosis is regarded as a recent discovery, it is far from recent, having been introduced in 1822 by Carson, an Edinburgh alumnus who had settled to practice in Liverpool (Cohen, 1963; Keers, 1980). The situation with respect to other treatments for tuberculosis is more complicated. The incidence of the disease began to decline long before control measures were introduced, even though the cause was unknown until Koch's discovery late in the 19th century. It was considered to be psychosomatic in origin and was treated by starvation and other measures aimed at quieting the passions. The modern approach was proposed by Bodington (Keers, 1980), born in 1799 in Warwickshire into a family that had been small landowners for 250 years. Educated at Oxford, he was apprenticed first at the age of 16 to a local physician and then a year later to another in London. He then studied at St. Bart's and was licensed in 1825, starting his practice in Birmingham, but soon moving to rural Warwickshire. His first publication was a critical comment in 1831 attacking the then-current treatment of cholera by bleeding and purging. In 1849 he wrote *On the Treatment and Cure of Pulmonary Consumption*, in which he denounced the accepted treatment with emetics, incarceration in closed rooms, and starvation. In its place he suggested rest plus moderate exercise, fresh (outdoor) air, a nutritious diet, and no medication except sedatives when needed. He took a house and received tuberculosis patients for his treatment. However, his book received little notice and no praise, and its review in the *Lancet* was notable even in those days for its scathing language. Discouraged, Bodington gave up his enterprise and finished his career as head of mental hospital. When he died in 1882, the *Lancet* obituary praised him as the unacknowledged originator of the sanatorium treatment for tuberculosis, which became and remained the standard treatment until the development of antibiotic therapy in recent decades.

The problem of lung cancer evidently troubled the leading clinicians of early 19th-century Dublin and London (Onuigbo, 1959), who recognized that its signs and symp-

toms were nonspecific. To some the progressive course of
the disease without response to treatment was suggestive
of the diagnosis, and the early occurrence of brain metastasis also aroused comment. Involvement of the cervical
sympathetic ganglia as caused by metastasis also was
known to practitioners more than a century ago.

In short, records indicate that the development of
concepts and recognition of syndromes of respiratory disorders proceeded actively in the early and middle decades of
the 19th century. Such an explosion of information occurred at a rate nearly equal to that associated with cardiology, and both were due to the combination of bedside
observation and post-mortem study.

Cancer and the Cell Theory

The subject of cancer concerned many physicians of
the early 19th century. A collaborative endeavor in 1803
led to the formation in England of the Institution for the
Investigation and Cure of Cancer, whose members hoped to
use the information being accumulated by clinicians and
pathologists to discover that elusive revelation of cause
that always seems to be the Holy Grail of cancer re-
searchers in modern medicine. Because of the lack of accomplishment, the Institution collapsed after a few years
(Triolo, 1969). Nevertheless, physicians still were required
to treat the condition, and although surgical approaches
were used from early times (Onuigbo, 1962), the treatment,
surgical or other, did not lead to any organized logical
formulations. Part of the problem resulted from the
marked differences in ideas about cancer which physicians
had held through the ages (Ackerknecht, 1958). An important hindrance to any advance was the concern of European physicians for theoretical considerations. For centuries medicine had perpetuated the superstition of body
humors, and despite the physical and mathematical concepts
brought forward to explain symptoms, such concepts still
were based on the assumption that humors really existed
throughout the body, although in local sites they might be
abnormally thick or thin, acid or alkaline, hot or cold, wet
or dry, or any combination of them. When pathologists

began to describe and define entirely local lesions, they were regarded as heretics and often scornfully called localists, solidists, or, in the worst cases, localist-solidists. Thus as late as 1846 when Warren in Boston performed the first surgical removal of a tumor under ether anesthesia, the event was hailed by some as a great advance in surgical technique, whereas others praised it only as a bold solidist approach.   The confused and - to some of us today - absurd conceptions of the nature of tissues will not be presented, since such concepts, based on incomplete and often erroneous data, have been discussed at length by others (Rather, 1969B, 1978; Rousseau, 1970; Belloni, 1971; Pickstone, 1973; Huard, 1974).   Virchow's application of the cell theory to oncology sidestepped much of this nonsense and was the most successful of all of his uses of the theory (Ackerknecht, 1958).

The slogan *omnis cellula est cellula*, which Virchow adopted rather late, was held earlier by others such as Remak and Kölliker and is called diplomatically the Remak-Virchow theory by one authority (Ackerknecht, 1958).   But Virchow's main accomplishment was the destruction of earlier dogmatic credibility by pointing out errors, a task at which he disregarded reputations.   He forced the great Rokitansky to withdraw his humoral concept of "crasis," a reformulation of Cruvilhier's early ideas about "cancer juice," which he used to explain cancer, among other things.   The cell theory that Virchow finally supported was far from Schwann's and Schleiden's erroneous ideas about cells, ideas that Virchow espoused for a long time. Schwann's formulation has been called a happy intuition, which it was, for it was not based on adequate data. When intuitionists' broad generalizations are accepted and details are required, inadequacies invariably are revealed. The early history of the cell theory illustrates that fact.

Part of the difficulty arises from the fact that we cannot be certain of what the observers actually saw.   In the case of Hewson, the 18th-century associate of the Hunters, there is little doubt that he saw and accurately described the red blood cell.   But what about the Frenchmen Milne-Edwards, Raspail, and Dutrochet?   Pickstone (1973) doubts that they could distinguish among cells, other structures, and the numerous artifacts resulting from poor microscope lens systems.   This is clearly the case with Milne-Edwards, but may not be with the others.   In Dutrochet's book, *Recherches Anatomiques et Physiologiques Sur la Structure Intime des Animaux et des Vegetaux et Sur Leur Motilité* (1824), the cellular structure of tissues and the fact that growth consisted of the formation of new individual cells were discussed.   In addition, he described what he called *endosmosis*, or the action of the osmotic force.   His illustrations were few and crude, but no more crude than some of Virchow's, which were done 40 years later.   How much of this was detailed observation and how much happy intuition stimulated by incomplete observation is unknown.   Raspail's idea of the fundamental nature of living matter certainly is based on a form of cell theory, as was shown by his *Nouveau Synthese de Chimie Organique* (1833).   Schwann's book published in 1839 had a specific section called *Theorie der Zellen*, so Schwann must be credited at least with naming the theory (Maulitz, 1971; Watermann, 1960).   When Purkinje reviewed that book he politely pointed out that he and his colleague had been studying cells for years (Kruta, 1971).   In fact Müller, who had taught both Schwann and Virchow, wrote the book *Ueber den Feineren Bau und die Formen der Krankhaften Geschwulste* (1838), in which he tried to distinguish the various forms of cancer both histologically and chemically.   He was much more successful with the former than the latter, and his observations actually were a basis of Virchow's extensive writings on the subject.

Many scientists objected to, and rightly so, using the word "cell" to designate the structure under consideration, but Virchow's use not only of the concept, but of the term, established them both unequivocally.   His brilliant lectures were an important factor in that acceptance (Wilson, 1944, 1947).   Virchow incorporated into his thinking two gross errors made by Schwann: that new cells developed from a hypothetical amorphous substance that Schwann called *phytoblastema* by a process similar to crystallization, although a number of leading workers could find no evidence of either the substance or the process (Wilson, 1944; 1947); and, concerning the very nature of the cell, that the wall was the important structure (hence the term "cell"), a view rejected by most others (but not at first by Virchow).

The contribution of Goodsir of Edinburgh, who in 1845 defined the cell as a functional entity, must not be forgotten. However, the confusion was not resolved until 1861, when Schultze defined the cell as a mass of protoplasm with a nucleus. (Purkinje had invented the term "protoplasm.") The title of Schultze's paper, "On muscle fibres and what has been called a cell," is revealing. Virchow's forcefulness and his enthusiastic following established a trend in studying tumors in term of cells, and Müller's previous observation of the embryonic undifferentiated appearance of some tumor cells gave direction to that study. Although it would be years before the technical developments introduced by Müller, Purkinje, and others would have their full effects on tumor study, the problem of cancer thus was given its present orientation. One early consequence of the spreading application of microscopy was the simultaneous discovery, by three different observers, of leukemia.

Such a recital of names and dates cannot convey adequately in the present what the contemporaries of early 19th-century observers believed. Information bearing that matter may be found in reports of the discovery of *Trichinella spiralis* in 1835. On February 2, 1835 a first-year student at St. Bart's, Paget, discovered the parasite in the tissues of a cadaver he was dissecting. Four days later he reported his findings before a local medical group, stating, as if it were a matter of common usage, that the worm was imbedded in "cellular tissue" (Campbell, 1969). It appears that the cell theory at least was accepted by the medical students. Paget continued his studies using a microscope borrowed from Brown, the botanist, who by then already had been recognized as an observer of the cell nucleus. Did Paget - and Brown - owe more to Dutrochet's 1828 paper than to those of the German microscopist of the 1830s? There is no way of knowing.

Infections

The fact that infections spread as epidemics has been noted recurrently in recorded history. Bubonic plague most often was regarded in this connection (Dols, 1976), but cholera could cause as much individual terror and general disorganization as the plague (McGrew, 1960). Although physicians were not in agreement concerning the mechanism of epidemic spread, there is no doubt that many of them, and some laymen, believed in contagion, for those who were able left an area at the approach of an epidemic. Exclusive of such signs and portents as comets and two-headed calves, the causes of infection most widely accepted were miasmas and animalcules. Although the belief in invisible living organisms as causes of infections existed in ancient Roman times, the majority of physicians believed in miasmas - putrid or poisonous airs coming out of rotting, swampy, or otherwise unhealthy soil. Nevertheless, the outnumbered so-called "animalculists" maintained their hypothesis against the more numerous so-called "miasmatists." Fracastoro and Kircher wrote about *contagium animatum* centuries ago; indeed, Kircher claimed to have seen "tiny worms" in the blood of people dying from the plague. Nevertheless, the 1546 theory of Fracastoro - like the later concepts expressed by Henle (1840) - had been dismissed for not providing *evidence* of an animalcular theory (Howard-Jones, 1977). The fact that Bonomo and Cestosi, pupils of Fracastoro, proved in 1687 that human scabies were caused by a mite that bored into the skin was not considered supportive evidence of the germ theory of disease. The first corroborative *evidence* of the animalcule theory resulted from a study of a disease of silkworms. Bassi, a lawyer and government official-turned-farmer, showed that material from diseased silkworms could cause that disease in others. The infectious agent later was shown to be a fungus. Those observations, published in 1835, were made by a man handicapped by failing vision, absence of formal training, and a lack of support from a learned organization (Major, 1944). Bassi's observations, however important in theory, had nothing to do with human disease. The application of the germ theory to human disease remained in the realm of hypothesis

(Bulloch, 1938; Shryock, 1972).   Nevertheless, even in America there were animalculists in Charleston, South Carolina, Philadelphia, Baltimore, and New York, who insisted on their ideas (Allen, 1947), as did Bartlett of New England.   In 1839 Schönlein suggested the fungal origin of favus, and two years later, independently, Gruby in Vienna proved it.   In the meantime, animal experiments with infected blood pointed more and more to the causative role of microorganisms (Bulloch, 1938).

Bacteriology came into existence as a science well before it became useful to physicians in the practice of medicine.   When Davaine apparently discovered the anthrax bacillus in the blood of infected animals, he started a controversy that became entangled in another controversy, the nature of septicemia (Bulloch, 1938).   The work of Pasteur clarified many issues not only in the nascent bacteriology, but also in biochemistry.   Subsequently his work, and that of his colleagues, increasingly became directed to bacteriology as a separate discipline.

Pasteur has been discussed widely as a man, a scientist, and a benefactor of mankind (Duclaux, 1920; Moschocowitz, 1948; Dubos, 1950).   His discoveries, which saved the silkworm and wine industries of France, evoked great enthusiasm that was not shared among physicians, at least those in countries other than France.   From 1859 through 1864 Pasteur participated in a celebrated debate on spontaneous generation.   The usual accounts emphasize scientific issues; but there were political issues as well (Farley and Geison, 1974).   The idea that his position (which varied over the years) was influenced by political and social factors that waxed and waned as the Second Empire waxed, throve, and collapsed in no way diminishes the importance of his experimental work, which, in science, is all that matters.   Pasteur's transformation from chemist to biologist and, finally, to medical scientist, brought him forcibly to the attention of physicians.   His work on the role of microorganisms in putrefaction directly influenced Lister's work on infections in patients, thereby leading to the discovery of surgical antisepsis.   Of even greater interest to physicians was Pasteur's use of attenuated organisms to develop vaccines against anthrax, fowl cholera, swine erysipelas and, then, most sensationally, rabies.   The

Pasteur Institute, established in 1888, continued Pasteur's research in the area of immunology and resistance. The work of Pasteur, a nonmedical scientist, gradually became of direct importance to clinical medicine; indeed, it gave medical practice an entirely new character. The observation in 1884 by Theobold Smith - that *killed* microorganisms are just as effective as *attenuated* ones in inducing immunity - further encouraged practical attempts to stimulate immune processes in medical practice.

At about the same time, other aspects of bacteriology as related to medicine were being explored in Germany. Koch, a graduate of Göttingen practicing medicine in a town in Posen, evidently was dissatisfied with the amount of help bacteriology was giving to clinical medicine. Almost singlehandedly he undertook the transformation of bacteriology along practical lines without, however, diminishing its status as science. He and his coworkers developed methods of staining, isolation and cultivation, and sterilization. In rapid succession German workers isolated a dozen bacteria and showed them to be causes of specific diseases. Koch's discovery of the tubercle bacillus provided his worldwide fame, and although it was of great help in diagnosing the condition, it proved useless for its treatment. When von Behring discovered how to make an antitoxin for the treatment of diphtheria, a disease commonly fatal until that time, there was much hope that the same approach could be used to cure most bacterial infections; but that hope was realized only with respect to tetanus.

Thus, the late decades of the 19th century saw the extraordinary growth of the science of bacteriology, but its content would not become of daily importance to practitioners for many more decades; in fact, there were many physicians who still rejected the germ theory of disease or suggested alternative explanations (Richmond, 1954a,b; Cassedy, 1962; Landing, 1962). Many prominent clinicians were reluctant to accept the idea that bacteria could be primary causes of disease (Philip, 1932). Virchow was also skeptical and, in fact, his skepticism was considered a hindrance to the acceptance of the clinical value of the new science of bacteriology. Finally, von Behring directed a 68-page blast at Virchow as a culmination of years of violent exchanges (von Behring, 1893).   American medical schools were slow to establish bacteriologic laboratories (Kramer, 1948).   The adaptation of discoveries made by bacteriologists applied not only to medicine, but to public health (Kramer, 1948; Rosen, 1958).   The public-health movement had languished until the findings of bacteriologists began to be used by public officials.   The benefits of those public health measures based on bacteriologic findings were easier to demonstrate than most others and, hence, gave the public-health movement of the late 19th and early 20th centuries an appearance of phenomenal momentum.

The widespread acceptance of bacteriology as a valid part of medical practice, in contrast to its clear place among the medicine-related sciences, actually came through surgery and not medicine.   It was Lister's work in Great Britain, and that of his followers in America, that originally gave bacteriology much of its support as a branch of clinical practice (Brieger, 1966).   It should be noted that Lister's work had its origin in his longstanding interest in inflammation.   Lister was born in Essex, England, the son of Joseph Jackson Lister, who became famous for inventions that perfected the microscope.   The elder Lister was elected Fellow of the Royal Society as a result of his discoveries.   Young Lister announced his interest in surgery while very young and actually began to study anatomy when he was 16 years old.   He entered the University of London and there obtained the bachelor's degree in 1847 and the medical degree in 1852.   He had been encouraged to do physiological work, chiefly on structures innervated by the sympathetic nervous system; but, when he became House Surgeon at the University College Hospital, he immediately came face-to-face with the dreadful facts of traumatic and postoperative infections (Edgar, 1961).   He resolved to try to lower the prevailing death rate of 20% to 60%, or more, and went to Edinburgh where he worked for seven years in surgery and in the study of the physiology of inflammation (Best, 1970).   Lister observed that in hospital gangrene a wound consisted of decomposing flesh full of tiny bodies, which he thought was a kind of fungus.   (This discovery came 17 years after Simpson's work on hospital cross-infection [Selwyn, 1965].)

By that time Pasteur had shown that fermentation and decomposition were similar in that they were caused by living microorganisms. Lister tried various approaches designed to destroy these organisms, finally deciding on carbolic acid, which worked well. In 1860 he became Professor of Surgery at Glasgow and expanded his studies of the suppurative process. Eight years later he returned to London, this time as Professor at King's College.

Lister published the results of his treatment with carbolic acid in the *Lancet* in 1867 and established antisepsis as a basis of successful surgery. Although his work was substantiated in many medical centers in Europe, in Great Britain his research first evoked bitter criticism. For example, Bennett, Professor of Physiology at Edinburgh and an expert microscopist, called germs imaginary, and most of the leading surgeons of Great Britain either attacked or ridiculed Lister. However, younger surgeons tried and succeeded with his methods. On the other hand, the military surgeons on both sides in the Franco-Prussian War ignored his work, and their patients paid for that neglect with their lives. By 1877, ten years after the publication of his method, there was widespread agreement about its efficacy. In the Russo-Japanese War 35 years later, the Japanese used Lister's method, and it proved its value once more. Lister's demonstration - under clinical conditions - of the validity and applicability of bacteriology was instrumental in the acceptance by many physicians of the germ theory of disease.

It is noteworthy that evidence, nearly as strong as Lister's, in support of a germ theory had been found in discoveries about childbed fever. In 1795 Gordon of Aberdeen showed that such a disease was transmissible (Porter, 1958). In Boston in 1843 Holmes called attention to Gordon's work, quoting several extracts from it, and then added his own supporting observations. However, Holmes did not know of the similar work of Simpson of Edinburgh in 1840, because it did not become published until ten years later (Selwyn, 1965). At that time Simpson called attention to Semmelweis' report, in 1847, which caused a furor in Vienna upon its publication not only because of its specific ideas but, perhaps even more so, because of the repressive atmosphere there. In any case, despite the strong and unanimous evidence of the transmissibility of puerperal sepsis, the then-current animalcular theory was too vague to be accepted in connection with childbed fever. In contrast, when Lister proposed his new clinical ideas, there was a body of scientific knowledge, however skimpy, which made them credible. That important principle - that clinical observations gain acceptance if explainable by whatever scientific material is available at the time - still is operative today. Although bacteriologic concepts were to play a great part in the development of surgical technique in the late 19th century, the large role of bacteriology in medicine did not come into full development until the mid-20th century. Before that time, although physicians had to integrate some bacteriology into their medical ideas, they did not have to take it into account in daily practice as frequently as they do now.

Clinical Pathology

Another nascent field - one that was to grow to monstrous size on inflated importance in the 20th century - was clinical pathology, perhaps more properly called laboratory medicine. In the middle decades of the 19th century serious efforts were exerted to utilize in clinical practice what the microscope revealed and what the simple chemistry of the time indicated. The works of Andral were outstanding, but there were many other studies being conducted, particularly in hematology (Verso, 1961, 1964, 1971). Counting methods for blood cells and color tests for hemoglobin were worked out laboriously. Examination of the urine emphasized the great variety of crystals that could be found after urine "stood." Heat coagulation was used to detect protein, and chemical tests were available for showing the presence of bile and glucose. Microscopy was used also to study the sputum (Finlayson, 1958). Textbooks of laboratory medicine began to appear (Foster, 1959, 1963), but the concepts, methods, and data presented in those books were used only rarely in clinical practice until the end of the century, and then sparingly at that. Nevertheless, leukemia was discovered independently and simultaneously by Bennett in England, Donne in France, and Virchow in Germany by applying microscopy to clinical problems.   Since the routine use of laboratory tests in medicine was unknown, the significance of the tests often was not considered by the practitioners of that era.

The future information explosion in bacteriology and clinical pathology was not anticipated and did not become burdensome to 19th-century practitioners.   It did affect those of the 20th century, at which time clinical pathology grew to such an extent that it often impaired, and in some cases destroyed, the doctor-patient relationship.

Deficiency Diseases

Reference has been made to London physicians who defined diseases of the kidneys, the adrenal glands and, although not widely appreciated, nutritional deficiency.   Deficiency diseases require additional comment.   Nutritional deficiency was not disregarded totally, for the writings on the dietary treatment of scurvy were well known before the start of the 19th century, and the fact that rickets and xeropthalmia were deficiency diseases also was suspected.

The history of beri-beri, another deficiency disease, is more complicated; moreover, it reveals the beginnings of the conflict outside Europe between clinical and scientific medicine.   That story concerns the career of Takaki of the Imperial Japanese navy.   Born in Kyushu, the son of a master carpenter, he began to study the Chinese classics at the age of eight, but soon showed a preference for medicine.   At 17 he went to Kagashima, the provincial capital, and became apprenticed to Ishigama, who had studied Dutch medicine at Nagasaki.   (Dutch physicians acquired their knowledge of acupuncture in Nagasaki, from which they brought it to Europe in 1682.)   A civil war having broken out, Takaki and his master went to Tokyo to serve in the army, at which point Takaki became acutely aware that his knowledge of medicine was poor.   When the new Kaisei Medical School opened in Kagashima in 1869, with Ishigama on the faculty, Takaki entered it.   In 1870 Wills, an Edinburgh alumnus, was invited to head the Kaisei medical School. Wills had been in Japan since 1861, and in 1869 was made Head of the Tokyo Major Hospital, which became part of the Faculty of Medicine of the University of Tokyo in 1870. Wills left the University in 1878 because the new medical school was determined to follow the German scientific model, not the English patient-oriented model; indeed, the new faculty included German medical scientists brought in from Germany. In the meantime Takaki's old master had become Administrator of the Tokyo Naval Hospital and, in 1873, he invited Anderson, a graduate of St. Thomas in London, to head it. Takaki joined the Imperial Japanese Navy as a surgeon in 1872 and in 1875 was sent to London to study at St. Thomas'. He had an outstanding record there, taking the highest honors. On returning home in 1880 he was made Chief of the Tokyo Naval Hospital. He established unofficial discussion and research groups there and then later at the Tokyo Hospital, a voluntary institution. All of the non-naval enterprises were supported by the Navy. (In 1891 Takaki's group became the Tokyo Jiku-Kai Jin Medical School, now the Jiku University Medical School.) Also in 1880 Takaki had studied the occurrence of beri-beri and had ruled out climate, weather, geography, crowding, clothing, and, in fact, all factors except diet. Persons who ate vegetables and meat did not develop the disease. He risked his status by sending out a ship on a long cruise. Under such circumstances the crew might have been expected to contract beri-beri, but they did not develop the disease because they were given officer's rations. He presented his findings in 1882, but could not say which element in food, by its presence or absence, had caused the disorder in the crews of previous cruises. The German-trained and German-oriented faculty of the University of Tokyo derided him, convinced, as were most high-ranking authorities everywhere, that the new science of German bacteriology held the secret of the cause of beri-beri. (Some clinicians were convinced that the disease was of dietary origin, albeit nonspecific [Carter, 1977].) The uncertainty regarding the nature of any dietary deficiency caused authorities to turn to the prevailing view that all diseases were due to bacteria. In accordance with that view, the Dutch government sent Pekelharring and Winkler to Java to study the disease, and their assistant was the German-trained bacteriologist, Eijkman. Although Eijkman remained, the other two returned to Europe, and stated that the disease was indeed of bacterial origin, but that they had yet to identify the organism. Eijkman's studies in animals showed that a diet of polished rice caused the disease, and his surveys of human populations supported this conclusion (Carter, 1977). By 1910 the conclusion was accepted by many; but, the bacterial-origin theory did not disappear. Some held that polished rice permitted the production of a bacterial toxin; in fact, Eijkman himself believed in a toxin at first. However, Grijns proposed that white rice lacked an essential substance. For years his conclusion received little notice, because the bacteria/toxin notion took a long time to die.

At that time there seemed to be only two deficiency diseases, scurvy and beri-beri, because Budd's work on rickets and Vitamin A deficiency remained ignored.

Industrial Medicine

Another aspect of early 19th century medicine that came to the fore concerned the effects of industrial changes on health. By then the Industrial Revolution was established and its result, the factory system, particularly with respect to cotton and woolen manufacturing, had not yet come under regulation. In England one of the medical leaders of factory-labor reform was Thachrah of Leeds who, after early education in the classics, went to London to study with Cooper and at Guy's Hospital. (His schoolmate was John Keats, who only a few years later was to die of tuberculosis.) After being licensed, he returned to Leeds to practice, but did poorly. He established a private medical school; however, it was refused recognition. Moreover, he quarreled with the established and respected physicians of the town and led a faction undertaking to remove their responsibility for medical education. A few years later all were reconciled and together formed the Leeds Medical School, on whose faculty Thachrah served. After fathering an illegitimate son, he married a woman other than its mother. The only child of this legal union died at a young age.   Having done badly in private practice, he became town physician to the poor and made recommendations for improving their deplorable housing.   At that time Leeds was becoming a great manufacturing city, attracting so many country people that the poor population grew phenomenally, increasing even more by the influx of many distressed Irish people after the suppression of the Irish revolt.   In 1831 Thachrah published a book entitled, *The Effects of the Principal Arts, Trades and Professions and of Civic States and Habits of Living on Health and Longevity*, which quickly made him famous; he published a revised edition a few years later.   It was a highly original work, one of the most original since Ramazzini's *De Morbis Artificium* (1713) and its later English and French translations and adaptations.   Thachrah's catalogue of diseases included inhalation of iron particles by machinists and cast-filers, lead poisoning among plumbers and house painters, arsenic poisoning among wallpaper stainers, mercury poisoning among mirror makers, and zinc-fume poisoning among makers of gilt buttons.   He considered intemperance "the great bane of civilized life" and noted the social degradation that it often caused among laborers. Although written in a warm and sympathetic vein, his book is free from the nauseating sentimentality and self-righteous indignation impairing the works of many reformers. Through it all Thachrah remained the calm, meticulous observer of the clinical manifestations of a social upheaval, the Industrial Revolution (Meikeljohn, 1957).   However, his remarks about the occupational hazards of doctors no longer apply:

> Anxiety of mind does more, I conceive, to impair health than breach of sleep, nocturnal exposure, or irregularity in meals.   The body suffers from the mind.   That sense of responsibility which every conscientious practitioner must feel - the anxious zeal, which makes him throw his mind and feelings, into cases of especial danger or difficulty - break down the frame, change the face of hilarity to that of seriousness and care, and bring on premature age.

Thachrah died at an early age of tuberculosis after a life of frequent and prolonged illness, but his work played an important role in the factory reform movement in England.   In America an attempt was made to avoid or circumvent the more awful horrors introduced by the factory system.   In fact, the Boston industrialists created new communities - whole cities - in the northern part of Massachusetts which were supposed to provide physically and morally ideal surroundings.   Apparently that was accomplished, although problems related to crowding still occurred (Rosen, 1944), initiating a debate in which Bartlett took place.   Despite the lack of any immediate decision, the debate probably did influence the factory laws here.

One disease that Thachrah's work did not discuss was necrosis of the jaw (called "phossy jaw" in England). The first writings on this subject were in 1845.   Factories for the manufacture of phosphorus-tipped matches by then had been functioning for 10 or 15 years in England, France, Austria, and Prussia.   In 1846 Vienna took the lead in promulgating regulations to control the hazards of the industry, and the document stating those regulations showed appreciation of that disease and the laws needed to prevent it (Proskauer, 1942).   The unending work of controlling and preventing industrial hazards was begun energetically well over a century ago.

Aging

In 1863 Maclachlan, Physician to the Royal Hospital for Veterans at Chelsea, wrote his book, *The Diseases and Infirmities of Advanced Life* because, he said, nothing much had been written on the subject in English.   An Edinburgh graduate, he had served in the Army with a Highland regiment for 12 years and then had been appointed Physician and Surgeon to the Chelsea Hospital for Veterans, serving there for 23 years.   His book is remarkably modern, for he mentioned elevated blood cholesterol levels, low urine specific gravity, low vital capacity, and softening of the bones:

Diseases accumulate with the progress of years.   The innumerable maladies that openly or secretly besiege the frame leave sequelae, are grafted upon each other, and present themselves associated and complicated in such wise as to diversify the character of the symptoms and modify the prognosis and treatment...it is in old people especially that the anatomist encounters the most singular modifications of structure, and the pathologist the most perfect and varied specimens of disease, benign or malignant, in the brain, heart, lungs and other viscera.

His observations, together with the material he collected from foreign writings, provided a broad yet detailed account of the aging of the body (Howell, 1973).   Senile dementia had been described in France by Esquirol in the 1840s, although ancient Greeks, and others in the interval, had commented on it.   The syndrome of senile psychosis later came to be considered a consequence of cerebral atherosclerosis, which it is not.

The scanty literature on the medical aspects of aging written before 1900 is in marked contrast to the voluminous printed material on prolonging life (Gruman, 1961). Those works have one thing in common: They all recommend moderation in all things, except, of course, moderation.   When Hufeland of Leipzig wrote his work on the subject in 1797, he coined the interesting term, "makrobiotic."

Comment

This account, however fragmentary, of the content of clinical medicine in the middle decades of the 19th century shows that there was an information explosion.   The magnitude of this explosion today is recognized easily, but its effects on the medical practitioners of the time only can be imagined.   It must have been stimulating, confusing, and disquieting in varying degrees simultaneously.   The 19th-century information explosion in medicine was much

less serious than the current explosion: the former consisting of material shown by practitioners to be of the
substance of medicine; the latter including masses of material not related to clinical conditions or misleading because
they are too artifactual to use.   The current situation
places unbearable pressure on today's practitioners: Not
only must they decide for themselves what is applicable
and what is not, but they must also be courageous enough
to stand by their decisions in this regard.   Any courage
that physicians might generate in this connection is likely
to be washed away by the near certainty of malpractice
suits.   Although the physicians of a century ago did not
have to face these peculiarly American difficulties, they
still had the problem of blending what was then the new
with what was at that time already the old.   Many could
not make the necessary mental adjustments, but many others could.   Regardless of whether they could or could not,
the younger ones soon would have to face more floods of
information.   Two new approaches were developing: bacteriology and clinical pathology, the former having major effects on clinical practice in the last decades of the century and the latter beginning to do so at the very end.
In the meantime, medicine as it was known, say, in 1850,
did not stand still.   Using the clinical and pathological
methods then current, it too was expanding rapidly.   Virchow's was the only recorded complaint of overwhelmed
physicans that I could find.

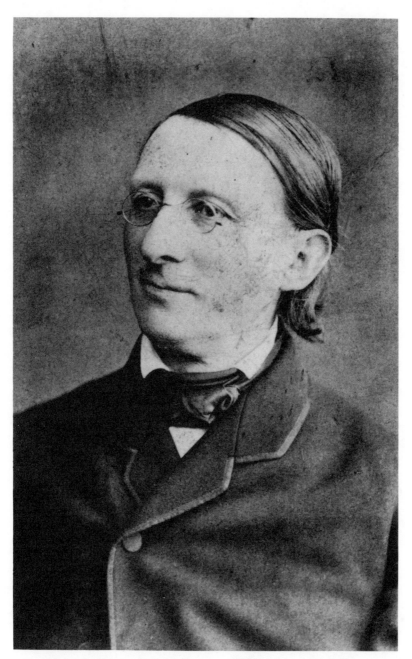

Karl Friedrich Wilhelm Ludwig, 1816–1895

Chapter 14: Medicine in Nineteenth-Century Germany

THE COURSE OF MEDICAL EVENTS IN NORTHERN ITALY, the Netherlands, Great Britain, and Ireland, France, the Austro-Hungarian Empire, and even America forms a consistent pattern. Even though this pattern is not completely uniform and the span of time involved is about 200 years, a sequence can be defined that agrees with the events that occurred. Regrettably this statement does not refer to what is now Germany. The reasons for the incomplete participation of that country in the medical developments that occurred in the rest of the Western World are undoubtedly many. In considering the events in the other countries, it was shown that the Baconian philosophy in England and the Locke-derived sensationist philosophy in France facilitated two processes that helped to free medicine from ancient superstitions. Those processes were the development of the practice of patient-oriented medicine and the study of medicine-related science. The philosophies of Bacon and Locke permitted the spread of the processes, but they did not invent them, for the two processes had begun in Northern Italy long before that time. If the Franco-English Enlightenment had any effect, it was attenuating the popularity of iatrochemistry and iatromathematics, although these two superstitions remained strong in the Netherlands and in Great Britain. Indeed, the decline of iatrochemistry in Edinburgh was accompanied by the rise of another superstition, the Brunonian, albeit for only a short time. In England and Ireland, the independence of the teaching hospitals and, in France, the relative autonomy of the hospitals are correlated strikingly with the rapid modernization of clinical medicine in those countries in the early 19th century. That did not occur in authoritarian Central Europe. Although German medical education of the late 18th and early 19th centuries did recognize the importance of bedside instruction, the level of that instruction was fixed where it had been in Leyden; that is, all history-taking and inspection (Choulant, 1920). Perhaps it was in-

nate conservatism that caused German medical teachers to
reject the new methods of auscultation and percussion, and
the mode of using pathological anatomy as the basis of
teaching; or, perhaps it was distaste for anything French
after their Revolution and the behavior of their Empire.
(However, in Germany some journals were published in
French, German not being considered sufficiently elegant.)
At any rate, for whatever reason, German medicine
strongly leaned toward dogma. This was by no means universal, for some influential physicians like Hufeland rejected dogma. Hufeland edited a journal in 1795 whose
policy emphatically stated that it would publish only those
papers based on observation. However, many leading German physicians, noting that earlier dogmas (*e.g.*, those of
Hoffman and Stahl) demonstrated a lack of utility, felt a
need for a new certainty in medicine. Curiously, Kant
supplied it, stating that if one knew the appropriate basic
facts, one could work out easily, by reason alone, all answers to all questions. It is confusing to find that he distinguished between reason and understanding. He declared
that the Brunonian superstition provided the one basic item
needed, and this pronouncement was received with enthusiasm, or perhaps relief, in Germany (Rosen, 1951; Risse,
1972, 1976). Such a fragmentary reference to that aspect
of Kant's philosophy certainly does no justice to his philosophy as a whole, but there is no need for a detailed
consideration of it at this time.

After a brief interval a new German dogma -
"Naturphilosophie" - arose, and it was given standing in
medicine by Oken, a biologist, and by Schelling, a Professor of Philosophy, who had studied natural science and
medicine. Oken's main thesis was that natural science
should be pursued as the study of the everlasting transmu-
tations of the Holy Ghost in the world. Schelling's view
was even more vague. That philosophy arose during a period not of Enlightenment, similar to that of Great Britain
and France, but during a period of *Aufklarung*, or elucida-
tion, of the philosophy of Kant and his successors, since
that philosophy was acceptable, albeit unclear. According
to a recent work (Engelhardt, 1976), there were actually
three kinds of "Naturphilosophie." One was based on
Kant's writings, and its concern was establishing the nec-

essary *a priori* considerations supposedly underlying all knowledge. A second type - metaphysical "Naturphilosophie" - had different aims, as expounded by Hegel and Schelling, who did not agree with each other. Hegel's basic premise was that all matter was appearance, as well as notion, and since the notion did not agree with the appearance, a process had to be devised to abolish the difference. That basic premise had no evident utility in either the theory or practice of medicine and, in fact, there was no likelihood that such an abstractly generated concept could be used to gain an understanding of any phenomenon encountered anywhere. That fact was not acceptable to Schelling, who claimed to have invented a system that gave certainty to clinical medicine. Schelling and his followers stated that the way to gain understanding about some phenomenon was to consider the phenomenon, then seek and study its opposite, combine the two - thesis and antithesis - and the *synthesis* would be the desired answer. Such a relatively simple, if unworkable, concept was complicated by Schelling's view that each being, living or nonliving, fulfilled the purpose for which it was created by individuation of its assigned role. All that had to be done was to discover the assigned role. A leader in their school of thought was the physician Kieser (Brednow, 1970). The followers of that brand of "Naturphilosophie" called themselves *"Gesellschaft Deutscher Naturforscher und Arzte,"* and their influence was localized to Germany. After the arrival in America of German refugees from the 1848 revolution, Philadelphia established a journal called *Zeitschrift für Naturforscher und Arzte*; but it lasted only for a short time. Years later, when he was a professor at Harvard College, Aggasiz recalled his experiences as a student and young researcher in Switzerland (then under Prussian control) when the "mania" of fanatics led to the invasion of "every center of scientific activity" in Germany by "Naturphilosophie." With Brown's superstitious system shown to be nonsense, and Schelling's brand of "Naturphilosophie" soon shown to be absurd, new ways of discovering and organizing information in medical education and practice became necessary. They were forthcoming.

Schönlein, who ended as Professor at Berlin, founded what was called the Natural History School, a system in which diseases were classified arbitrarily into groups following the Linnaean method. Although Schönlein was evidently a good thinker (combining chemical and hemotologic studies with percussion and auscultation), he was neither a good physician nor a popular teacher. He was gruff most of the time or else shied away from all contacts with others. Whatever he and his pupils gained from their up-to-date methods of examination, they lost by trying to make their findings fit the Procustean classification upon which he insisted. His dogma lasted only for a brief period.

Although medical specialties are not discussed in depth in this work, German psychiatry in the first half of the 19th century is of particular interest. The concepts of German philosophy, particularly that of "Natur-philosophie," were given particularly prominent roles in the branch of medicine concerned with mental disease. It is useful today to think of the German psychiatry of that period as a continuum (although the philosophers then would disagree). In the case of Kant, if one grants him his definitions and axioms, it is possible to understand what he says, without necessarily accepting all or any of it. At the next level in our arbitrarily constructed continuum, that of Hegel, the situation is different: One is never sure whether or not one is being victimized. Fortunately his tenets are not important to clinical medicine. At the third and lowest level (or perhaps the highest if one goes by the content of hot air), that of Schelling and his followers in medicine, the content quickly reveals itself as an indigestible mixture of sentimental and theological dogma blended, and a philosophy intended to be speculative but actually in the realm of fantasy. The most persistent promoters of that system of ideas in the field of medicine were certain psychiatrists who, because of that habit of thought (or perhaps merely of expression), have been called "Mentalists" (Marx, 1965; Mora, 1975; Dewhurst and Reeves, 1978). Common to all was the reference to mental diseases as diseases of the soul. It is probable that such a style of thought was, to some extent, a predictably absurd reaction to the absurdities of the iatrochemists and iatromechanists of the 17th and 18th centuries.   Stahl, a leader of the vitalist school making the body subservient to the soul through the medium of a hypothetical (and undefined) vital force, refused to remain buried.   His explanation - "the collective processes of life cannot be comprehended unless we comprehend its purpose.   The purpose can be no other than the soul" - was hardly an explanation.   It was a slogan, and it became the justification of those who followed him.   It was recognized more than a century ago that Stahl's dogma was the first in modern times to claim to bridge the gap between philosophy (a speculative pursuit) and physiology (an observational science).   The gap was closed by having physiology absorbed by philosophy, retaining only its name.   Thus Stahl's *Theoria Medica Vera* (1707) was still the answer to medicine's problems for many German physicians.   Under that scheme there could only be diseases of the soul.   Such speculation did not lend itself to clarity, precision, or even logic, as recent accounts of it show (Marx, 1965; Mora, 1975; Dewhurst and Reeves, 1978).   Of course not all philosophers or psychologists accepted the notion.

Despite its reliance on introspection (a treacherous method), psychology was making important advances.   One such advance was Schopenhauer's conclusion in his treatise on the Will, that much thinking was unconscious, a conclusion that later stimulated the development of interest in "unconscious cerebration" in the British literature around 1850 (Altschule, 1977).   Later in the century, the idea of unconscious thinking was combined with the idea of the Ego into the notion of something sometimes called the Subliminal Self, a creature within each of us that runs things in its own way, is indifferent to what is going on around it, and does not bother to let anyone know what it wants to do.   That scary notion (more properly part of a grim fairy tale) became important in Viennese and American psychiatry.

Another development was the concept of the Ego (*das Ich, le moi*) in the writings of some of Germany's chief psychologists, such as Herbart and Beneke.   Ego-psychology became part of medicine in 1845 when Gresinger wrote a fine textbook of clinical psychiatry, all the more remarkable for having been written in terms of the then-

emergent ego-psychology.   As originally developed, the
concept of the Ego was that it was an abstraction, that
is, a functional state of the mind, analogous to other abstractions such as renal glomerular function and cardiac
conduction-system function.   The original fundamental utility of ego-psychology was to distinguish what was "I" from
what was "not-I."   Regrettably, the concept has been per-
verted in several ways.   One group - today's most influential American educationists - teaches that the "I" is infinitely more important than the rest of the Universe, or
the "not-I."   (This is reminiscent of the belief of some
American Indian tribes that the center of my Universe is
where I am.   The borrowing by influential thinkers of
ideas of American Indian tribes is an established procedure,
for a good part of Freudian dogma was enunciated using
certain notions of the Huron Indians.)   A truly regrettable
perversion of ego-psychology has been to make the ego an
independently functioning entity with remarkable powers
and attributes, unrelated to any known physical substrate.
(Here we find that the soul-psychology of early 19th-cen-
tury Germany never died; it merely slumbered and actually
came to thrive in America.)

When the "Naturphilosophie" that had dominated
medicine and biology during the first four decades of the
19th century finally was recognized for what it was - a
mass of absurdities - the creation of a system of philosophy explaining everything about life, non-life, or anything
else was taken over by men trained in the sciences.

The philosophical system that has been given the
name "Scientific Materialism" is important in this historical
account because it exemplifies the hold that experimental
science had on some minds outside science.   Because science played a large part in the thinking of all radical and
most liberal people of education, it had an important role
in medicine, but was not limited to it.   The fact that the
findings of experimental science pervaded fields as removed
from medicine as philosophy, religion, and politics tells us
that the reductionism announced by strongly worded statements of physicians in 1848 was merely part of a much
broader German phenomenon.   While most of the writing
published in the field of "Scientific Materialism" fell into
the decades after 1850, the three men most active in that

field started their efforts before 1848, taking the metaphysical stand that the then-current science was all that was needed to explain everything in the universe, including the nature of God, if any. They were all strongly anticlerical but not antireligious. Evidently, the movement grew out of criticisms advanced against Hegelian philosophy in the 1840s by Feuerbach, and apparently, it had an enormous effect on the thinking of university students and some of their instructors.

The quarrel arose over Hegel's ideas about consciousness. Hegel's *Phanomenologie des Geistes*, which discussed the certainty of sensation, claimed that all sensation was selective, a product of thought. The reaction to that view was led by Feuerbach, who argued that in cognition sensation was as primary as thought. The Scientific Materialists insisted that all thought and all sensation must be explained in terms of biology, chemistry, and physics and, hence, that all psychological matters, including consciousness, must be so explained. Since data proving those suppositions were lacking, the leading Scientific Materialists, who were all physicians, created fanciful analyses of the forces of nature to support their viewpoints. They did not agree with each other in most details, but they all agreed that religion was incompatible with natural science; however, they were not atheists, as were Marx and Engels. The importance of Scientific Materialism for German medicine was its reductionism, the belief that all manifestation of life must be explained in terms of chemistry or, more appropriately, physics. Not only were the three leading Scientific Materialists physicians, but the idea that reductionism must be adopted immediately was strong within the academic medical community and for a time after 1848 influenced medical thinking in Germany.

A more rational, and for a time successful, revolt came about through the efforts of three men - Wunderlich, Rosen, and Griesinger - who originally were classmates and who worked together to some extent thereafter. They invented what they called "The Physiologic Medicine School." All three were students of medicine at Tübingen, and after graduation Wunderlich taught there until he was called to Leipzig to succeed von Oppolzer in 1850. The three young men founded the *Archiv für physiologische Heilkunde* in

1842, a journal, like its creators, dedicated to the replacement of the medical philosophic systems then dominating Germany by a medicine based on data from the
medical sciences.   They not only attacked Schelling's
"Naturphilosophie," but also denounced Schönlein's "Natural
History School of Medicine."   Their journal was short-lived
because only a small amount of physiologic data was available for use in formulating or supporting concepts in clinical medicine.   All three men were good clinicians, with
Griesinger probably the most remarkable.   Wunderlich's
main interest was temperature regulation in man and animals, and in the pursuit of this interest he made thousands
of measurements of body temperature in patients with
fevers.   His monograph on the subject, published in 1868,
still is regarded as an outstanding contribution to the understanding of fever.   An unexpected effect of his work
was the initiation of the great antipyretic movement in the
pharmaceutical industry, which resulted in the development
of the first synthetic remedies used internally.   Another
unexpected effect, albeit an undesirable one, was that
physicians began to treat a patient's chart instead of the
patient himself, thereby weakening the doctor-patient relationship; however, that kind of practice, unforeseen in
Wunderlich's time, did not become widespread until the
mid-20th century.   The School of Physiologic Medicine
merged with, and became submerged by, the School of Reductionist Medicine, which had been created in Berlin in
1849 in connection with the political revolution of that period.   It declared that medicine had to be viewed only in
terms of physics and chemistry.

In Germany and Austria, unlike in France, the armed
revolution of 1848 failed.   Some revolutionaries fled to
America and other countries, which thereby were enriched.
One such revolutionary was Krackowitzer, a graduate of
Vienna and an assistant in its surgical clinic (Boas, 1948).
He became a captain in the Academic Legion in March of
1848, participated in the fighting in Vienna, and fled to
Germany when that city was retaken in October by the
Croatian regiments.   He was appointed Clinical Assistant in
Surgery at Tübingen but, fearing extradition to Austria,
came to America in May of 1850, settled in New York, and
became a leading practitioner there.   Many more Germans

and Austrians left their countries years after the revolutions (Rosen, 1974).   One of the most notable of the refugees was Jacobi, a graduate of Bonn in 1847.   When Krackowitzer joined the Communist League, organized by Marx and Engels, and became an active propagandist, Jacobi was imprisoned, but managed to escape to America. He began practicing in New York in 1853 and, in 1857, started lecturing on childhood diseases at Columbia's College of Physicians and Surgeons.   In 1860 he was appointed the first Chair of Pediatrics in this country.

Moritz Schiff affords another example.   He was born in Frankfort-on-Main in 1823, a member of a family that has given the world a number of famous scientists, as well as that great New York philanthropist, Jacob Schiff. After preliminary education in his home town, Moritz Schiff studied medicine at Göttingen, taking his M.D. degree there in 1844.   He then studied for a time in Paris with Magendie and others.   Returning to Frankfort in 1845, he passed his licensing examination but pursued his main interest, the physiology of the cardiorespiratory and nervous systems.   Subsequently, he studied with Tiedemann at Heidelberg, where Kussmaul was a fellow student.   When the fighting started in 1848, Schiff, encouraged by Tiedemann's oldest son, joined the revolutionary army as a surgeon.   Both were captured by the Prussians.   Young Tiedemann was shot, but Schiff, condemned to death, managed to escape with Vogt, the man who was later to become Marx's main revolutionary rival.   A few years later, a professional post in experimental pathology became vacant at Göttingen, and Schiff applied for it.   His qualifications were outstanding, and the faculty favored him enthusiastically.   However, the minister of education refused to appoint him, apparently because he feared that Schiff might insert some of his radical ideas into his medical teaching (Friedenwald, 1937).   Schiff instead took the post of Professor of Microscopic Anatomy and Pathology at Berne, and then in 1863, that of Professor of Physiology at Florence.   In 1876 he took a similar post at Geneva, where he remained throughout his life.   His experimental work was outstanding in its quality, ingenuity, and subsequent influence on physiology.

It is clear that the events of 1848 caused the loss of a considerable number of outstanding physicians in Germany as well as Austria. It is also probable that a number of excellent medical teachers were denied the opportunity to teach, thereby resulting in a significant loss to German medicine. In sum, medicine in Germany was affected adversely, while that in America and other countries was enriched.

Another circumstance forming German medical thinking in and after the 1840s was the development of certain Utopian viewpoints. It has been mentioned already that German doctors participated in the idealistic revolutionary movements of the 1840s, in which the emphasis was on the reform or destruction of intolerable political systems. Some physicians also supported the idea of a reform of the social system as well, more specifically either the abolition of capitalism, leading to state ownership of the means of production - socialism - or else a communist revolution in which all property would belong to the state, with people rewarded only for their work and laborers alone given political or social privileges or rights. Whereas socialism carried the idea of democracy with it, communism did not. (Marx referred to democracy as "a cesspool.") No one pattern of thought can be found among the revolutionary physicians of Germany in the 1840s and later. Some wanted only political democracy with, in some cases, a strong leaning toward nationalism - the political unification of the German states. Other physicians adhered to the socialist ideal and a few, like Jacobi, were communists, at least verbally and temporarily. (It is easier to desire a social system that does not exist than to accept one that does.) A few physicians associated or corresponded with communists but did not necessarily adopt their views.

Much of the Utopian thinking of German physicians then was committed to progress through technology, which differed from the ideal of progress through political or social reform or revolution in that the desired political and social progress were to be secondary but inevitable results of technological developments. The notion that man's nature is improved by making it possible for him to feed, clothe, and amuse himself with little work, or by permitting him to own or have the use of a great multiplicity of objects regardless of his need or desire for them is one of the most prevalent human superstitions.   Its application to medicine was adhered to generally by young German physicians of the 1840s, many of whom, as a matter of faith, turned toward technology as the prime, and perhaps the only, motivational force in medical advances (Schipperges, 1968).   When carried to its logical extreme, as was done by some German (and today American) physicians, it led to the conclusion that the fruits of technology, while not always beneficent, were far superior to the fruits of any other product of human thought or activity.   When put so simply, the idea sounds crass and foolish, and few persons of intelligence and sensibility, physicians or others, could adhere to it.   However, when the idea is reworded without its implications, it becomes acceptable and desirable in the minds of many physicians.   By then saying that all biological science including medicine can progress only if studied by the methods of physics and chemistry - which happen to be technological - we are agreeing with a considerable number of German physicians of the 1840s and earlier. The strong hold that technological Utopianism had on many German physicians was made justifiable by the rise of a new German philosophy, "Scientific Materialism," in the period under discussion.

   That belief in the physicochemical nature of biology and medicine was part of a broader belief, *reductionism*, which held that biology was best considered as chemistry, chemistry as physics, and physics as mathematics.   Such a general system had nothing but simplicity to recommend it to medicine.   (Surely, Einstein's statement that mathematics had nothing to do with reality rendered the chain of sciences created by reductionism irrelevant.)   Reductionism in 19th-century medicine was not a new approach. Strictly speaking, Hohenheim's attempt to make everything in the universe, including medicine, a branch of his own version of chemistry was an early example.   Another reductionist period occurred in the 17th and 18th centuries, when some academic physicians and other prominent members of the profession forced physiological and clinical phenomena into patterns dictated by available data in chemistry and physics.   (Today the medical writings of iatrochemists and iatrophysicists are regarded with amazement or amusement.)

Reductionist systems were destroyed by observational medicine and experimental science. It is ironic that the latter stimulated another wave of reductionism, that of 19th-century Germany. However, that was not to be the last, for today we are in the midst of another wave both in biology (Ayala and Dobzhansky, 1974) and in medicine. The phoenix-like reappearance of reductionism is an astonishing phenomenon that becomes less so when we realize how many of our ideas have recurred repeatedly during the last 2,000 years.

Early 19th-century Germany was fertile soil for the development of reductionism. Few American readers can appreciate the hold that philosophic writings had on the minds of the educated. Those reform movements stimulated by the Peace of Vienna in 1815 spread to involve philosophy which, in fact, had nothing to do with the repressions of the period. Philosophers became reformers not only in their own fields, but in everything. Many were carried away by their logical powers and rhetorical eloquence, to an extent unimaginable by Americans today. Reforming German philosophers of the 1840s and 1850s have been described as men who "gave themselves up to the illusion that they sat at the loom of history" (Hornack, 1900).

It is true that professional scientists themselves ignored that broad philosophy; they were content to construct a reductionist system that would apply only to physiology and biological chemistry. It remained for those trained in science, but not great practitioners of it, to create the new philosophy. The three men - Buchner, Moleschott, and Vogt - whose writings comprised most of the body of "Scientific Materialism" were holders of the M.D. degree, although only one practiced for a long time and another only briefly. Vogt had the distinction of being the recipient of Marx's most vituperative scorn. He even called Vogt a product of the middle-class, the most insulting epithet that a Marxist could utter. The "Scientific Materialists" also were attacked by conservatives. The chemist von Reichenbach insisted that chemistry and physics were not really fundamental to life.

What was fundamental, in his opinion, was a force that he called the "Od" (not to be confused with the "id," invented by embryologists in the 1890s and later adopted by Freud).

Vogt, Moleschott, and Buchner were products of the German university milieu as it existed in the decades after the Peace of Vienna and the restoration of the old *status quo*. Vogt was born in 1817, the eldest son of a liberal medical professor at Giessen. There were a number of churchmen in his father's family, despite which young Vogt developed a vitriolic hatred for the church that lasted throughout his life. His mother's family had been a source of trouble to the police for years. One of them had participated in a student riot that broke up a government celebration in 1817, was imprisoned, and then exiled. His younger brother conspired with other members of a group called the "Geissener Schwarzer" to assassinate a government official. He escaped to Switzerland, but left when he became convinced that agents of the Holy Alliance were pursuing him. He came to America and joined the Harvard faculty, becoming the first Professor of Germanic Philology there. Other relatives had less dramatic roles in the revolution of 1830. Vogt himself received his secondary education in Giessen and then entered the university there, soon achieving an outstanding reputation as a drinker, duelist, and brawler; however, later he settled down and studied chemistry there with Liebig. His father and uncle were suspected, probably correctly so, of implication in the revolutionary attempted seizure of the Federal Diet at Frankfurt in 1833. The father had to leave the University in 1834, so young Vogt stayed behind with Liebig, becoming involved in helping radical students escape from the police in 1835. Eventually he fled to Strasbourg, where a considerable number of radical exiles had congregated. He then went to Switzerland and studied at Bern, taking the M.D. degree there in 1839. He worked with Agassiz at Neuchatel for the five years before Aggasiz left to become Professor at Harvard, during which time he was not very productive.

Vogt then spent the years 1844 through 1847 in Paris, where he wrote the first of his famous materialist articles. He returned to Giessen as Professor of Zoology, on Liebig's recommendation. He was elected Delegate to the Frankfurt National Assembly, an organization with dubious claims to legitimacy. When the revolution of 1848 in Germany collapsed, he again was forced to leave Germany. After some wanderings, he took the Chair of Geology and Paleontology at Geneva, where he stayed until his death. He spent many of the years after 1850 writing popular books aimed at showing that a life in science was a good one, although he had hoped earlier that the revolution of 1848 would set science on a new, correct road. Throughout his life he remained a target of anyone who opposed materialism. He lost friends in Germany when he declared that Prussia's attack on France, and the resulting annexation, was outrageous; nevertheless, his books were highly popular for many years. He never practiced medicine.

Moleschott, another of the three medical leaders of the new philosophy, was markedly different from Vogt. He was born in 1822 in Holland, the son of a Catholic physician who had lost his faith but who did not consider himself an atheist. His early schooling emphasized the classics and other literature. Young Moleschott was sent to one of the schools in Leyden, but when the family's Catholicism proved to be an obstacle, he and his brother were sent to the *gymnasium* in Cleves in Germany. Here his education further emphasized the classics and introduced him to German philosophy. Thereafter Moleschott decided to study medicine and was sent to Heidelberg, where his teachers included the physiologist, Tiedemann (whose son was to die in the 1848 revolution). He entered the University in 1842, committed to the study of science, especially physiology, as the basis of medicine, a view held by his father. Although still interested in German philosophy, he turned to Feuerbach's version of Hegelian dogma, for Feuerbach insisted that religion, too, should be based on science. (How that was to be accomplished, he did not say.)

At the University Moleschott must have been regarded as peculiar, since he did not carouse or duel, but instead read Goethe and philosophy, and played Beethoven. He did his thesis work under Henle and took his M.D. degree in 1845. He then worked in Utrecht under the famous chemist, Mulder. Mulder was an unusual man. Born in Utrecht in 1802, he studied at the University there, receiving the M.D. degree in 1825. He practiced medicine and lectured on botany and chemistry at Rotterdam. His biochemical researches soon made him famous, and he was called to Utrecht as Professor of Chemistry in 1840. He established biochemistry in Holland and had many famous students, among them Donders and Pekelharring. Extremely sensitive to criticism, Mulder never forgave or forgot an imagined slight. On one occasion, when Liebig mildly questioned one of his statements, Mulder furiously wrote an article entitled, *Liebig's Question Put to the Test of Science and Morality.* On several occasions he became "overwrought" and had to retire for a time. Moleschott, however, was one of his favorites. It is possible that Moleschott's later vituperation regarding the exposition of the materialist doctrine was learned from Mulder.

Since Moleschott was not satisfied with the intellectual life of his native Holland, he returned to Heidelberg in 1847 to become Lecturer in physiological Chemistry. He wrote the section on nutrition for Tiedemann's physiological text. When angered by the treatment of a friend at Leyden, he wrote a long article denouncing Holland and recommending its absorption by Germany. Moleschott continued his research on nutrition and published his own text in 1850. He then wrote a popular scientific work, much of which was erroneous, but appealing to the widely held view in Germany that science was the optimal means for helping mankind understand everything. Moleschott believed that his version of nutrition would reveal the nature of the bond between body and soul, stating that "Without phosphorus, no thought," and deprecating the German dependence on potatoes. His works were received enthusiastically by materialists in general until he published a work in 1852 stating that all life, in whatever form, was simply matter in motion, with humans, like other animals and plants, participating in the life cycles of other organisms. Moleschott also attacked Liebig's vitalism, thereby satisfying the then-current German taste for invective. He also attacked the idea of free will and, to the horror of many, the idea of consciousness as separate from matter. His only praise of Christianity was that it recommended love. He held that only socialism could better distribute the resources of social reforms; communism could not. His recommendation that corpses be used to fertilize fields was too much for the university administration. In 1854 he was warned to watch his tongue, whereupon he resigned. Although unemployed, he was able to live on the income from his scandalous writings until 1856, when on the recommendation of Virchow he succeeded Ludwig as Professor of Anatomy and Physiology at Zurich. After five years he went to Turin, took Italian citizenship, and became a senator some years later. Gradually he spent less time in physiologic research and more in politics. Marx detested him. Except for the sensational effects of his writings in the 1850s, he would be forgotten today. He practiced medicine very little.

The third physician-materialist who scandalized Germany in the 1850s was Buchner, the son of a physician-graduate of Giessen who had served in Napoleon's armies. Buchner's older brother Georg was one of the earliest communists and today is remembered as the author of *Woyzeck*. While a student at medical school in the 1830s, Georg had become involved in radical activities and fled to Strasbourg. He then went to Zurich as Lecturer in Anatomy and died of typhus a few years later. The father, while sympathetic to criticisms of religion, would not tolerate attacks on the political order. Buchner had his early schooling at Darmstadt, where his father practiced and dabbled in mathematics and physics, although he showed more aptitude for literary studies and philology. In 1843 he entered Giessen University to study philosophy and literature. He then decided to study medicine in order to learn more about God's nature through His handiwork, rather than to be a practitioner. In the middle 1840s he and his younger brother became active in radical student affairs, and during the revolution of 1848 they joined in the publication of a radical periodical. He joined the volunteer corps, of which Vogt was head, but did not fight. In 1848 he also took his M.D. degree, writing his dissertation on reflex activity. In it he not only attacked Hall for not having taken a strong stand in favor of materialism, but also attacked the notion that consciousness was an essential part of nervous activity. His thesis was accepted with the examiner's comment that it did not rep-

resent necessarily the committee's views.   Buchner lost a
good deal of his enthusiasm for revolt when the revolution
collapsed. He returned to Darmstadt to practice medicine.
Four years later he took a post as Assistant in the Medical Clinic at Tübingen, where he also lectured, all of
which he found depressing.   In 1852 he began his treatise
on the "Od," the force that he believed pervaded all nature, much like Mesmer's magnetism.   Having read some of
Moleschott's materialistic writings, he resolved to follow
his lead.   In his own work, after praising himself for his
courage and honesty, he brought together and summarized
the philosophic works of all those materialist writers who
had based their convictions on the fragmentary, erroneous,
and misinterpreted science found in their works.   Accordingly, his writings became the "bible" of materialist philosophy.   In subsequent editions he seemed to have lost his
self-confidence, and later he became deeply depressed.
His writings brought denunciations from many sources, and
he lost his job at Tübingen.   Upon his return to practice
in Darmstadt, he usually was depressed, pessimistic, bitter,
and self-critical.   He came out of his depression after a
time, married, and wrote a sort of retraction of his earlier
stand, in which he examined materialism critically.   When
Prussia went to war, Buchner served as a physician to the
wounded.   After 1870 he toured the world, giving lectures
in 32 American cities, among others, and talking mainly
about free thought and impartial truth while attacking the
injustices of capitalistic society and militarism.   However,
he opposed both communism and socialism and came out
strongly in favor of love.   (He even spoke of hydrogen
loving chlorine.)   Buchner was regarded as the great pop-
ularizer and justifier of natural science of late 19th-cen-
tury Germany.

These three physicians, who could not survive in the
academic medicine of mid-19th century Germany for political reasons, today would seem sinful in their misuse of the
then-current physics and chemistry, which they attempted
to make the basis of an all-encompassing philosophy.   Their
motivation seems to have been a strong "do-good" impulse,
an impulse that also led them into revolutionary politics
and action.   We may suppose that their extended use of
physics and chemistry was an expression of their urge to

remake society.   Physicians not taking this broad view of the uses of physics and chemistry seemed to fare better. A question arises about the role, if any, of the Marx-Engels group in mid-19th-century German medicine, although today some Marxists insist on such an influence.   Clearly Marx thought that whatever was wrong with medicine, or anything else, was the fault of the middle class.   According to him, being a city-dweller, being self-employed or in a managerial post, living an ordered life, and not being engaged in manual labor destroyed whatever good qualities someone could have.   He wrote that the middle class "have stripped the halo of every occupation hitherto honored and looked up to with reverence and awe."   Among the professional people he felt to be degraded by the replacement of the fine old aristocratic ideals by the filthy mores of the newly powerful middle class were physicians and scientists. According to this orthodox Marxian view, anything that might be wrong with today's medicine can be the fault only of employers or other members of the middle class. Hence, specific criticisms of medicine are not necessary in the Marx-Engels *corpus* because Marxian dogma, by saying that anything bourgeois or capitalistic must be evil, has given the true believers a way to solve any problem needing a solution.   According to some of today's Marxists, the capitalist system specifically engenders sickness and does little to prevent or treat it (Novarro, 1976).   (Publications of that sort, which average one *non sequitur* per page, are of no value in this book.   Examination shows no evidence that Marxism directly influenced or was influenced by ideas about the nature of medicine which developed in the 1840s, despite the claims of his medical disciples.)

A belief in the importance of chemistry and physics in medicine, of course, was not restricted to 19th-century German medicine, for it had been a recurrent feature of medical theory.   Modern medicine, comprising bedside observation and physical diagnosis fused with pathological anatomy to create the early French version of clinical practice.   Experimental physiology and chemistry then were incorporated as soon as they were developed, and when Magendie carried out his experiments on animals, he inevitably saw how some of his studies resembled the phenomena of physics and chemistry.   Magendie certainly was aware of the concept of vital spirits, vital forces, or whatever other term was used to distinguish the living from the nonliving. However, rather than trying to prove or disprove their existence, he simply stated that instead of presuming a vital force, one should invoke it only when physics and chemistry cannot explain a phenomenon (Pickstone, 1976). The implication was that vital forces should be invoked when physics failed, but it remained for Dutrochet and his immediate successors in France in the 1820s to clarify the role of physical forces.

Dutrochet is significant not only because of the nature of his own work, but because he served as a model of sorts for the fanatical reductionists of Germany in 1848. However, it is interesting to note that while Dutrochet was moving ahead in his application of physics to biological phenomena, absurd debates on the existence of vital forces were going on in England, involving philosophers, theologians, physicians, and scientists. Of course, the philosophers and theologians were steadfast in their beliefs, certainly justifiable, since no significant evidence to the contrary was proffered (Temkin, 1963). Whereas the natural sciences were used in Germany to refute or destroy religion, in England the sciences and religion were considered to be mutually supportive parts of a single truth. Cambridge and its scholars, both resident and graduated, pursued this idea so energetically that they became the focus of that concept, although many other Victorians participated (Cannon, 1978).

Bell's comment on Paley's *Natural Theology* (1836) is noteworthy, since it called attention to the utter failure of the exact sciences in advancing the science of life. Bell maintained that their methods were so inadequate that good minds seeking answers to questions about life had to be satisfied with false analogies taken from the world of the nonliving objects accessible to study by physical scientists. They "cease from inquiry and leave science stationary. The mathematical and mechanical physicians long retarded the true knowledge of Physiology," wrote Bell. However, defining life was not easy, he said. Noting that living things do not putrefy, he (like John Hunter) adopted a definition based on the differentiation of "living matter which is subject to a controlling influence which resists the chemical agents, and produces a series of revolutions, in an order and at periods prescribed; the other dead matter is subject to lapse and change under chemical agency and the common laws of matter." However inadequate this definition of life, the validity of Bell's comment about the physical sciences must be recognized.

Philosophical, or perhaps theological, reasoning did nothing to clarify the relationship between physics and chemistry on the one hand, and biological functions on the other. An attempt must be made to trace the thinking that developed among Dutrochet and his followers in France in the 1820s, and the reductionism of the Germans 20 or 30 years later.

Dutrochet's life exemplified remarkable adaptability to change. He was born in 1776 in the Touraine, the son of a noble family. During the Revolution his father left the country, and the family's wealth was lost. After his early schooling, which ended in 1781, he did little except hunting. A decade later he decided to study medicine and natural sciences and went to Paris in 1802, where he completed his formal studies in 1806, but maintained a scholarly interest in the sciences. He then entered the army and served in the Peninsular Campaign, a notably dirty war. Placed in charge of a typhus hospital at Burgos he soon contracted the disease. He returned to France in poor health, was discharged, and went to live at Chateau Renault, which belonged to his mother's family. He did his research there until his mother's death in 1833, after which he moved to Paris. Much of his research concerned plants as well as animals, and around 1820 he developed ideas resembling a cell theory. His reputation grew greatly after he formulated the concept of osmosis in 1826. (It should be noted that physicists had come close to the idea a half-century earlier [Maluf, 1943].) At first Dutrochet held that osmosis could occur only through a living membrane, but when he found that a nonliving membrane could serve as well, he was pleasantly astonished. The phenomenon of osmosis was considered explainable by the science of physics, as was true of some other biological phenomena discussed in France in the 1820s. Dutrochet and his colleagues - Blainville and Fodera in Paris - formulated a view of living matter which recognized no barrier between living and nonliving. They held that living bodies had properties that occurred in nonliving bodies, but were more complex in form because they were more numerous and more complexly combined in action. They further maintained that a new physics would have to be developed because the old was inadequate. Their concept of living matter could be called vitalism only by greatly stretching the definition of the word. The concept was, in effect, an expression of materialism, at least as regards animal bodily function. Decades later Bernard gave that concept of living matter the support of his authority. In fact, Ludwig, who modeled himself after Müller, the greatest of Germany's physiologists at midcentury, said much the same thing (Frank and Weiss, 1966).

French biological materialism was more restrained in language and logical in conception than the German scientific materialism that erupted around 1848 (Temkin, 1946b). Before that time Ludwig already was using physics and chemistry to extend the range of explanations of living phenomena (Rosen, 1936b). Regrettably his writings in that area did not adhere to the guidelines he himself professed in his Introduction to *Textbook of Human Physiology*, guidelines that were enunciated by the French physiologists of the previous decades and intended to supplant the errors. There were two methods used to make phenomena of living organisms seem to adhere to whatever physicochemical concepts were current at any given time. One was to make inadequate or erroneous physicochemical data seem applicable by the free use of inference, supposition and, when the occasion demanded, *non sequitur*. The other method was to make the conditions of observation so artifactual that the biological phenomenon being studied could but resemble the recognized physicochemical phenomena. The former was used by Ludwig, although he was a great physiologist and did much to advance the subject in other ways.

Ludwig was born in Germany near Cassel in 1816, at the end of the Napoleonic wars. His father, an army officer, had been wounded in action and forced to retire, obtaining a government post in Hanau. Young Ludwig received his early education there and then entered the University at Marburg, where he quickly developed a reputation for turbulence and fighting. He was forced to leave for a time, but ultimately returned and took the M.D. degree in 1839. Two years later he became Prosector under Pick and a year later was granted the right to teach, which was occasioned by his thesis on renal function. Ludwig described renal function in terms of the physical theory of diffusion under pressure, a theory that he later discussed more fully in his articles on osmosis in 1849 and 1856. In 1846 he became Professor at Marburg and held that post for three years, after which he went to Zurich. While at Marburg he developed expertise in anatomical dissection and, through the influence of the chemist Bunsen, in physical and chemical theory. He became more and more well known as he created devices and methods that permitted physiology to become quantitative. He invented a kymograph, flow meter, blood-pressure recorder, and devices for perfusing isolated organs. He visited Berlin in 1847 and became closely allied with von Helmholtz, Brucke, and duBois-Reymond, the three physiologists who were to make the reduction of physiology to physics and chemistry (chiefly the former) an article of revolutionary faith in 1848. In 1855 he was appointed Professor of Anatomy and Physiology at the Josef Akademie in Vienna and in 1865 took the newly created Chair of Physiology at Leipzig. His development of new methods created one of the great institutes of physiologic research there. He and his students pursued his aims, largely by the invention and perfection of measuring and recording devices. (It should be noted in passing that some of his earliest devices introduced artifacts that future workers eliminated [Hoff and Geddes, 1959].)

His brilliant, ingenious mind and his keen interest in individual teaching maintained his Leipzig Institute as the center of Western physiology in the second half of the 19th century. Students from all over the Western World came to work with him, and these pupils, together with the manner in which he himself organized and presented his material, made him, in collaboration with Bernard, the creator of modern physiology (Rosen, 1936b; Schoer, 1967). As he said about his relations with the three Berlin reductionists, "We four imagined that we should constitute physiology on a chemico-physical foundation, and give it equal scientific rank with physics, but the task turned out to be much more difficult that we anticipated" (Maluf, 1943). As he made more and .more physiological observations with his quantitative methods, he paradoxically found fewer and fewer that could be explained by the then-current physics and chemistry. He recognized that discrepancy, and trying to prove the reductionist hypothesis ceased to be the primary motivation of his work. However, the noisy pronouncements of the "Berlin 3" kept the reductionist movement alive, ultimately drawing Virchow into it.

The physiologic physics of 1848 Germany had its origin in an exaggerated response to the earlier and blander French version. In 1841 Müller in Berlin received a copy of an earlier French work on electrophysiology and asked his pupil, duBois-Reymond, to study the phenomenon. It occupied him for the next 40 years and made him the spokesman of the reductionist movement. By 1847 duBois-Reymond and Brucke had been friends for years. Von Helmholtz joined the group in 1845, all three of them being students of Müller in Berlin at the time. As early as 1841 duBois-Reymond wrote about the desirability of showing that the phenomena of life are essentially the same as those of physical phenomena, and in 1842 he wrote, "Brucke and I have sworn to make prevail the truth that in the organism no other forces are effective than the purely physico-chemical." They were both 23 years of age at the time. A year later duBois-Reymond published *Untersuchengun über Thierische Elektricitat* and made it not only the repository of his observations, but the manifesto of his revolutionary movement (Cranefield, 1957b). The American Morgan, a graduate of Columbia University's College of Physicians and Surgeons, worked with duBois-Reymond and published an English version of the book. However, despite the many experiments he carried out, duBois-Reymond was no nearer establishing his creed at the end of the century than when he started. "He had at that time, one may say with all charity, outlived himself" (Magnus-Levy, 1944). Brucke, never an enthusiastic propagandizer, contented himself with pursuing physiologic research. Ludwig, initially an enthusiast, eventually devoted himself more to physiologic research and less to propaganda.   Von Helmholtz, the last of the group, took a different course in his career.

Von Helmholtz was born in Potsdam in 1821, the son of a teacher at the local *gymnasium*.   It was believed that his mother's ancestor was William Penn.   His early interest was physics, but lack of money made him enter the Army Medical School in Berlin.   He became part of Müller's circle of young physiologists.   As a 26-year-old army surgeon he found ample time to pursue physiological studies, one of which was the measurement of the heat produced by a contracting muscle using a thermocouple.   In 1850 he measured the speed of the nerve impulse, and a short time later published his great paper on the conservation of energy.   He studied the physics of vision and in 1851 invented the ophthalmoscope.   He also turned his attention to acoustics and other sensory subjects.   He was Professor of Physiology at Koenigsberg from 1849 to 1855; at Bonn from 1855 to 1857; and at Heidelberg from 1857 to 1870.   Then, in 1871, he left medicine to become Professor of Physics at Berlin, holding that post until 1894.   Thus, 24 of his 46 years of professorships were spent in physics (Gruber and Gruber), 1956.   His departure from medicine relieved him of the necessity of proving his original thesis, that life was explainable entirely in physicochemical terms.

A question arises about the fact that the Ludwig-duBois-Reymond-Brucke-von Helmholtz creed never established itself.   For one thing, some eminent physiologists, such as Pfluger, refused from the very first to accept its far-reaching (or perhaps far-fetched) concepts.   In fact, the movement was nothing but another philosophical system based, like the "Scientific Materialism" of the period, on the fragmentary and partly erroneous physics and chemistry current in that era in Germany.   Unlike that metaphysical system, the biophysical reductionist dogma avoided discussion of God, the soul, and similar considerations, but it still was a philosophy (Cranefield, 1966; Galaty, 1974) created in part to dispute the previously accepted German *"Naturphilosophie."*   Perhaps von Helmholtz' loss of enthusiasm for reductionism was the result of his growing skepticism of dogmatic systems that "promise to solve all riddles."   His lecture, *"Das Denken in der Medizin,"* given before a convention of German army physicians in 1877, delineates his skepticism (Luckhardt, 1968).

Although the roles of physicochemical reductionism and "Scientific Materialism" diminished in 19th-century Germany, their effects lasted, those on psychiatry of particular interest. For one thing, proving the invalidity of the soul's force in thinking required that some other force(s) be established. In a completely unexpected fashion the writings of Schopenhauer and his successors seemed to fill that need. Schopenhauer's *World as Will and Idea* (1818) stated that will, blind and unconscious, was the prime motivating force in human behavior. Man, according to such a view, was a pawn not of wholly exterior forces, but of his own unconscious will. That notion was adopted and expanded by Hartmann in 1861 with his *Philosophy of the Unconscious*. Those who were loathe to give up the idea of an executive soul could accept the "scientific" view of an executive unconscious will. The idea was accepted so completely by English physicians and psychologists that a number of them fought with each other around 1860, each claiming to have discovered it. (Today Freud's disciples claim that *he* discovered it around 1900.) Unconscious cerebration was not neglected in America. William James accepted Schopenhauer's and Hartmann's view of the primacy of an unconscious mind, but declared it to be that part of the mind with which we commune with God, proving that it was after all a kind of Soul. It is interesting to contrast this statement, loaded with portentous Germanic profundity, with that of Holmes, who also believed in the reality of the Unconscious Mind (as well as in a Superego). Holmes declared that the conversation of women proved the existence of unconscious thinking. The concept of unconscious thinking came to play a large and usually dogmatic role in European psychiatry of the late 19th and early 20th centuries.

The other psychiatric element resulting from the German revolutionary movement in medicine was quite different: the contribution of Griesinger. Griesinger was not only one of the greatest internists of all times, but also one of the greatest psychiatrists of the 19th century. Born in Stuttgart in 1817, the son of a hospital administrator, he had his early education locally and in 1834 en-

tered the University of Tübingen to study medicine. He
had grown up with and was a close friend to Wunderlich
and Rosen. All three were at Tübingen together and became attracted to the physiology being taught only by
Müller at that time in Germany.

Griesinger also distinguished himself by his independence of mind, his absence from classes, and his participation in the forbidden revolutionary political activities of
the students. He was expelled from Tübingen in 1837 and,
despite the objections of the German government, went to
Zurich, where he took the M.D. degree in 1838. He spent
a year in Paris attending Magendie's lectures and visiting
the hospitals, and then returned to Germany to practice.
He worked at a mental hospital for two years and, after
more travel to Paris and Vienna, joined Wunderlich at
Tübingen in 1843. While there he published his remarkable
textbook of psychiatry (1845), in which he based the entire discussion on the ego-psychology of Benecke and
Herbart. The book evidently was admired widely, judging
by the frequency with which it was plagiarized by other
German authors. It went through several editions in German, French, and English and was to become one of the
foundations of American psychiatry of the period after
World War I. Griesinger was given a professorship at Kiel
in 1849 but left after a year to go to Egypt as Director
of the Health Service, Dean of the Medical School, and
Personal Physician to the Viceroy. After two years he
left, and in 1854 he became Professor of Medicine at
Tübingen, and in 1860 at Zurich. At Zurich he taught not
only medicine but neurology and psychiatry (Marx, 1970,
1972). He wrote authoritative works on malaria and typhus, and typhoid and relapsing fevers, as well as establishing the relationship between hookworm infestation and
anemia. (Earlier it was called miners' anemia, bricklayers'
anemia, St. Gothard-tunnel anemia, and Egyptian or tropical anemia; for a time it was called Griesinger's anemia.)

He described Griesinger's sign - edema of the mas-
toid process in patients with cavernous sinus thrombosis.
Pulsus paradoxicus was called "Griesinger-Kussmaul's sign,"
and muscular dystrophy, "Duchenne-Griesinger's disease."
In 1841 he and Wunderlich together founded *Archiv für
Physiologische Heilkunde* to speak for the school of physi-

ological medicine.   He was editor of that journal from 1846 to 1848.   In 1864 he went to Berlin as Professor of Psychiatry, also teaching neurology.   In 1866 he established the *Archiv für Psychiatrie und Nervenkrankherten* and tried to reform German psychiatry on a neurological and psychological basis, but the Berlin psychiatrists refused to follow his lead.   He died two years later (Marx, 1970, 1972).   Two peripheral manifestations of the medical revolution in early 19th-century Germany - the interest in unconscious cerebration and Griesinger's formulation of ego-psychiatry - created American psychiatry more than a half-century later.

Even more important for 19th-century medicine was another peripheral manifestation of earlier German changes: the nature of medicine as envisaged by Virchow.   Virchow had great influence, most of which was good.   He was born in Pomerania in 1821 and was said to be Slavic in appearance, as were many Pomeranians.   Educated locally, he entered the medical school in Berlin, obtaining the M.D. degree in 1843, and subsequently became Prosector in Pathology at the Charité.   He had a brilliant, active mind and an acid tongue.   Accordingly, he was given to strong statements.   Many of them were unfortunate, although they were overlooked or minimized in the laudatory articles written about him (Wilson, 1947; Plaut, 1953).   He was greatly influenced by some other German physicians of his or earlier times and, in particular, he openly admired and generally recognized the physiological school of medicine. Less well appreciated was his debt to the writings of Jahn, a co-founder with Schönlein and Stark of what they called the *"Naturhistorische Schule,"* which replaced *"Naturphilosophie"* with an equally irrational speculative system. However, a number of Jahn's ideas were worthwhile and were adopted by Virchow (Pagel, 1945).   One was the idea that disease was nothing but modified normal life, that physiologic and pathologic phenomena are basically similar. Jahn also held that disease was a local phenomenon, at least at first.   Here Virchow followed Goodsir's more explicit view that the cell was the local unit of bodily function.   Jahn also mentioned the cellular structures described by the precursors of Schleiden and Schwann.   Virchow's active mind recast these older materials.

The breadth and volume of Virchow's activities were phenomenal (Ackerknecht, 1953; Rather, 1958).   In 1847 he founded *Archiv für Pathologische Anatomic und Physiologie*, much of the first issues of which were comprised of his papers.   A large part of his own early material was exhortatory rather than informational, the first issue of the journal containing strongly worded statements about pathological physiology being the future of medicine.   In 1848, like many other young academics, he participated in antigovernment demonstrations but did not fight.   In 1848 he also founded a short-lived political and sociological journal called *Die Medizinische Reform*, in which he expressed in so many words his idea that medicine was a social science, an idea he later did not emphasize.   Also in that year the government sent him to Silesia (seized a century earlier from Austria) to study the typhus epidemic there (Tridan, 1964).   In terms of the data collected, the report is excellent; in terms of recommendations, it is less so.   For immediate control of the epidemic he recommended certain administrative measures, but evidently was unaware of Lind's hygienic recommendations of a century earlier.   For long-term prevention of the disease he merely repeated the manifesto of the revolutionary groups then active: full and unlimited democratic government, local partial self-government, free education, education of girls, separation of Church and State, reform of taxation, and also the sending of government experts to improve agriculture and introduce industry.   He did not in this report state his later view that the people should receive an education in the basic sciences in order to make them more moral.   His liberal social beliefs, which he never hesitated to enunciate, diminished his popularity in Prussian government circles, and he was discharged from his teaching job in 1849.   However, he quickly was given the Chair of Pathological Anatomy at Wurzburg, where he served for seven years.   His brilliance as lecturer and teacher led to his recall to Berlin in 1856 as Professor of Pathology and director of a new institute erected for him.   He also served in the Prussian legislature in 1862 and, after the creation of a united Germany, in the Reichstag from 1880 to 1893.   He was against the middle class and for industrial laborers.   Moreover, he took every opportunity to repeat his radical beliefs in the most spirited terms, and Bismarck, who had his own ideas of social reform *via* pensions, social security, and state medicine, is said to have become so annoyed with him as to wish him out of the way, although he never did anything about it.   In Berlin Virchow helped secure a new sewage system and also became the head of so many learned and political societies that one wonders how he was able to adapt his thinking and behavior to all of them.   However uncomplimentary Bismarck's opinions about Virchow might have been, there was no doubt about the high opinions of Virchow held by the scientific and medical-academic community.   To them he was a constant and perpetual hero.   When in the Franco-Prussian War the Natural History Museum in Paris was shelled, French journalists called the Prussians a barbarian Mongol race.   Virchow thereupon recorded the skull measurements and hair and eye color of 6,000,000 German school children to prove that they were ethnically Aryan and not Mongol.   Over half of his 2,000 publications were on the subjects of anthropology, archaeology, and politics.

Virchow's record in medicine produced a mixed picture.   His work on thrombosis was first-rate, demolishing the superstition held by Cruvielhier and other French authors that it was the basic lesion in disease.   (Many inflammatory lesions have thrombosed blood vessels in and near them, but that is no reason for assuming this process to be primary.)   His observations of stroke clarified many ambiguities (Schiller, 1970); his destruction of the superstitious belief in the primacy of nervous-system function in all disease was a valuable service (Rath, 1959), although by that time he was whipping a very feeble, if not quite dead, horse.   Today his greatest claim to fame is his *Cellularpathologie*, and the circumstances of his writing it are worth discussing.

Virchow had been a pupil and ardent admirer of Müller, the great Berlin physiologist.   As early as 1846 Virchow wrote in his report to the Prussian Minister of Culture and Education that pathology as morbid anatomy was too static and should become physiological (Rather, 1966).   In the first issue of his *Archiv für Pathologische Anatomie und Physiologie* he stated strongly his conviction that the future of medicine was pathological *physiologie*

(Temkin, 1947; Klemperer, 1958).   But where was the physiology of disease to be found?   His answer to this question was in the use of the microscope.   Shortly before Virchow published his admirable *Cellularpathologie* certain events had occurred.   Goodsir had formulated the idea that the nutritional function of the body was in the cells (as Virchow recognized), and Remak had shown that cells always came from other cells (Pagel, 1945).   Perhaps most important of all was Kolliker's publication of *Mikroskopische Anatomie* (1850-1854) and *Handbuch der Geweblehre der Menschen* at about the same time (Zuppinger, 1974).   He did his work at Wurzburg, where Virchow had served as Professor of Pathology for seven years.   Kolliker, in his quiet way (he is rarely mentioned today), created with his two monographs the science of microscopic anatomy in its first organized, systematic, and extensive form.   For the next 50 years they served as the main, and at times the only, sources of material in that field.   Not only were they used, but they were copied and plagiarized widely. From the beginning, and well into the 20th century, microscopic anatomy was considered a branch of physiology, one that gave a different, but at least as equally valid, picture of the function of body tissues as did the experimental physiology of the French (like Magendie) and the Germans (like Müller).   Microscopic anatomy had the advantage that it could be used *post hoc*, that is, after the death of the organism.   It was the answer to Virchow's expressed need for a physiologic component of pathology, and Virchow, with characteristic energy and enthusiasm, took advantage of it.   If he had not written his *Cellularpathologie* when he did (a few years after Kölliker published his phenomenal treatises), somebody else would have done so.   It is doubtful, however, that many of his contemporaries could have done it so brilliantly.   There is no question that the time of cellular pathology had come, and Virchow announced it spectacularly, although he himself was surprised by the success of his book.   Although modesty was not one of his virtues, he did not see himself revealed by this work as the new Messiah.   The Preface of the *Cellularpathologie* was addressed, in part, to practicing physicians who were told sympathetically that they could not be expected to keep up with the massive amount of current medical literature, but that they would be brought up-to-date by the contents of his lectures. (This kind of statement must sound familiar to today's American practicing physicians who are persuaded, or perhaps forced, to listen to lectures on some basic science as a means of making them more up-to-date in the way they practice medicine.)

Virchow's great contributions to medicine cannot be denied, but they are balanced to some extent by the harm he did. He was considered infallible by many physicians - perhaps by himself - and he put forward a number of massive errors in his habitual forceful manner which retarded progress for a time. When forced by facts that controverted some theory of his, he might simply have left the room. He was wrong in opposing Cohnheim's demonstration that leukocytes went through blood capillary vessels in inflamed areas. Even after Langenbech showed that cancer spreads by migration of cells *via* the bloodstream (Rather, 1975), Virchow insisted that the tumors spread by secondary development *de novo* from hypothetical, and never demonstrated morbid tissue juices. (This was interesting because sometime before then he had demolished Rokitansky's view that morbid fluids and even abnormal molecules might be responsible for disease.) Virchow insisted that the two main types of tubercles represented different diseases despite Villemin's demonstration that they were the same. Virchow refused to accept Weismann's concept of "germplasm," a concept that survived Virchow's criticism (Churchill, 1976). Von Behring's discovery of diphtheria antitoxin was received so coldly by Virchow that von Behring felt constrained to write a 60-page polemic against him in a medical journal. As was perhaps typical of the time and place, the argument disintegrated into hair-splitting definitions of words of peripheral importance. Early in his career Virchow would have therapeutics based on nothing but cellular pathology. It was not clear how this was carried out, although he was in active practice at the time. At any rate he wrote less and less about this type of treatment and finally stopped writing about it entirely (Ackerknecht, 1970).

It is not unknown for scientists, like others, to make mistakes in their work and to adhere stubbornly to them.   If these mistakes have ill effects, the blame for them must be put on those who believed.   Although the effects of most of Virchow's scientific errors were not long-lived, one of his errors did last for some time and had serious adverse effects.   When he said that medicine was like a fortress, the central redoubt being experimental science, with clinical practice and even pathology as mere outposts, he made a serious error.   There were few, if any, Germans who took him seriously; regrettably, there were a number of Americans who did.   Although Virchow held that experimental pathological physiology was the "genuine theory of medicine," he stated clearly that the definition of the problems that experimental science was to solve could come only from clinical medicine and pathology.   On the other hand, he stated equally clearly that medical practice could do little that was worthwhile unless informed by theory.   He wrote in the first issue of *Archiv*, "The standpoint we propose to adopt and which already manifested in this first issue is simply that of natural science.   Practical medicine as applied to theoretical medicine, and theoretical medicine as an embodiment of pathological physiology, are the ideals toward which we shall strive."   Now, after more than a century of progress in the laboratory sciences related to medicine, we know that Virchow's formulation was not only overly optimistic to the point of naïveté, but also was seriously in error concerning the nature of medicine.   His errors may be understood as owing to inexperience and to the fact that he was writing during a time of marked enthusiasm about revolutionary changes, "What is a revolution without a manifesto?"   Nevertheless, his formula required that the content of the laboratory sciences related to medicine should be connected to what patients experienced and should not take its direction from theories in the sciences themselves.   Virchow's demurral has not been adhered to by many laboratory scientists on the faculties of today's American medical schools.

The reason for the markedly enthusiastic acceptance of experimental physiology as the true basis of medicine in Germany is only partly clear.   For one thing, bedside medicine did not play as important a part in Germany as elsewhere (von Brunn, 1963).   It is also probable that the

Germans' enmity toward everything French after Napoleon's wars influenced their thinking; for example, whereas Great Britain, Ireland, and America accepted physical diagnosis by means of percussion and auscultation as a great advance, many German physicians and medical teachers scorned it (Choulant, 1920). Von Helmholtz noted that many physicians at midcentury held that these methods of examination were "a coarse mechanical means of investigation which a physician with a clear mental vision did not need; and indeed it lowered and debased the patient who, anyhow, was a human being by treating him as a machine" (Gruber and Gruber, 1956). The widespread but far from universal rejection of the currently accepted methods of medicine in Germany created a need and left an opening for another approach. Owing to circumstances that prevailed at the time, that new approach came to be based on physiochemical reductionism.

In contrast to what happened in Germany, the Revolution of 1848 in Vienna changed only the form of the curriculum (Billroth, 1924) and seemed to have little effect on its content or theoretical formulations.

In Germany, by the early 1880s, ideas about medicine espoused by Virchow and Cohnheim - medicine as physiology based on physiochemistry - came to have a separate existence. It took the name of *innere Medizin* in medical societies, textbooks, and journals (Bean, 1982). That name, unfortunately, has been translated as "internal medicine" in America. The word *innere* has many meanings in addition to "inner." It also means "intrinsic" and "core," and in Germany from the 1880s until after World War I it was used to designate the essence of medicine, as distinguished from the mere practice of medicine. Reductionist medicine began to lose its standing in Germany around World War I and now seldom is mentioned there. In Germany today, when the subject arises, that kind of medicine is likely to be referred to as another one of those awful American imports.

Chapter 15: Some Aspects of Relations Between Chemistry and Medicine

PREVIOUS CHAPTERS DISCUSSED THE CHEMICAL INTERESTS of some leading clinicians. In particular, the intimate role of chemical thinking in medical theory was presented for that period when many leading clinicians, including de le Boë, Boerhaave, Willis, Cullen, and others, were iatrochemists. Van Helmont, the Capuchin friar-turned-physician, had a key place in this development. Wildly imaginative in his thinking, he nevertheless did call attention to the function of digestive juices. He was, however, a man of unpredictable opinions, criticizing members of various schools for using metaphor and poetic liberty in likening digestion of food in the stomach to the cooking of food in a pot. The Helmontians attacked Willis' metaphor of life as a burning oil lamp, and of fermentation of the blood as a cause of illness. Van Helmont considered the reasoning about living things from what happened *in vitro* as mere metaphor. He even rejected the macrocosm-microcosm system of analogies that made up much of Renaissance medicine, calling the comparison "poetical heathenish and metaphorical, but not natural or true" because man was created in the image of God, and not of the whole corrupt world. By and large his influence on medicine was negligible except for one thing: his support of Paracelsus, although he differed from him in detail.

It is probable that medicine was influenced by chemical factors long before records began to be kept. Although chemistry, as we know it today, started its development in the 17th and early 18th centuries, it is important to recognize that its precursor, alchemy, and early medicine were related closely. The dependence of treatment by alchemy in the ancient and medieval world is appreciated widely. What is not known is that the reverse was also true: Medical theory influenced alchemical thinking (Crosland, 1962). Thus some alchemists wrote about treating base metals to improve them as if they were applying a remedy in a sickness. (Some alchemists believed that since gold was perfect, it had to comprise a balanced mixture of the four primary Galenic qualities, just as health in the Galenic system was considered to be the result of a balance of the four humors. In fact, in some of the ancient Arabic alchemical literature a synonym for gold was "the healthy one," and silver was called "leprous gold.") Facts such as these attest to the antiquity of the relationship between chemistry, whatever its concepts and content might have been at any time, and medicine, whatever *its* concepts and content might have been at the same time. A transfer of concepts and content in both directions between chemistry and medicine is clearly the normal relationship between the two. Such was the case even before chemistry had become chemistry (as we know it) and clinical medicine (as we know it) had appeared on the scene.

The manipulation of natural substances, most of them of botanical origin and some of animal or mineral origin, has been associated with medicinal therapy, at least as far back as there are records. The earliest medicinal preparations seem to have been simple mixtures of such substances, but by the era of ancient Greece and Rome more complicated operations were performed. Thus in ancient times Dioscorides and Pliny the Elder used extraction, decoction, and even distillation in their efforts to improve the substances they believed to have medicinal properties. Later the alchemists who sought to make the philosophers' stone, or to create gold from base substances, used a variety of chemical processes, including distillation. Lull's writings refer to these operations (Kocher, 1947; Debus, 1968). However, only after the growth of interest in inquiry and experiment at the start of the Renaissance, soon followed by the development of printing, were systematic works on the use of chemical procedures published. Two men, Gesner and Brunschwig, made the notable contributions, and their works were read widely. Another man, Paracelsus (also known as Philippus Aureolus Theophrastus Bombastus von Hohenheim), was lecturing and writing (but not publishing) on chemistry either unknown to those two or unrecognized by them. The history of that period has become confused due to the creation in recent years of the cult of Paracelsus among some Swiss and German historians of medical thought.

Paracelsus was born near Zurich in 1493, the son of a physician who was also an alchemist interested in making gold from base metals. In 1502 the boy became an apprentice in the Fugger mines, where he learned the processes involved in smelting metals and also observed the diseases of the miners. (He wrote a well-known tract on the latter subject some time later.) At the age of 14 he started his wanderings. There is no evidence that he earned a degree anywhere, but he did serve as a barber-surgeon in several armies. A crude, ill-mannered, offensive person, he was unable to remain long in any one town, although he hoped to settle down in his 30s. Whenever an opportunity presented itself he declared himself the greatest physician of the era, far superior, in fact incomparably so, to any other. He despised Galenic remedies, which were mainly botanical, and recommended extracts or distillates of them, as well as of inorganic substances. He strongly favored compounds of metals like antimony and mercury. In 1527 he was called to Basle to treat the famous Frobenius, who had a stubborn ailment that other physicians had failed to cure. We do not know what it was, but since syphilis was a widespread epidemic in Europe at the time, it is not surprising that a mercury compound cured the illness. Paracelsus became Personal Physician to Frobenius' friends, including Erasmus, and through them was appointed City Physician of Basle, giving him the right to teach at the University. He announced that he would have nothing to do with the works of Hippocrates, Galen, and Avicenna and threw a book that was purported to contain the works of Avicenna on the bonfire on St. John's Day. His behavior did not increase his popularity among the students (the faculty had always disliked and ridiculed him). Frobenius died in October of 1527 and Paracelsus, now without his protector, fled after a dispute with a churchman over money. He wandered about Europe, writing most of the time and lecturing when he could. His recommendation of a mild salt of mercury for treating syphilis outraged the powerful Fuggers, who controlled the market in guaiacum, the generally recommended (and useless) treatment for that disease. The Faculty of Medicine at Leipzig forbade the publication of his book on the subject. He then wrote *Paragranum*, a long, wandering, confused, and redundant work in which he likened the world to a chemistry laboratory and the creation of the world to a chemical separation by the Great Chemist in the Sky. (Descartes was later to liken Him to a Celestial Watchmaker.) As regards his ideas of medicine, several anecdotes claimed that he cured some persons, but the only known review of his clinical methods revealed that all whom he had treated died. Paracelsus himself died young, at the age of 48. His cultists claim that he introduced many new remedies, but the available evidence, at least from England, shows that a chemical medical revolution was underway before his works became known there (Kocher, 1947; Multhauf, 1954; Debus, 1965, 1968, 1972). His exact role in Continental medicine is not clear, but it certainly is not as important as his cultists state. At most, his contributions to clinical medicine were his writings on syphilis and the diseases of miners. The remarkable book on chemistry written by Brunschwig was published in England in translation in 1527; Gesner's in 1552. Neither mentioned Paracelsus. The English physicians who were chemically oriented regarded Gesner as the one who had stimulated the growth of chemistry in England. English medical works published as late as the late 1660s including some that discussed distillates, balsams, and tinctures, did not mention Paracelsus but did refer to Lull, Gesner, and Brunschwig (Kocher, 1947). Paracelsus' cultists claim that what he had introduced into England was flourishing decades before English physicians had ever heard of him. In fact, his works began to be published only after his death in 1541, a sizable collection having come out in 1590; but, masses of his writings remained unpublished for years, and some still are unpublished. Some physicians who searched for effective medicines and did not find them in previously available sources turned to Paracelsus' remedies, and hence he had some influence on the practice of medicine. Except in a few cases, Englishmen vigorously rejected Paracelsus' theories on the nature of man, the universe, God, and whatever else aroused his interest. Although his views influenced medical practice somewhat, they had little effect on the development of the iatrochemical theory that permeated medical education in the 17th century.

The growth of interest in chemistry's relationship to medicine in the 17th century, at least in England, is best understood if the part played by two physicians is recalled. One of them was Fludd, the second (or perhaps the fifth) son of a Kentish knight who served at one time as financial officer to Queen Elizabeth's military. Born in 1574, Fludd entered Oxford in 1591 and received the bachelor's and the master's degrees in 1596 and 1598, respectively. He spent the next six years traveling on the Continent, returning to Oxford with an excellent reputation as a chemist. He was granted both the M.B. and the M.D. degrees in 1605. At first the College of Physicians refused him a license to practice, but a short while later granted it, although the examiners were not convinced fully of his competence. A few months later he was accused of anti-Galenic utterances, but when his accusers failed to appear at the hearing, he merely was admonished and not punished. Elected a Fellow of the College of Physicians, he again was admonished for insolence. Nevertheless, a year later he was elected a censor for several years. He practiced in London in style, with an apothecary in his own house and a secretary to record his ideas on anything he happened to think about at odd hours. Like Paracelsus, he had his own description and explanation of the cosmos, based on the assumption that the Scriptures contained the basis of all speculation and all true science. He became a Rosicrucian, joining them in their promise to produce a universal reformation of the world. Although reputed to be learned in chemistry, he made no contribution to medical chemistry, but did write, under various names, highly speculative works that evoked the criticism of astronomers like Kepler and physiologists like Gassendi. More a talker than a doer, he nevertheless was reputed to be an alchemist, or even a magician. He exemplifies a trend toward mysticism among some physicians and expressed an interest in chemistry. In these respects he resembles Paracelsus, although he is far more logical in thought and precise in expression.

The other English physician appropriately discussed here is Harris. Although he was not, like Fludd, a contemporary of Paracelsus, he lived and practiced later, at a time when Paracelsus began to have a following in England. Born in Gloucestershire in 1647, he went to Oxford and took his bachelor's degree there in 1670. Shortly afterward he joined the Church of Rome and had to resign his Oxford fellowship. He went to France to study medicine, received the M.D. at Brouges in 1675, and started to practice medicine in London the next year. In 1679, during the excitement about a papist plot in London, he gave up the Catholic faith and shortly afterward was granted an M.D. degree at Cambridge. He was elected to the College of Physicians and thereafter held a number of its offices. His first medical book was *A Rational Discourse of Remedies Both Chymical and Galenical* (1683). In it he discussed the six great remedies then recognized: mercury, antimony, vitriol, iron, Peruvian bark, and opium, all remedies drawn from both Galenic and Paracelsan sources. He derided gold boiled in broth, a recommended medicine at the time. (Was it the forerunner of today's Jewish mother's chicken soup?) He was Physician to Charles II and after him to William III and Mary. A friend of Sydenham, he showed little of his clinical expertness, despite which he continued to publish clinical works, some of which clearly were based on Sydenham's observations. His last work, published in 1727, was a theological treatise. Harris exemplifies the position taken by a number of English physicians who accepted some of Paracelsus' recommended medicines but ignored his physiological, cosmological, and theological speculations. Harris pointed out that in the second half of the 17th century "by degrees physicians grew Chymists, and the Chymists became physicians."

At the end of the 17th century Boerhaave stated that medicine had to be based on science, by which he evidently meant chemistry. That kind of statement could safely be made at that time, since there was no way of testing it, and in fact there was considerable disagreement about what the content of chemistry was. Except for the observation that the urea in urine was probably the degradation product of digested meat, there were no reliable data on the chemistry of man. Since the fanciful iatrochemical concepts were unable to be tested, either by ex-

periment or by comparison with what should occur in disease, those concepts could have been - and were - used
freely in teaching. During the 18th century the data of
chemistry increased in some areas, depending on the methods developed for studying it, and many physicians were
interested in it. As time went on, however, the 18th-cen-
tury physicians became convinced increasingly that chemistry was of little or no help in the practice of medicine.
Of course physicians had to know enough not to mix incompatible substances in prescriptions, but otherwise
chemical knowledge had no practical status (Crellin, 1974).
Even enthusiastic chemist-physicians admitted that chemistry was no better than "amusement," no matter what
might be its theoretical importance. However, the Industrial Revolution was making chemistry highly important in
metallurgy, ceramics, and dyeing, and persons in those industries needing to learn chemistry could do so only by attending the lectures in general chemistry given by physicians. Such courses also were supported strongly by medical and apothecary students. The reason for that support
was that chemistry came to be joined to Latin, Greek, music, poetry, literature, and the pictorial arts as proper pursuits for those considering themselves members of a
learned profession (Crellin, 1974). Chemistry in that sense
was coupled with natural history, an ill-defined conglomer-
ation of biological and geological sciences. In 1759 Oliver
Goldsmith, a failed medical student (at least he had no
degree) wrote, "Were I poor, I should send my son to Leyden and Edinburgh.... Were I rich I should send him to
one of our own universities. By an education received at
the first, he has the best likelihood of a living; by that
received in the latter, he has the best chance of becoming
great." The fact that he was in error is not the point.
The point is that those statements expressed what he believed. The contents of the chemistry lecture courses
given - only by physicians - at Leyden, Edinburgh, Oxford,
and Cambridge showed that the lecturers were more concerned with the subject as a distinct science rather than
as an ally of medicine.
   A main preoccupation of many 18th-century chemists
was what was called the "animalization" of vegetable matter; that is, the process whereby vegetable food turned

into animal flesh. All of them, except Boerhaave who was Dutch and Beccari who was Italian, were Frenchmen - Hauberg, Lemery, Venel, Berthollet, and de Fourcroy. All believed that if that problem could be solved, the benefits would be immeasurable. Physicians would know how diet caused disease and how it might be changed so as to cure it. The analyses of animal and plant materials by distillation, extraction, digestion, and so forth, created a vast amount of information, but it did not provide answers to the doctors' questions. However, it did stimulate biologists to try to classify plants and animals on the basis of their chemical constitution (Goodman, 1971), but that attempt also failed. One of the early hypotheses was that only animal tissues contained protein, and that notion persisted until the end of the 18th century despite the fact that Beccari in Italy had discovered the protein gluten in wheat around 1700. Not until de Fourcroy in 1791 and Vauquelin in 1802 showed that protein was, in fact, a constituent of plants did chemists and biologists give up their hypothesis. Nevertheless, the hope that chemistry ultimately would establish criteria for distinguishing plants from animals was not abandoned. In the 19th century studies with this aim were continued in new directions, but they failed (Goodman, 1972). For example, after chlorophyll was established as a main pigment in plants, its presence in some animals also was demonstrated; after starch was held to be a product of plant metabolism, Bernard showed that a closely related substance, glycogen, was produced by the mammalian liver; after chitin was shown to be an insect substance, it was then found in mushrooms. (This led one ingenious biologist to suggest that either insects were flying mushrooms or mushrooms were sessile insects.) An extreme chemical view of the difference between an animal and a plant was expressed by Boussingault and Dumas, who in 1844 defined an animal as an oxidizing, and a plant as a reducing, organism. (This is but one example of the narrowness of outlook often imposed by competence in a basic science.)

Studies in plant and animal chemistry followed different paths for some time, more owing to the stereotypy of the human mind than to the nature of the subjects. Thus in the 1830s and 1840s botany seemed to be fanatically preoccupied with the size, shape, and color reactions of starch grains in plants, as revealed by the microscope. Schleiden, in language said to be typical of him, wrote in his article in *Flora* in 1840,

> We Germans have had the triumph of seeing the French, after making many easily avoidable detours, on account of superficiality in the work, reach the position already attained by Fritsche 10 years before, and now the whole phantasy dreamed up out of the air in the manner of Raspail is being thrown into the literary lumber room.

The "Raspail phantasy" referred to by Schleiden (today called the discoverer of the cell theory) was Raspail's observations on and descriptions of cells in his 1829 paper. Among other things, Raspail had already shown that the cytoplasm of plant cells contained protein. Regrettably, he was unable to pursue his observations because his activities connected with the 1830 Revolution resulted in a long incarceration. Two friends of his, without troubling to acknowledge their debt to him, in 1842 claimed this discovery as their own and showed that the metabolic activities of plant cells, like those of animal cells, depended on proteins. Sometime afterward in 1866, Haeckel published *Generelle Morphologie der Organismen*, in which he came to the remarkable conclusion that the cells's nucleus was responsible for the transmission of hereditary qualities, whereas the cytoplasm was concerned with adaptation of the cell to its surroundings (or, in complex plants or animals, the *milieu interieure*.) That book stimulated research on the different chemistries of the nucleus and the cytoplasm. However, men like His and others resented the microscopists' concept of organization, which seemed to impede the biophysicists' aim of reducing physiology to the molecular level (Olby, 1969). Before this, scientists like the Englishman Beale objected to the biophysicists' view of life and introduced vitalistic concepts into, of all things, discussions of staining reactions. At the same time men like Miescher were confirmed in their biophysical approach because they considered the chemical conclusions of the microscopists, which were based on crude staining techniques, to be too inexact to be accepted (Olby, 1969). Although the purported usefulness of chemistry usually was regarded with skepticism by medical practitioners in the late 18th century, the application of the new methods of chemistry to mammalian biology produced material that later would become useful to medical practitioners.

The early leader of this approach was von Liebig, with his epoch-making work of 1842 entitled, *Organic Chemistry Applied to Normal Physiology and to Pathology.* In it he not only classified the organic nutrients and summarized the then-available knowledge of nutrition, but he described new methods chemically analyzing organic compounds; established the empirical formulas of many compounds, some of which he had discovered; established the theory of "radicals" in chemistry; propounded the hydrogen theory of acids; and actually created agricultural chemistry. His own work, and that of his students, dominated biochemistry during most of the 19th century. Another German, von Hoppe-Seyler, carried the subject forward. Originally an assistant to Virchow, he became Professor at Tubingen and then at Strasbourg. His monumental work, *Physiological Chemistry* (1877-1881) was published in four parts: (1) general biology; (2) special physiologic chemistry, including the digestion and absorption of nutrients; (3) blood, respiration, and lymph; and (4) the organs of the animal body and their function. Although published a century ago, it remains a modern book.

In one sense von Liebig's writings constitute a source of confusion: he insisted that his application of chemistry to the study of life phenomena had to be conducted and interpreted in accordance with the scientific principles of physics and chemistry. In another, he stated that "everything in the organism goes on under the influence of the vital force, an immaterial agency, which the chemist cannot employ at will." He used the term "*Lebenskraft*" as if it were a specific kind of energy, saying at the same time that the words "vital principle" must be considered having equal validity to the terms "specific" and "dynamic." He added cynically that in medicine "everything is specific which we cannot explain, and dynamic is the explanation of all which we do not understand" (Lipman, 1967). At the time von Liebig was active, the terms "specific" and "dynamic" often were used loosely, because the sciences that employed them were fragmentary in content and vague and variable in concept. It is evident that von Liebig was handicapped severely by the inadequacies of the physics and chemistry he hoped to use to explain his observations. Suffering from the disorder that seems endemic in scientists, he assumed that current scientific data, however incomplete, artifactual, and erroneous, must be the procustean bed in which biology must lie. Von Liebig further assumed that whatever he could not explain in living things must be owing to "*Lebenskraft*," or "vital force." He was forced to engage in a certain amount of tightrope-walking, implying that "vital force" was evident in physiology, but not in test tube chemistry. Thus he believed that "vital force" was evident in physiology, but not in test tube chemistry. Thus he believed that "vital force" explained the digestion of food and its assimilation into the tissues of an animal; moreover, it explained growth, locomotion, and various defense mechanisms. He regarded it not as a metaphysical concept, a manifestation of a soul of some kind, but rather as part of the framework of scientific law, which acted in harmony with the known laws of the sciences. For example, he held that when the amount of "vital force" in an organism exceeded the amount necessary to maintain it, growth would ensue. Von Liebig's discussion of the subject reveals the inadequacies of the scientific material used by 19th-century reductionists and makes it clear that attempts to define the phenomena of living organisms on the basis of inadequate data is not an invention of the 20th century. Surprisingly, except for those determined reductionists reacting violently to any mention of vitalism, medical scientists, if they objected at all, merely criticized von Liebig's general concept of force; hence, some physicists made serious efforts to study his concept of force in an attempt to give it precision. In those discussions von Liebig's vitalism largely was passed over (Lipman, 1966), but the materialists would not let the matter drop.

The influence of von Liebig on nutrition and metabolism extended through much of nutritional biochemistry. After he and his pupil Wohler showed what the end-products of the utilization of food were and the circumstances in which they were formed, a second stage ensued. In this period von Voit and von Pettenkoffer (one of von Liebig's students) conducted studies on nutritional balance, showing how the amounts of protein, carbohydrate, and fat broken down in the body could be calculated from the amount of nitrogen found in the urine and that of carbon dioxide in the expired air. Von Voit's pupil, Rubner, demonstrated the caloric equivalent of the nutrients. That school of physiologic chemistry created the basis of the modern understanding of the macronutrients, carbohydrate, protein, and fat. Regrettably, the emphasis on the macronutrients encouraged some physicians and nutritionists to ignore the micronutrients, whose existence, but not (their) nature, was known to clinicians. Ignoring the micronutrients led to adverse effects before the error was recognized. Again, we see how preoccupation with a basic science, the study of which requires narrow specialization, leads to a narrowness of outlook that can have deleterious clinical effects.

One other comment might be offered on the subject of 19th-century medical biochemistry, and this refers to its role in the rise of German scientific materialism at mid-century, some leaders of which were chemists.

It is interesting that an American medical school was a leader in the trend of appointing nonphysicians as Professors of Chemistry in such institutions. The medical school at the University of Pennsylvania, the first in our country, was founded by, and for most of its early years staffed by, Edinburgh men, and the same could be said about the College of Physicians and Surgeons in New York. Perhaps stimulated by Cullen's interest in chemistry at Edinburgh, these two schools early established professorships in chemistry. The chair having become vacant at Pennsylvania in 1818, Hare, a layman, was elected to fill it (Klickstein, 1953). This was done with the advice of Hosack of New York, who stated that a physician was preferable, but not essential, for teaching the subject to medical students (Klickstein, 1954a). Today biochemistry is taught at many American medical schools by nonphysicians - or atrophied physicians.

At first Germany led the way in biochemistry, but the work of English scientists began to come to the fore by the end of the 19th century. Although in England biochemistry had long since taken the road toward becoming an independent discipline, it continued to be pursued in Germany in, or in association with, medical institutions. In England, the efforts of Hopkins and his many students finally led to its status as a discipline independent of medicine (Young, 1963; Kohler, 1978, 1979).

As biochemistry developed appropriately as an independent scientific discipline, proportionately less of it became applicable to medicine, and even less useful to it. In the early years of the 20th century the number of chemical determinations which could be carried out on a patient's urine, blood, or other body fluids amounted to a few dozen. The number of determinations that were essential to the diagnosis, or necessary in following the clinical course, were perhaps one-tenth that number. Subsequently, however, as biochemical determinations proliferated and were simplified in performance, numerous biochemical tests were introduced into medicine. Unfortunately many of the modern tests, especially those relating to enzyme activities, have had to be made highly artifactual in order to give readings of a readily measurable magnitude. Accordingly, these tests only can be used empirically and cannot be used validly to define physiologic states, a fact that usually is ignored. Today a significant number of tests performed on patients do not describe, as now interpreted, physiological states accurately. Even worse, they allow for - and in many academic centers encourage - the treatment of the patient's chart instead of the patient.

On the other hand, the contributions made by chemistry to medicinal therapeutics are enormous (Poynter, 1963). The remarkable advances in treatment afforded by chemistry also have given us increased numbers of undesirable side effects. The result being the necessary balancing in each case of the risk of giving a drug against the risk of not giving it.

Chapter 16: Some Aspects of the Relationship Between Physiology and Medicine

LONG BEFORE PHYSIOLOGY BECAME ESTABLISHED as the science of the function of living organisms, medicine as conceived and as practiced had strong functional implications. This was true even in the most ancient days, when demonic possession was believed to be the mechanism of disease: the demon entered the body and changed the way it functioned, and cure was the resumption of normal function, owing to expulsion of the demon. When, after the establishment of Greco-Roman civilization in the Mediterranean and associated areas, the humoral concept became established, it persisted for 1,000 years through the authority of Galen's works. Even during the Dark Ages, when most of the writing was done by the clergy, and hence was religious in content, the evidence is that most medicine was Greco-Roman, barring, of course, the medical service of the poor, which was in the hands of quacks (MacKinney, 1937). Although the clergy, who believed that illness was God's punishment for sin, did not believe that they should interfere actively, many of them, such as St. Isidore of Seville, did not disparage medicine. Practice at that period was comprised of blood-letting, diet, and giving herbs, and on the few occasions that pathologic physiology was mentioned, it was humoral in character. There was no way of knowing to what extent the sick were helped by the medical treatment based on humoral physiology. Some died of it (*e.g.*, Emperor Otto II, who died of excessive purging). The prevailing humoral physiology was in part inferential and mostly speculative. Its inferential component was based on the then-current notions of anatomy, as expounded in Galen's works.

The late Middle Ages and early Renaissance witnessed a growth in surgery, stimulated by the remarkable amount of trauma that seemed to be part of daily life. The surgeons needed to know anatomy, and Galenical anatomy was wanting. The need for an accurate system of anatomy stimulated dissections by a number of surgeon-anatomists, culminating in Vesalius' *De Fabrica Humani Corporis* in 1543. It is interesting to note that Vesalius' teacher at Paris, Dubois, was a fanatical Galenist who called Vesalius mad and who insisted that the differences between Galen's anatomy and Vesalius' only were due to the fact that man had changed between the writings of those men. The new anatomy destroyed the inferential basis of Galenic physiology and, in addition, created uncertainty and skepticism about the rest of Galen's system.

Perhaps the first casualty in the search for a new physiology dictated by the destruction of Galen's was Servetus. A heretic in many ways, he recorded in his book *Restitutio Christianismi* (1533) that the blood in the pulmonary circulation was carried to the lungs, where it was mixed with air and then returned to the heart. It is unlikely that Calvin, his persecutor, realized the significance of this observation, and he had Servetus burned at the stake for his heresies, together with his book, only two copies of which have been found since. Harvey's discovery of the circulation a half-century later further emphasizes the errors of Galen's physiology.

The weakening of Galen's hold on physiological thinking created a void that was filled quickly by two superstitions: the iatrochemical and the iatromechanical. For example, Descartes analyzed what he considered to be the bodily functions as if they were products of delicate machines. Borelli published his *De Motu Anamalium* (1680), in which he analyzed locomotion, breathing, and digestion in mechanical terms and produced some ludicrous errors. Mechanics proved insufficient and, since Borelli had thrown out Galen's "animal spirits," he had to invent the "*succus nerveus*," or "nerve juice." A little later Baglivi adopted the iatromechanical superstition, and a century later Pitcairne in Edinburgh still adhered to it. It is worthy of note that Baglivi, the enthusiastic iatromechanist, was an excellent bedside teacher; he left his iatromechanical theories behind when he entered the clinic. It cannot be emphasized too often that the pursuit of unproved or even erroneous ideas in physiology and chemistry did not exclude effective clinical performance, which required only that the patient, and not the current content of some laboratory science, was the court of last resort.

The strong acceptance of iatromechanical physiology in England was a notable phenomenon (Brown, 1970, 1977; Valadez and O'Malley, 1971). After an initial period of rejection or ambivalence, the mechanical explanation of physiology was accepted, especially in academic quarters. The acceptance of that superstition was held by some to be a manifestation of the Scientific Revolution, an attempt, however premature and unjustified, to achieve in medicine what had occurred outside it, the mechanization of the world picture. That explains why the iatromechanical theory was acceptable, but not why it was accepted, a question perhaps answered by the demonstrated need for a new synthesis after the decline of the Galenic system. Iatromechanics could not last, for it could not survive the spread of observation in biology which had been stimulated by the success of observation in astronomy and physics.

Although those superstitious systems did not survive, they filled a need for those physicians unable to tolerate uncertainty and needing the feeling (surely not a belief) that they fully understood the mechanisms of what they were doing clinically. Such systems were pushed aside by observations that were made in animals and humans in health and disease, for physiology as an experimental and observational science was pursued regularly during the entire 17th century. However, speculation was still a large part of the physiological thinking of the time, but at Leyden, particularly during the time of de le Boë, many of the speculations were tested by experiment in the laboratory. De le Boë encouraged the work of a number of younger physicians, and Leyden became a place of great activity in physiological research. Swammerdam and de Graaf are the most famous names of that period, but there were many others.

The first outstanding general work on modern physiology was that of Haller, one of Boerhaave's pupils at Leyden, and a universal genius in his own right. He was born in Berne, Switzerland, in 1708. His mother died shortly afterward, and his father not long after that time. He was delicate and probably rachitic, but he showed enormous capacity for study. By the time he was nine years old he read Greek, Latin, Hebrew, and Chaldean. For his own interest he wrote biographies of more than 2,000 notables, and presumably derived inspiration from the lives of some. He began his medical studies at the age of 15 in Tubingen, then went to Paris and finally Leyden to complete his studies. He had to leave Paris suddenly when the police raided his dwelling in search of a corpse (which they found) that Haller stole and was in the process of dissecting. After two years at Leyden, Haller started his travels, taking annual walking tours in the Alps and writing romantic poetry based on them. Historically he is better known, at least in Switzerland, as a poet, novelist, theologian, and political scientist than as a physiologist (Beer, 1947). His strict moralistic writings are particularly interesting in the light of his confession that, later when his marriage proved unhappy, he found consolation with the servant girl. At the age of 19, after his graduation from Leyden, he visited London, whose medical scene was connected strongly with Leyden's. His comments on the sights, sounds, and way of life of London were perceptive, particularly in the sphere of politics. He was high in his praise of English science, especially biology. He became acquainted not only with the physiologists, but with Swift, Addison, and other literary figures.

On his return to Basle he began teaching of anatomy and physiology. In 1736 he was appointed Professor of Anatomy, Surgery, and Botany at the newly founded University of Gottingen and served there for 17 years. At Gottingen, Haller pursued studies chiefly on the sensibility and irritability of tissues. At the age of 45, his homesickness for Switzerland and his hopes for a career in politics led him to resign at Gottingen and return to Berne. There he was given a minor municipal post, but soon gained a reputation for political wisdom which caused many government officials to seek his advice. He continued his animal experimentation at home and, in addition, continued to accumulate literature on physiologic matters, a habit he acquired while attending Boerhaave's lectures at Leyden. All of this material was collected in his *Elementa Physiologiae* (1759-1766), a work including his own research on circulation, which went much further than Harvey's in that it permitted the creation of the first general conception of hemodynamics. He also worked on the physiology of wound-healing. Much, but not all, of that physiology was inferential; that is, based on the interpretation of anatomical findings in health and disease. However, he was an expert anatomist, and his descriptions of physiologic phenomena in terms of anatomy usually were sound and, in any case, evocative.

Despite Haller's importance as a physiologist, his career was mainly that of public servant. His last years were filled with philosophical and religious doubt. He took refuge in morphine for his physical pains and in the Bible for his moral pains. His phenomenally productive work probably offered him distraction from both. He died in 1777.

Haller intended his work to be an account of all that was known in the field, but he recognized that what was known was quite inadequate for a sound understanding of bodily function in health and disease. Therefore, his work became an indicator of what had to be learned, and as such it stimulated and directed physiologists who followed him. By the end of the 18th century, physiology was clearly in a growing stage, and the first 50 years of the 19th century brought forward some outstanding scientists: Legallois, Magendie, and Flourens in Paris; Muller in Berlin, with his pupils, von Helmholtz, Brucke, and duBois-Reymond; Heinrich and Weber in Leipzig; Hall in London; Ludwig in Berlin, Vienna, and later Leipzig; Purkinje of Breslau and Prague; Pfluger in Bonn; and Bernard in Paris. (Since excellent histories that explore these and other men in detail are available, there is no need, if it were possible, to repeat that fine material. Only a few of them will be discussed because of their particular interest to medical practitioners.)

Magendie was the leader of physiology in France during the golden years of French medicine which ended around the middle of the 19th century. The son of a Bordeaux physician and revolutionary (who at times during the Revolution occupied high positions and at other times a jail cell), young Magendie began his medical studies in Paris at the turn of the century without, however, neglecting the fashionable salons of the period. In 1808 he passed the M.D. examination of the Imperial University, established two years earlier by Napoleon. He did outstanding research and soon attained high position. His work was important to practitioners for several reasons: (1) His pharmacologic studies introduced a number of alkaloids into medical practice. (2) He was strongly against vitalism and declared that "vital spirits," "animal spirits," Galenic "faculties," and van Helmont's "archaeus" were all excuses for ignorance. (3) He insisted that facts and facts alone should be presented and that the facts available in physiology were so few and scattered as to prevent generalizations. (4) His writings stimulated a search (vain, in my opinion) for a general philosophy of life and of knowledge (Olmsted, 1944; Temkin, 1946a; Albury, 1974). (5) He established specifically the function of the anterior and posterior nerve roots (Cranefield, 1973), a finding later claimed by Bell.

Muller was probably the greatest biologist in Germany's early history. Born a cobbler's son in Coblentz in 1801, he early distinguished himself for his passion for study. He won scholarships that permitted him to go to Bonn University, where he gained the M.D. degree at the age of 21. After two years of research at Berlin, he returned to Bonn as Assistant Professor and immediately started numerous studies in a wide variety of fields - anatomy, comparative anatomy, embryology, and physiology (Koller, 1958). One of his contributions was the logical classification of the lower organisms. Aside from his work on the embryology of the genitourinary system (Mullerian ducts), he was of interest to physicians because of his *Handbook of Physiology*, published in two volumes in 1833 and 1837. Like Haller's, it was a compendium; unlike Haller's, its many gaps were filled with vitalistic explanations. The year 1848 was a trying one for Muller, for he witnessed three of his closest students - von Helmholtz, Brucke, and duBois-Reymond - come out in violent criticism of his vitalistic, as well as his other scientific, ideas. At that time he was Dean of the Medical School at Berlin, where he tried to keep the students' demonstrations within tolerable bounds and to persuade both sides to discuss matters calmly. He failed in this and became deeply depressed, remaining so for a year. Afterward, he traveled and made observations on oceanic life, but his spirit was deflated and his life became restricted to work and associations with a few friends, including the former student, von Helmholtz.

Another physiologist who made crucial contributions was Purkinje. Like Rokitansky, Skoda, and von Hebra, he was a Czech in the Austro-Hungarian Empire, but he was not welcome there, for as an adult he was a Czech nationalist and involved in working for Bohemian self-determination. Also, he was a Freemason, dedicated to the ideal of universal freedom. He was born in 1787 in Bohemia, and after early education took holy orders and entered into a teaching career. He decided to enter the medical school at Prague, receiving the M.D. degree in 1819. His political opinions made it impossible for him to be given a position anywhere in the Austro-Hungarian Empire, but he was appointed Professor of Physiology and Pathology at Breslau, perhaps through the influence of his friend Goethe. The faculty there voted against him, but they were overruled by the German Minister of Education. He was received coldly at first because Slavs, in general, were scorned, and there were few of them in the German academic world. However, Purkinje's evident brilliance, together with his friendliness and urbanity, ultimately made him friends everywhere. He stayed at Breslau for 27 years. He was an expert histologist, developing new methods and making a number of discoveries in many aspects of physiology. (He coined the term "protoplasm" in 1839.) His discoveries included the observation, two years before Schleiden and Schwann, of the similarity of plant and animal cells. In 1823, long before Galton, he pointed out the importance of fingerprints. Soon after arriving at Breslau, he instituted laboratory training for students at the University, initiating the system by building a laboratory in his own house. The results were so striking that the German government built an institute for him at Breslau in 1842 and had the system copied elsewhere. After the Revolution of 1848 the repressive atmosphere in the Austro-Hungarian Empire was lifted, and in 1850 at the age of 62, Purkinje was made Professor of Physiology at Prague, where he taught often in the Czech language until the age of 82. He remained a political optimist until the end of his life.

The greatest physiologist of the 19th century was Bernard. He was born in 1813 in the Department of Rhone, the son of a small grower and winemaker. His early education was at a Jesuit school, where he became chorister. He wrote a farce called *La Rose du Rhone*, which was produced with some success in Lyons; but he made his living as a pharmacist's assistant in that city. His next play was a five-act tragedy about King Arthur, but he found little encouragement or opportunity for a literary career there, so he went to Paris in 1832. A critic read the play and acknowledged his aptitude for dramatic poetry, but suggested that a professional career might be more secure, whereupon young Bernard entered the medical school. He seemed to be no more than moderately interested in clinical medicine, but his associates found him uncommunicative and hence had no idea about his interests and ambitions. Nevertheless, what he saw at the bedside guided his research on laboratory animals, while his early work in literature gave him a clarity, precision, and euphony of expression, making his work accessible even to those with meager scientific backgrounds. In 1839 he served an internship as a student and in 1841 became assistant to Magendie, who at once recognized his genius in the planning and execution of experiments using relatively intact animal preparations. He took his M.D. degree in 1843, at the age of 30. He made many outstanding discoveries: the cerebral factor in the regulation of sugar metabolism; the formation and role of liver glycogen; the concept of internal secretion; pancreatic secretion in fat digestion; the function of vasomotor nerves; and the fact that carbon monoxide was a poison because it bound hemoglobin. Because of such discoveries, he was appreciated early (Holmes, 1974) and became famous later. His marriage, however, was a failure, and even his children were estranged. By 1854 he was given the new Chair of General Physiology at the Sorbonne and in 1858 succeeded Magendie as Professor of Physiology at the College there. He never held a faculty position at a medical school - nor did Magendie, Bert, and the other great French physiologists - since physiology was considered an "accessory" science, not a "basic" one, for medicine.

The low esteem in which physiology was held was shown by the deplorably poor laboratory facilities he had to use until 1869, when Napoleon III had new ones built for him (Schiller, 1966). In 1860 he had a severe relapsing illness, not diagnosable today, which forced him to withdraw from active work. When his mind was separated from his day-to-day studies in the laboratory and the preparation of lectures based on that work, it turned toward the philosophical basis of his way of life: The result was *Introduction to the Study of Experimental Medicine* (1865). Previously localized to physiology, his fame became more widespread, he gained honors and, a little later, adequate laboratory facilities. There is an irony in that, for it was his fame outside of physiology that gave him a physiology laboratory after many years of deprivation. The work is the finest exposition ever written of the experimental method in physiology and has been discussed widely as such (Henderson, 1927; Olmstead, 1935; Hoff, 1962; Schiller, 1967). Outstanding as that treatise is, it is not without faults. For example, when he stated that experimental pathologic physiology must be the basis of medicine, he was expressing a then-current view that was incorrect. It is true that pathologic physiology, experimental or otherwise, is an excellent means of indicating mechanism, and hence it is important in therapeutics; but it can do no more than suggest etiology. This is in contrast to other accessory sciences, such as bacteriology, toxicology, and nutrition, which can, where applicable, indicate not only etiology and prevention, but also therapy, to a great extent. Nevertheless, Bernard did not go so far as Virchow, who defined medicine as nothing but pathologic physiology, with the clinic and the autopsy room as mere "outposts."

Perhaps Bernard's most famous formulation is that of the *milieu interieur*, a constant composition of the extracellular fluid that protects the highly organized and sensitive mammalian cells from the effects of large changes in environmental conditions. That concept, however, is accurate to only a limited extent. For example, whereas the concentrations of most inorganic ions, including the hydrogen ion, are highly constant, the concentration of one of them (*i.e.*, phosphate) may vary markedly for brief periods. In the case of the organic substances, whereas uric acid, urea, and creatinine concentrations are constant, those of sugar, fatty acids, and cholesterol concentrations are not. We must remember that Bernard did his work at a time when physiology was not far from its infancy. In the history of a science broad generalizations are easy to make and at such times laws are easy to formulate. Such generalizations and so-called "laws," however, always prove to be limited in their applicability. Different tissue cells have different degrees of susceptibility to changes in their environments and, hence, the need for a constant *milieu interieur* is always relative and is variable from tissue to tissue. Normal ranges are broad, and there is no absolute boundary between sick and well. Despite these deficiencies in some of Bernard's generalizations, he remains the greatest physiologist in history for his elegant experiments, conceived with disciplined imagination and planned and interpreted with unfailing logic. The direction of his work at first always was to clarify previously unexplained situations encountered in medicine, not to examine some current theory.

Toward the end of his career Bernard began to deviate from those patterns when he paradoxically widened his horizons and focused more closely on certain phenomena. He began a course of lectures on general physiology - the fundamental phenomena common to living organisms - but he never finished them (Hoff, *et al.*, 1974). Despite the incompleteness of those last lectures, we must recall two principles relevant to this subject which he had stated a decade earlier. One related to vitalism. Here he enlarged upon the views of earlier writers when he pointed out that the physiologist and the physicist differed not as regards the principles that guided their research, but only with respect to the complexity of the conditions on which they made their observations. The goal was the same in the physicochemical and biological sciences, but "it is much harder to reach it in the latter because of the mobility and complexity of the phenomena we meet." He emphasized that fact especially in relation to cell function (Holmes, 1963). Bernard's statement should never be forgotten by physicians, especially those who try to reduce all the phenomena of human illness to current physicochemical concepts derived from *in vitro* or other oversimplified systems. Another of his comments was that all living organisms, including men well or sick, existed in equilibrium with *their* environment:

> There always comes under consideration the *body*, in which the phenomenon takes place, and the outward circumstances or the environment which determines or invites the body to exhibit its properties. The conjunction of these conditions is essential to the appearance of the phenomenon. If we suppress the environment the phenomenon disappears, just as if the body had been taken away....Indeed, if we absolutely isolate a body in our thought, we annihilate it in so doing; and if on the contrary, we multiply its relations with the outer world, we multiply its properties.

The last statement, although he did not intend it, has strong psychological implications with respect to the personality.

In the meantime, in many parts of Europe, physicians, many of whom had never heard of Bernard (indeed some lived before he was born) were making physiological observations on their patients, and in some instances, on animals as well. Some of these observations will be discussed later.

A number of men had described studies on the gastric juice of men and animals removed from the body and had argued about the mechanism of its action (Bates, 1962). However, it was Helm of Vienna who, first in a brief note in 1801 and then in a book in 1803, described his observations on a woman with a hole in her stomach (Kisch, 1954). We know little about Helm except that one of his sons later became Professor of Medicine at Pavia in Austrian Italy, and still later Director of the Allgemeine Krankenhaus in Vienna. Helm took his work seriously but modestly. After mentioning the physiologists whose work on animals had preceded his, he wrote:

If these men had taken care of my patient, they would have done better than I did. I confess my inferiority, and would not like by this paper to elevate myself to the level of these scholars. I merely did not wish to miss this favorable opportunity, and regarded it as my duty to communicate my observations, in order to light a candle in a field where unpenetrable darkness prevails and to replace hypothesis by irrefutable facts in medicine. To clear the path which leads to the truth, to turn isolated observations through experiments and investigations to real experience by analogy and induction, that is the cumbersome but beautiful task of the practitioner among the physicians.

Sublime speculations at the desk will not advance a practical science like medicine the slightest amount, even in centuries, and thousands will pay for them with their lives.

If my laborious experiments should contribute in the least degree to enlightening us concerning one dark problem in animal economy, should they help even one single human being to alleviate his suffering through selection of food which is easy to digest, should they perhaps inspire only physiologists and chemists to a more adequate investigation of the process of digestions, so important for the animal organism, then I feel a hundred times rewarded for every trouble and every expense and I shall be happy to the very end of my days knowing that I have contributed my share to the welfare of mankind.

It is certain that natural science and chemistry have advanced practical medicine and will advance it more than millions of concepts contrived and concocted at the desk.

He might have added, in explanation of his last three lines, that the sciences in medicine are often helpful in patient-oriented studies, but less often do anything for theory-oriented experiments.

In his book Helm described how mechanical irritation (*i.e.*, poking his finger into the hole) affected secretion. He noted the changes in food placed in the stomach, in particular the curdling of milk. Helm's work was neglected in Germany and Austria; however, Waterhouse, then at Harvard, became aware of it through his friendship with deCarro in Vienna. A year after the work was published, Waterhouse mentioned it in, of all places, his lecture advising students on how to keep their bodies healthy by not drinking or smoking (Kisch, 1955). Waterhouse also described Helm's work in a letter to the periodical *The Medical Repository*. In the meantime, back in 1803, James Young, a medical student at Pennsylvania, wrote his thesis on gastric digestion, having done his work in animals (Bates, 1962). Young concluded erroneously that the acid in the juice was lactic. Beaumont's observations on a man with a hole in his stomach were published in 1833, and his many studies especially emphasized the role of many factors on gastric secretion and on the color of the mucosa through the gastric mucosa. Beaumont is an example of an intelligent, mentally active army medical officer stationed in a remote isolated post, who nevertheless found stimulation in a medical phenomenon that presented itself. His work received wide attention in Germany (Rosen, 1943), less in England, and very little in France. With the passage of time, appreciation of Beaumont's work, but not that of Helm, has grown all over the world.

Prout, who was at Guy's Hospital with Bright, Addison, and Hodgkin, stated that there was hydrochloric acid in the gastric juice, a discovery he had first made in 1824. Thus the observations made on patients by practicing physicians in the 19th century were the beginning of our knowledge of gastrointestinal function, and the technology of the 20th century advanced our knowledge of that function in health and disease, and in response to treatment. The part played by active practitioners in this process is notable, but not surprising. Gastroenterology is an example of the way in which medicine adapts and utilizes technology in a manner that need not impair the doctor-patient relationship and, in fact, may improve it.

Data on the physiology of respiration also were being accumulated by physicians in practice. Hutchinson modified Lavoissier's so-called "gazometer" to produce the water spirometer, whose design has not changed significantly in over a century (Spriggs, 1971). Hutchinson also defined the various subdivisions of the lung volume much as they are defined today. A few years later Salter, using respiratory tracings, defined the pattern of normal and abnormal respiration in humans (Neale, 1963). His interpretations of respiratory mechanisms, particularly in asthma, are remarkably modern after 125 years. Artificial respiration by means of an iron lung was developed almost simultaneously by Dalziel in 1834 (Baker, 1971) and a little later by Higgison (Gray, 1972). Afterward improvements were made by other practitioners before the end of the century (Baker, 1971. In the 20th century, particularly in its second quarter, medical practitioners chiefly in Germany at first and then in America published their findings in diseases like emphysema and pulmonary fibrosis (in which radiographic data may not be very helpful). Here, too, conducting the tests required not only the proximity to, but the cooperation of, doctor and patient, and, if anything, enhanced the relationship between the two. The other phase of respiratory function clinically in use today relates to the blood gases, a physiologic function having its origins in the 18th century, when Black in Edinburgh discovered carbon dioxide and Lavoissier in Paris noted the respiratory function of oxygen. Although in the previous century Boyle had obtained air from blood by means of a vacuum pump, it was not until Gustav Magnus, Professor of Physics and Technology at Berlin, began his studies that the modern era began. He obtained blood from horses and from "commoners who for a small sum permitted themselves to be bled." In his first experiments Magnus merely bubbled pure hydrogen through blood and collected the gas, which then demonstrably contained carbon dioxide. Then he used a mercury vacuum pump and demonstrated the presence of both oxygen and carbon dioxide (Breathnach, 1972), showing that arterial blood contained more oxygen than did venous blood. He concluded that uptake of oxygen by the blood was accomplished by diffusion in the lungs, subsequently giving off carbon dioxide. Over the next few decades improvements were made in the method, improvements associated with the names of Ludwig and Pfluger among the well-known German physiologists. Paul Bert in his book published in 1878 claimed that the invention was really French, and he also noted the snob-appeal of a foreign label. In his *Barometric Pressure, Researches in Experimental Physiology* (1878) he wrote

> The invention of the mercury pump is usually attributed to German technicians and with the love of foreign advertising customary to us we often decorate this instrument with the name of 'Geissler pump.' The truth is that the invention belongs in principle to M. Regnault.

As a member of Gambetta's party after the defeat of France by Prussia, Bert hardly could be expected to avoid an opportunity of criticizing Germans. He inveighed against "the charlatanism of decimals which leads to claim exactness for the thousands in a number which is wrong beyond the units, [a charlatanism] common on the other side of the Rhine."

Changes continued to be made which, in the present century, led to the widely used van Slyke apparatus, developed in America. It was accurate but cumbersome. In the last few decades electronic methods have come to the fore and are used widely for studying blood obtained by puncture of an artery.

Respiratory measurements early came into use in the study of energy production in humans and animals. Lavoissier was the first to measure oxygen uptake and carbon dioxide production in humans as affected by work, food, and temperature, using a copper helmet over the subject's head. Before 1800 he measured those gases in a guinea pig and related them to the heat production of the animal as determined in a calorimeter. In the 1820s a prize was offered in Paris for the best article on the subject, and a number of French investigators responded to the challenge by writing excellent monographs. Around

1849 several Frenchmen developed a closed-current apparatus for measuring the gas exchange in humans. Fifty years later that was done in Germany by Hoppe-Seyler and ten years after that in America by Benedict and his co-workers. After this a vast literature developed. Open-circuit methods were simpler to use and the work, with such a device, by Voit and Pettenkoffer beginning in 1868 became expanded into the studies of the effects of different foods, starvation, and overfeeding. The data of Voit, Pettenkoffer, and later Rubner, made the Munich and Berlin schools of metabolism famous (Magnus-Levy, 1947). Much of our understanding of the effects of different foods on energy production in humans grew out of this work (as did the popular parlor game of counting calories), which led to the invention of the basal metabolism test (no longer performed).

The history of physiologic studies on the cardiovascular system presents a varied picture. At about the same time Struthius made the first estimates of blood pressure in humans, and Harvey showed that the blood moves in a circulatory system, with the heart as the pump. However, the forces that caused the blood to circulate were not explained fully. Although it was easy to understand how the force imparted by the heart to the blood pushes it through the arteries and capillaries, the mechanism by which the blood returns against gravity from the legs and lower body to the heart was unknown. In the early 19th century two English physicians, David Barry and James Carson, showed that the negative pressure in the chest sucked blood "up" from the lower body (Cohen, 1963; Breathnach, 1965). The problem of studying the cardiovascular system in humans engaged the attention of medical scientists around the middle of the century. Although Vierordt developed the first externally applied device for studying the arterial pulse, reported in his *Die Lehre vom Arteriepuls* (1855), the apparatus was cumbersome and not highly reliable. It was Marey who made this approach widely applicable with his own device (Nichaelis, 1966; Lawrence, 1978).

Marey was another of the unusual men who made French clinical medicine famous. He did his work at a time when the reputation of French medicine was said to have gone into eclipse, a period also of Bert and Brown-

Sequard, who worked in it and are recognized today as farsighted pioneers. Marey was born in Beaune in 1830 and at an early age exhibited his highly intelligent interest in two areas - animal biology and mechanics - which he later united brilliantly. He entered the medical school at Paris in 1850, not with the primary intention of becoming a medical practitioner, but with the idea of combining his two interests. Nevertheless, his clinical training in large measure determined his research activities. Convinced of a need for increased accuracy in the detection and appraisal of physical signs, he turned his attention first to the recording of cardiovascular phenomena in humans. He devised an apparatus that, when strapped to the wrist, carried the pulse impulse to a rotating drum on which the impulses were recorded. Such an apparatus was intended to be only a pulse-counter, but its use soon broadened, and it was applied to measuring pulse-wave velocity and, more particularly, abnormalities in pulse-wave form. After receiving his M.D. degree in 1860, he continued his work on the mechanical recording of vital phenomena, improving his apparatus and broadening the scope of its use. His appointment as Professor at the College de France gave him more and better laboratories for his work in humans and animals, and permitted him to acquire a group of devoted assistants. In the meantime, his tambour sphygmograph, an instrument of easy use, low inertia, and freedom from artifact, was used in clinical studies, notably in England, on the abnormal pulse-waves encountered in disease. The results obtained with Marey's device were received enthusiastically by some physicians. Others declared that the tracings taught them nothing they did not already know, a response typical of the closed mind.

Many men contributed to the development of cardiovascular physiology in animals in the 19th century (Wiggers, 1960). Much of the advance was made possible by Ludwig's development of the kymograph, although initially the blood-pressure curves obtained with it were artifactual (Hoff and Geddes, 1975). Marey and others greatly improved the accuracy of the tracings. Chauveau devised a method of catheterizing the cardiac chambers of a horse, and he and Marey published remarkable tracings of the pressure changes in the ventricle and auricle during the cardiac cycle.   Marey also invented a device for recording electrically the action currents of the heart (Geddes and Hoff, 1961).   The tradition of the study of cardiovascular dynamics in animals was continued brilliantly in the 20th century by Heymans' group, Wiggers, and others.   In the first half of the 20th century, after the development of appropriate methods by physicians working in physiological laboratories, hundreds of clinicians wrote hundreds of articles on the physiological disturbances of the cardiovascular system encountered in its diseases.   These have been collected elsewhere (Altschule, 1954).

The autonomic nervous system plays an important part in visceral function, a concept whose role in the development of the modern understanding of the autonomic nervous system as it related to physiology began with the writings of Willis 300 years ago.   Willis anatomically divided the peripheral nervous system into two portions: One was concerned with the voluntary motion, and the other with involuntary motions, such as those of the heart and the abdominal viscera (Ackerknecht, 1974).   The term "sympathetic" was applied to the involuntary nervous system because at that time there was a belief that processes acted on each other within the body by sympathy, whatever that was.   Such an idea suggested that at least part of the autonomic nervous system, the sympathetic, was the medium whereby emotions induced, or were manifested by, changes in visceral function (Altschule, 1976).   Since some of these emotions might not be perceived consciously, many physicians of the mid-19th century believed that one function of the sympathetic nervous system was to express some aspects of unconscious cerebration.   In contrast, at about this time, von Feunchtersleben in Vienna was propounding the dogma that the "ego" was making known its wants or decisions by bodily manifestations that were symbolic expressions of the "ego's" thoughts (Altschule, 1976). The accumulation of writings on the action and mechanism of action of the sympathetic nervous system was due to the efforts of most of the leading physiologists of Europe, principally Germany.   A considerable portion of the physiologic literature of the 19th century consists of their controversies, not about "what," but rather "how," an action occurs.   The vagal portion of the autonomic nervous system created special problems. Whereas the prevailing view in the past was that nerve impulses *did* something, those who studied vagus function found that it *inhibited* something (Hoff, 1940). Although that was known to French physiologists around 1800, it was the work of the Weber brothers that clarified the situation. In the late 19th and early 20th centuries, the works of Gaskell and Langley in England unified and clarified the vast amount of available data and conceptual material. Following the discovery of the neurotransmitters and their different receptors enlarged our understanding of how certain drugs worked. While all of those positive contributions were being made, a number of academic physicians, unable to resist their inner need to generalize, gave us the concept of diseases due to an imbalance between vagal and sympathetic activity (Ackerknecht, 1974). Those are best forgotten except as examples of what always happens all around us - creation of broadly applicable dogmas to explain what is not explainable. Leaving such peculiarities to one side, since they do not represent an important part of medical data, the great benefit of today's medicinal therapeutics imported by the physiologic research on autonomic function should be recognized.

It is evident that physiological thinking, since it is based largely on data obtained in studies of whole animals or at least whole organs or tissues, has always been close to clinical thinking. This is true because physicians, although often concerned chiefly with one organ or system, must nevertheless deal with the patient, an entity certainly different from, and perhaps greater than, the sum of its parts. When physiology removes itself from its traditional area of whole organisms, organs, or tissues, it separates itself from clinical medicine and deprives the latter of the use of physiologic data, while at the same time suffering from a lack of the stimulation given it by observations made in sick people by practicing physicians. This most emphatically should not be taken to indicate that knowledge of physiology (and its related chemistry) is all that a practicing physician needs to know in order to be a physician.

Chapter 17 Changes in American Attitudes Toward French and German Medicine After the American Civil War

THE HIGH LEVEL OF EXCELLENCE OF FRENCH MEDICINE that developed in the first half of the 19th century did so despite the marked changes in political climate occurring at that time. The defeat of Napoleon I was followed by the restoration of the Bourbon monarchy, with its extreme conservatism and its reliance on the Jesuits to define educational policy. There was a purge of those medical teachers and hospital staff members known or believed to be out of sympathy with the aims of the new regime. Despite such turmoil French medicine continued to prosper during the 14 years of Bourbon rule, in part because some outstanding physicians, such as Laennec, were themselves conservative, and many took no strong stand either way. However, the Bourbon monarchy was abolished forever in 1830, when the "bourgeois king" Louis Phillippe took over the government. French medicine continued to prosper and the names of many famous French physicians of that era are remembered today. French medicine was considered to be leading the world, and hundreds of Americans and other foreigners interested in the study of medicine went to Paris. However, the frequent alterations in the political regime naturally had an unsettling effect after 1848. That year the revolution, created by the more or less liberal middle class and participated in by more radical elements of the population, seemed to offer hope of social and economic liberalization under a republic. However, in the first election for the presidency of France, Louis Napoleon made himself a candidate. (The radical Raspail was a candidate also.) Napoleon won easily, helped by the memories of past glories; in addition, the newly enfranchised peasants, conservative by nature, voted predominantly for him. He was elected and two years later had himself voted Emperor, with the title Napoleon III.

Adverse effects in academic medicine became evident almost as soon as Napoleon took office. For one thing, political polarization became marked, as shown by the physically rough handling received by Bernard from radical students because he was conservative in politics. Evidently they considered his conservative politics more important than his scientific greatness.   There were faculty changes as well.   For example, Orfila, a great physician, was forced to give up his post as Dean of the Faculty of Medicine.   Orfila had an interesting history, graduating in medicine in Spain and, despite anti-French feeling generated in Spain by the atrocities of Napoleon's campaigns there, being sent to Paris for additional study.   He remained there, using his outstanding chemical talents and knowledge to create the science of toxicology as a new branch of medicine.   His qualities as scholar, scientist, and teacher were recognized widely, as were his personal qualities of integrity and humanity.   Nevertheless, Napoleon III forced him out.

Napoleon's policies resulted in marked decreases in the support of medical sciences.   Despite Bernard's recognized greatness worldwide, his laboratory was shamefully inadequate, while at the same time Napoleon was spending large sums on his disastrous military adventures: the Crimean War, the support of Maximillian's attempt to seize Mexico, and finally the greatest disaster, the Franco-Prussian War (not initiated by Napoleon).   The collapse of France was followed by the revolt of the Communards while Paris was under siege.   Twenty thousand people died in Paris during the fighting and famine, and the Parisian academic world was harmed seriously.   When Paris medicine declined, French medicine as a whole declined, for although there were schools in other cities in France, most were not nearly as famous as that of Paris.   Moreover, one of France's finest schools, Strasbourg, was lost to Prussia.

Even before the events of 1870 and 1871, in fact in the 1850s, American physicians and students in Paris showed their disenchantment with the regime of Napoleon III by volunteering to serve in the *Russian*, not the French, army in the Crimean War.   Although economic recovery in France was rapid after Sedan, French medicine did not recover, and the attraction that Paris medicine had held for American students was diminished permanently.

The Americans' disadvantage - the different language and lifestyle - in France had been offset in the past by the advantages afforded by training in French medicine. Those advantages largely were gone because the stimulating atmosphere of vigorous clinical development due to new approaches in the 1830s and 1840s was dissipated when such new approaches became old.

This is not to say that French medicine had come to a complete standstill or had regressed. Far from it. For example, Trousseau was a great clinician in an earlier style and was recognized as such during his lifetime. His systematic clinical works were translated into other languages and were especially popular in America. On the whole, however, French clinical medicine had few followers in America. In addition, modern neurology was created by a remarkable group of clinical neurologists trained also in the neuropathology then being developed. The contributions of Charcot, Duchenne, Marie, and others are memorialized in the names of the syndromes they defined. No American neurologist could claim expertness in that specialty unless he had been trained in Paris, but neurologists were few in America. Similarly, the field of psychiatry in France gave us Pierre Janet, one of the greatest physicians who had ever studied the clinical phenomena of mental disorders. His high standing in the opinion of today's American psychiatrists is shown, for example, by the fact that they uniformly ascribe his comments on neurosis to Freud. (This syncretism, whereby the local deity acquires the virtues and powers of all predecessors, commonly occurs in religions of all sorts.)

One of the most interesting aspects of French psychiatry almost has been ignored totally. French psychiatrists of the last decades of the 19th century used the recording methods of Marey and others to study the changes in circulation and respiration occurring in association with emotion. Binet and Courtier, in effect, created psychophysiology. Some of their tracings showing changes associated with *angoisse* are remarkable in themselves and also because they emphasize that facial expression may be a poor indication of what a person is feeling. Their observations were received with general indifference. The French psychophysiology of the time was the study of the bodily physiologic changes associated with feelings and emotions and should be distinguished from the physiologic psychology of Wundt, Fechner, Ludwig, and von Helmholtz, which involved functions such as sensory modalities and voluntary reactions.   The latter was received skeptically by British psychologists (Daston, 1978); the former was ignored, not only by the British but also by most of the rest of the world, a notable exception being Mosso in Italy.

The leader and, in fact, creator of much of the new neurology and psychiatry was Charcot.   Born in 1825, he obtained the M.D. degree at Paris in 1853.   Nine years later he became Physician to the Salpetriere and, starting with a small number of patients with neurological disorders, he created the greatest neurological clinic the world had yet seen.   He made notable contributions to the understanding of hysteria as well.   In addition to his work in neuropsychiatry, he made important studies on diseases of the liver, kidney, and lungs.   Although outwardly serious from his student days and seemingly lacking in sociability in his maturity, he held weekly, eagerly anticipated social events for his associates and students.   A man of great sensibility, he refused to experiment on animals.   When combined with his clinical perceptiveness, his skill as an artist produced remarkable drawings of his patients and historical pictures of critical scholarly discussions of matters related to medicine.   He was also co-author of a monograph on demonomania (Guillain, 1959).   He achieved great fame as the physician who, alone or with his students, was the first to describe a great number of neurological disorders.   That should not make us lose sight of his contributions as a medical thinker, as opposed to a medical theorizer:

> Symptoms, then, are in reality nothing but the cry from suffering organs.   The condition of the patient is only an accident in the history of the disease, just as each of us is only an accident in the history of humanity.   How is it that, one fine morning, Duchenne discovered a disease which probably existed in the time of Hippocrates?

Disease is very old, and nothing about it has changed. It is we who change, as we learn to recognize what was formerly imperceptible. It is the mind which is really alive and sees things, yet it hardly sees anything without preliminary instruction. In the last analysis, we see only what we are ready to see, what we have been taught to see. We eliminate and ignore everything that is not a part of our prejudices.

Clinical medicine is made up of anomalies, while nosography is the description of phenomena that occur regularly. What we look for in the clinics is almost always exceptional; what we study in nosography is the rule. It is well to know that, in the practice of medicine, nosographer is not always a clinician.

His comments on the nature of medicine are so completely different from those that make up the *Ideengeschicht*, which occupies so much space in medical historical writings, that they rarely find their way into them.

Unlike neurology and psychiatry, a good part of the other French contributions to medical science was ignored or given little attention until the end of the century, or even later. That curiously deferred recognition of French research is seen in both physiology and bacteriology and helped divert attention from French clinical medicine. In physiology the work of two men - Paul Bert and Brown-Sequard - who followed Bernard exhibits that characteristic.

Bert was born in 1833 in Auxerre in Burgundy, the son of a lawyer who had become a civil servant and a Bonapartist politician. His mother was the daughter of a civil servant of Scottish descent, and her grandfather had established the family fortune by buying church properties seized during the Revolution. (Years later in 1880 Bert was accused of being the greatgrandson of a thieving monk, whereupon he sued for slander, won the suit, and donated the money he won to establish a prize in history.) Bert's mother died of tuberculosis when he was only 13, and his only brother died of that same illness. He himself, though sickly, was full of energy and mischief. He started to study engineering, but his father, who seemed to be something of a tyrant, forced him to change to law. Bert led the frivolous life of students of the period, spending much time in the Latin Quarter, where he achieved local renown as a composer of romantic melodies; nevertheless, he completed his studies at the age of 24. He then went to Algeria to hunt for a few months and on his return to Paris did nothing for a time until his father allowed him to study medicine. He was interested particularly in comparative anatomy, and three years later, in 1860, took his diploma in natural sciences, writing a thesis on respiration which he defended against the views of Bernard. The two, however, became close friends. Later he took the M.D. degree, writing a thesis on tissue grafting, for which he won a prize. Although urged to marry an available wealthy woman and go into practice he decided instead to pursue a career of science, becoming Bernard's assistant. He married an 18-year-old Scottish girl in 1865, and the marriage was a happy one. Bert was Professor of Zoology at Bordeaux for a few years and later became Professor of Physiology in Paris, a post he held until 1885. In addition, he was active in politics, and after the fall of Napoleon III, he was sent to Lille as Prefect to reorganize its government. He served in the Chamber of Deputies for some years, as Minister of Education for two, and as Resident General in French Indochina in 1886. He died in Hanoi of dysentery after six months of effective service there.

Bert's work on tissue grafting in animals, had it been the sum of his research work, should have given him an excellent reputation, for his studies were designed to establish not merely the possibility of transplantation but, as befits a disciple of Bernard, the influence of the tissue milieu on that phenomenon. His work on the role of barometric pressure in physiology was even more outstanding. In fact, the studies of Jourdanet on mountain sickness stimulated Bert to extend his own studies on respiration to the effects of atmospheres with low and high barometric pressures. He published papers on that subject between 1870 and 1885, but the essentials appeared in his monograph of 1878, which contained a historical review of the subject followed by his new data. He showed that when the barometric pressure falls, the oxygen tension of the air breathed, and that of the circulating blood, likewise falls; an increase in barometric pressure has the opposite effect. At very high pressures, the body is poisoned by the oxygen, and it is oxygen tension rather than oxygen percentage which determines the effect. Moreover, decompression sickness is due to the release of nitrogen from its dissolved state in the blood. All of that work was forgotten until it was resurrected in World War II and served as the basis for studies on the hazards of high altitude and undersea existence.

Bert's extensive and prominent political activities in the early days of the Republic evidently overshadowed his outstanding qualities as a researcher in physiology (Ackerknecht, 1944). His interest in politics had begun long before the Revolution of 1870, but his activities in government had to wait until the fall of Napoleon. He lived only 16 years after that event, and he spent them in the pursuit of his two main interests, physiology and government; but, it was the latter that kept him in the public eye. The neglect of his monumental work on upper atmosphere and underwater physiology was perhaps as much due to the fact that in 1880 there was no air travel and little effective diving to bring to everyday attention the hazards of these activities. (Such highly practical research is an example of what is today called "project-oriented," with no project yet in existence to give it current importance.)

One wonders what Bert imagined of the future. Was he a science-fiction fanatic like his countryman Jules Verne? His political, educational, and governmental activities showed him to be fully at home in the real world, but also demonstrated his hope for a better future. It is ironic that in Germany Virchow's generally ineffective liberal political activities made him a hero, whereas in France Bert's highly effective liberal political activities led to the criticism that he had discarded science for politics. Of course, that was not true, for Bert was a greater scientist than politician. It is also ironic that

Bert's name is not included among the great French physiologists: Magendie, Bernard, and Brown-Sequard.

Brown-Sequard is the last of the French physiologists to be discussed. His mixed career exemplifies many points mentioned previously: that physicians attracted to physiologic research still could be attracted to clinical practice; and, that the nonmaterial rewards of research could outweigh the intellectual and material rewards of practice. Moreover, it illustrates the fact that the penchant of leading French physiologists was to conduct disease-related studies rather than the theory-based studies of those who were more interested in defining the nature of life or establishing some theory about it. Perhaps aspects of Brown-Sequard's personality influenced his decisions at times. He was born on the island of Mauritius, then called Isle de France, a French possession 550 miles east of Madagascar. His mother was the daughter of a French trader and government official who had settled there. She married Charles Edward Brown, a captain in the American Merchant marine who was born in Philadelphia of Irish parents. The British took possession of the island by treaty in 1814, having conquered it the year before in reprisal for its use as a pirate base for attacks on their Indiamen. Thus Brown-Sequard, although American-French by heritage and totally French by upbringing, was a British subject by birth. His father was lost with his ship on a voyage to India before his son's birth. The widow was poor and took in sewing, and young Brown-Sequard worked as a clerk in a store as he grew up, but disliked it. When he was 21 his mother took him to France so that he could finish his education, and once there he decided to study medicine. For some time his mother kept a boarding house for students, until her ill health finally terminated that enterprise. When she died he added her family name to his, making his own Brown-Sequard.

Brown-Sequard took his M.D. degree in 1846 with a thesis on the physiology of the spinal cord, a subject which was to interest him for decades. The poverty of his student days was little ameliorated after his graduation. Although interested mainly in physiology, he took work under Larrey in a military hospital in 1849 and distinguished himself in the treatment of numerous cholera victims there.

However, his work in physiology was recognized by his election as one of the secretaries of the *Societe de Biologie*. In 1852 after the *coup d'etat* by Napoleon III, Brown-Sequard, perhaps uneasy about the possible adverse effects on his career of his republicanism, went to New York City where he taught French and practiced medicine. He married the first of his three wives, a niece of Daniel Webster's wife. He then returned to Paris to pursue his research until 1854. At that point he was refused a professorship at the Museum of Natural History, largely because of opposition from the other professors. He left France again, this time for practice in his homeland, Mauritius, where he served well during a cholera epidemic. In 1855 he was given the Professorship of the Institutes of Medicine (today called pathological physiology) at the Virginia Medical College in Richmond. However, his antipathy toward slavery and his inadequate working conditions drove him away. The next year he was back in Paris pursuing his physiological research. Among other things, he removed the adrenal glands in animals to study the effects of the procedure and likened those effects to the human disease. That work was conducted in a rented laboratory, where he also gave private lectures on neurophysiology to medical students. His many lectures and his monograph on epilepsy and other diseases gave him a worldwide reputation. In 1858 he started the *Journal de Physiologie* to which he contributed frequently, without apparently diminishing the numbers of his papers in other journals. A year later he was made Chief at the Queen Square Hospital in London, where he lectured on clinical neurology and neurophysiology. He also held famous lectureships in England from time to time, and his talks were published in leading journals. In 1864 Harvard gave him the Chair of Physiology and Pathology of the Nervous System.

Brown-Sequard gave the opening lecture of the academic year at the Harvard Medical School on November 7, 1866. As was customary, the class had it printed at their own expense (Brown-Sequard, 1867). That speech emphasized the practical value of knowing physiology and chemistry, a value clearly exaggerated in the light of knowledge of those subjects in 1866. By today's standards his most valuable comment was the following:

But it is said that scientific researches are long and difficult, and they bear fruit only after hard and prolonged labor; and that therefore a busy practitioner, and still more a busy student, cannot do anything for science. There is certainly some truth in this; but let me ask you a few questions:-

Are not the busy practitioner and the student in a hospital constantly in presence of facts which have not yet been discovered, and which can easily be discovered?

Are they not constantly the witnesses of phenomena disproving great theories which, by being false, are obstacles to the progress of science?

Only a man who was a clinician as well as a laboratory scientist would understand that most of the ideas responsible for opening new fields of study for laboratory scientists were suggested by those bedside observations recognized as out of the ordinary by some medical practitioner.

He held that Harvard post until the death of his wife. The provincialism of Boston caused him to return to Paris in 1867, where he gave the course in Comparative and Experimental Pathology at the Faculty of Medicine, but was not given the professorship because he was an alien. With Charcot and Vulpian he founded another journal, *Archives de Biologie*. (We are familiar with Charcot's name but not Vulpian's. Vulpian should be remembered for one of those typically French researches with long lead-times before exploitation. A century ago, when he cut the adrenal glands of animals and showed that the cut surfaces turned red, he was actually describing the first step in the change of catecholamines to melanin, a process now recognized as crucial in the function of the brain.)

Despite Brown-Sequard's enthusiastic following among students and his worldwide reputation as a neurologist and neurophysiologist, he again left for New York City to practice medicine (and marry another American woman). Vulpian not only was given Brown-Sequard's course, but the professorship that accompanied it, one which was denied to Brown-Sequard (Schiller, 1966). After traveling to London and Geneva, Brown-Sequard returned to paris where, on the death of Bernard, he inherited the Chair as Professor of Experimental Medicine at the *College de France.* He spent the rest of his days in France, receiving its highest honor in the biological sciences, election as President of the *Societe de Biologie.* His output of experimental findings remained high, although the quality deteriorated.

Brown-Sequard made adrenal gland extracts for injection, and he is often referred to as "the father of endocrinology;" but, his experiments were controlled poorly and failed to support his ideas conclusively. Moreover he marred his standing with overenthusiastic reports of sexual rejuvenation induced by extracts of testicular tissues. On the whole, Brown-Sequard's contributions to neurophysiology and clinical neurology, together with those of Charcot and his famous co-workers in clinical neurology and neuropathology, made France the leader in the field of neurological diseases into the 20th century.

While the great French physiologists Bernard, Bert, and Brown-Sequard were working in shamefully inadequate laboratories that had no space or facilities for training students or visitors, the situation developing in Germany was quite different. There, the success of Purkinje's institute in Breslau stimulated the various German states, separate until after 1870 and in many respects competitive with each other, to establish their own institutes for physiological work conducted almost entirely on animals or parts of them. The men who headed these institutes are recognized today as the creators of quantitative studies of the functions of the organs and tissues. The institutes had excellent facilities not only for the senior scientists, but also for large numbers of students at various levels of training. By the 1870s the men trained in those laboratories were well on their way to filling posts created in response to the explosion of interest in physiology which was occurring. Unlike the French physiologic institutes, which were isolated somewhat from the milieu of medicine, those in Germany were part of the medical educational structure, much to the benefit of physiology and, to some extent, medicine. Although much of the work being done in the German institutes was theory-based rather than patient-oriented, such institutes at that time remained connected with university medical faculties. Accordingly, the view spread that German medicine was the most innovative and, hence, the best in the world. The fact that some outstanding physiologists had to leave Germany for political reasons after 1848 merely hastened the spread of German ways.

There was no question of the German physiologic brilliance, but there were serious doubts about its applications, which often were in accordance with the dogmas of Scientific Materialism. For example, when Erni became Professor of Chemistry at the University of Vermont College of Medicine, his introductory lecture in 1857 defended that view by emphasizing the physician's need for scientific training. Moreover, he stated that the era of a truly rational system of medicine was approaching, and that every student in the near future would need a thorough acquaintance with Science as the only sure and true basis upon which to build. Since medical students tended to pay more attention to surgery, obstetrics, and practical training, Erni had to defend the place of chemistry in the medical curriculum. He noted that some professional men of the "old school" considered chemistry an idle and useless handmaid of medicine, often sneering at the revelations of a microscope as applied to physiology or pathology. Erni believed that every disease was attended by chemical changes, and that the profession had advanced from that time when physicians ascribed supernatural forces to medicines, to the present, when it was known that the effect of a medicine was directly related to its chemical properties. Although what he said undoubtedly was true, he omitted - as others of his opinions always did - the fact that there was too little available chemical data to permit the creation of a scientific medicine.

The scientific aspects of bacteriology, however, remained isolated from medicine, in terms of locus and interest to medical practitioners. Pasteur's early interest in bodily immunity did have practical results in his attenuated virus vaccine for rabies. The heat-killed vaccines developed by Theobold Smith made it possible to immunize people and animals *before* they contracted an infectious disease, but the treatment of those already suffering from the disease was not at hand. Laboratory studies by Rous, Bordet, von Behring and others showed that toxic bacterial substances were the actual causes of symptoms in many diseases. Von Behring's discovery of an antitoxin that neutralized the toxin produced by the diphtheria bacillus was highly important. Similar attempts in other diseases were not successful, although much was learned from studies done at the Pasteur Institute and from those of Ehrlich and Wasserman in Germany. The discovery by Charrin and Roger in 1889 that the serum of immunized animals caused clumping of the offending bacteria was developed by Widal, a Paris physician and later Professor of medicine in Paris, into the well-known Widal test for typhoid fever. As he described it in 1896, the test consisted of mixing a patient's serum with a known culture of typhoid bacilli and, if clumping occurred, it proved the diagnosis in the patient. Widal previously had shown that animals could be immunized against typhoid fever using a vaccine of heat-killed bacteria, and that approach was adopted widely to prevent typhoid fever and related infections in humans. In 1901 Bordet and Gengou first described the complement reaction, an evidence of an immune process, and Widal proved its success in humans (Hunter, 1963). In 1900 Widal and his associates developed not only the method of staining exudates from patients, but also tests like the Widal test for other diseases. In 1902 Richat discovered anaphylaxis, a type of hypersensitivity reaction, and this, too, was an outgrowth of earlier theoretical work on immunity. Arthus, another Frenchman and a graduate of Paris who had worked for a time at the Lille Pasteur Institute, did pioneering work on immune processes which resulted in his discovery of what is known today as the "Arthus phenomenon." He published his great monograph, *De l'Anaphylaxie a l'Immunite*, in 1921 (Sigerist and Longcope, 1943). However, Arthus also should be remembered for his comment, "Seek facts and classify them and you will be the workmen of science.

Conceive or accept theories and you will be their politicians."

Such examples show that the interest of Pasteur and his students in immunity to disease eventually played important roles in clinical medicine. Nevertheless, the actual treatment of people suffering from bacterial diseases moved slowly despite those studies on immune protective processes made by Bordet, Ehrlich, Wasserman, and others. Only years later, if ever, did their laboratory studies become usable in medicine, an extremely frustrating fact, since the work of Koch and other mostly German workers had identified the bacterial causes of many diseases, and it was hoped that these diseases would be conquered. Clearly another approach was needed.

Koch and others tried to cure bacterial diseases in experimental animals by injecting antiseptics such as bichloride of mercury, but that soon proved useless, since any chemical that killed the bacteria also killed the animals. However, studies made by protozoologists provided a clue to a new approach. In 1880 the French Army physician Laveran discovered malarial parasites by direct microscopic examination of blood specimens. Since they were *animal* parasites and not bacteria, the idea of directly poisoning them arose. (Actually quinine had been used for centuries to kill the malaria organism in patients.) In 1902 Laveran and his colleagues at the Pasteur Institute showed that the blood of animals infected with trypanosomes could be cleared of the organisms temporarily by giving them an arsenic compound, sodium arsenite. That observation stimulated Ehrlich to study diseases produced by trypanosomes, using infected animals sent from the Pasteur Institute. Ehrlich was interested greatly in using dyes as stains, and he had learned much about it from his uncle, Weigert, the great stain chemist. Ehrlich and Shiga injected the infected animals with different dyes and in 1904 found one, trypan red, which was effective, but not always so. The testing of already available or newly created dyes went on frantically. Thomas at Liverpool showed that an organic compound of arsenic was more effective against the organisms than sodium arsenite. That compound was relatively nontoxic and, hence had been given the name "atoxyl." Using his considerable chemical knowledge, Ehrlich made variants of atoxyl and tested them on animals infected with both trypanosomes and also the spirochete of rat-bite fever, which resembled the organism causing syphilis. Ehrlich's aim was to find the chemical cure for syphilis, which he accomplished on the 606th attempt, calling the effective compound "606" or "salversan" (Goldston, 1940). At the same time he was developing staining reactions for the white blood cells, a matter of great importance, since the Russian Metchnikoff, working at the Pasteur Institute from 1880 onward, had shown the role played by those cells in fighting infection. Ehrlich contributed ingenious hypotheses regarding the process of immunity and also the manner in which chemical remedies worked. From that time the science of the chemotherapy of infectious diseases proceeded along the lines laid out by Ehrlich, and the results are well known today (Jacobs, 1940).

Ehrlich's brilliant ideas and propensity for dramatic expression helped disseminate his findings. His discovery of Salvarsan deserves every praise; however, it was development, not research. His theories of immunity were useful formulations but were oversimplified representations of what was happening. His greatest contribution - the one for which he should be famous - was the discovery of the cell-staining methods that permitted the recognition of the different kinds of blood cells, with their differing functions in the body economy. He created an entirely new science, one far broader than he envisioned. Moreover, although Ehrlich worked in a separate institute, his dramatic pronouncements attracted the attention of physicians, and his discoveries became known to them.

Although this account of the differences between French and German medicine in the second half of the 19th century is condensed, it is neither oversimplified nor exaggerated. The contrasts between the struggle of the medicine-related laboratory sciences in France and the enthusiastic government-mediated stimulation of those same sciences in Germany are evident. In addition, the highly visible immediate usefulness of the products of German science, especially the creation of impressive (but evanescent) theories, differs from the less evident immediate usefulness of many products of the great French physiologists.

In addition, the sociopolitical events in the two countries were markedly different.

In France the succession of forms of government - empire, Bourbon kingdom, Orleanist kingdom, republic, second empire, and finally republic - created problems of political loyalty among the faculties and tensions between students and some of the faculty.   Under the final republic, a succession of constitutional and political crises kept France in a highly unsettled state, despite its remarkable economic recovery after the war with Prussia.   All of those factors dissuaded many foreigners, especially Americans, from turning to France for studies in medicine and medically related sciences.

In Germany progressive science was leading the world in new directions and, accordingly, foreigners were encouraged to go there for study.   At this time the newly created government of the united Germany, as a matter of policy, created scientific showplaces with its universities and institutes.   Huge amounts of money were poured into the universities in Berlin and, craftily, Strasbourg, which the German government wanted to make the finest of any, apparently to show the world, and more particularly the French, what German culture meant.   To all of this must be added the fact that at that time in America there were thousands of refugees from the failed German and Austrian revolutions of 1848.   Several American cities virtually became German, and others had German newspapers, clubs, hospitals, and schools.   Refugee Germans participated actively in American life.   Their record in the Civil War was admirable and their political and cultural influences great. To a large segment of the American population, German was a second language, and in some rural areas it was the only language.   In contrast, the number of French-speaking people in America numbered only a few thousand, with perhaps a majority speaking a Cajun *patois* (in Louisiana) or a Canadian French dialect (in northern New England). The circumstances favored a large migration of Americans to the German-speaking nations of Germany and Austria. While Germany was expanding the role of medicine-associated sciences, Austria maintained its position as a clinically oriented medical culture, a fact noted by Bigelow, Professor of Surgery at Harvard University, in his address to the Massachusetts Medical Society on June 7, 1871 (Bigelow, 1871).

The superiority so obvious in French medical science, and to whose valuable teaching the German school owes much, has gradually yielded to the rapid strides of more recent German progress.

Paris, once the Mecca of the medical student, has yielded to the predominance of the German in science, as in arms, partly through the original indirect influence of the common school, - because, while France means Paris only, Northern Germany is covered with centers of intellectual activity and production, so that, to enumerate them all, one has to go down to towns of the third and fourth rank.

The barren fields of speculative hypothesis and arbitrary assertion have been fairly replaced by the precise results of induction from observed phenomena; and when we consider the multitude of able minds and the vast labor thus for years concentrated upon the facts of health and disease, we shall be astonished neither at the amount nor the character of the progress of medical science in Germany during this period, nor at the advantages which the German schools offer at this moment to the medical student.

To the foreigner, the especial attraction of Vienna - as of Paris formerly - is, that the student who desires instruction upon any one of twenty or twice twenty different, yet distinctly medical or surgical subjects, of every-day use to the practitioner, can, with half a dozen of his friends, induce an able teacher, for a moderate compensation, and with every facility for clinical or anatomical illustration at command, to exhaust the subject for their particular benefit. The knowledge is exactly what you want, imparted when you want it, and by a teacher with whom you are brought into close personal relations. But it is an error to confound the idea of this medical knowledge proper with any vague notion of a higher education and a higher science to result from extended collateral study. Let us distinctly bear in mind that the American medical student abroad commonly has little to do with either Physiology or even Chemistry, unless he pursues it as a special branch of study, and for some purpose other than the practice of medicine.

Bigelow's comments were corroborated emphatically by subsequent events (Bonner, 1963). The American physicians, trained largely without laboratory experience, were fascinated by the outstanding reputations of German and Austrian physicians and medical scientists, as well as by the new freedom of learning and teaching. Prior to 1850 the German universities, combined, had less than 24 American students; however, that number rose rapidly thereafter, and other foreign students followed suit. It has been estimated that 1,500 American physicians and medical students received much of their training in a German-speaking university between 1870 and 1914, a majority coming from the Eastern States, and a few from the South. Most were postgraduates. A minority spent their time in the laboratories of Leipzig, Strasbourg, Breslau, or Heidelberg, usually entering academic medical life back in America; but, the majority did *clinical* investigations at Berlin or Vienna, perhaps with those interested in specializing preferring the latter.

As the end of the century approached, Berlin's popularity as a clinical teaching center increased, but it never equaled Vienna's. Regarding the medicine-associated sciences, Breslau and Leipzig were outstanding, and Strasbourg even more so. The proliferation in Germany of laboratories devoted to medicine-related sciences and attached to clinical services was remarkable. It seemed almost to take on the character of an evangelical movement; much of the impetus apparently had come from the great naturalist von Humboldt, who believed strongly in the need for laboratories and libraries connected with the university facilities.   He founded the University of Berlin in 1810, largely because that city already had some notable libraries and collections.   The growth of the movement outside Berlin was slow at first.   However, Liebig was able to persuade the Hessian government to provide a fine laboratory, equipped for research and teaching, at Giessen in 1826.   Purkinje later was given a physiological institute at Breslau, Muller had his at Berlin, and Ludwig at Leipzig. Virchow took the Chair of Pathology at Berlin in 1856 only on condition that he be given an institute there.   After 1872 Hoppe-Seyler had one for physiological chemistry at Strasbourg, Pettenkoffer one for hygiene at Munich, and Koch for bacteriology at Berlin (Rosen, 1965).   Those given clinical appointments also demanded facilities for research and teaching.   Naunyn, when appointed at Konigsberg, demanded adequate experimental laboratories with appropriate budgetary support.   Von Giessen at Munich was given attached laboratories for chemistry, physiology, and bacteriology, plus a library and examination rooms.   The idea that clinical services had to have scientific laboratories became the established mode in Germany.   All were state-supported and contrasted with the privately supported Pasteur Institute established in France in 1886 (although Ehrlich in Germany had a privately endowed institute).

On the whole, approximately two-thirds of the Americans went only to Vienna, and another 20% only to Berlin.   It should be noted that while the Americans disliked the German students, as contrasted with Austrian students, they praised the professors (Bonner, 1963).   The Americans considered the German students unappreciative of what was offered to them and stubbornly insistent on their own selfish, arrogant ways.   This discrepancy between the human qualities of teachers and students is a puzzling phenomenon, and although it has been discussed (Bonner, 1963), it never has been explained.   Was it the cause or the consequence of the German insistence on science *vs.* the Austrian attention to clinical practice? Whichever it was - perhaps both - it nevertheless indicates a defect in the German medical educational system. The quality of any educational system is determined first by the students, next by the faculty, then by the facilities, and last of all by the curriculum. The German university medical educational system had the second and third of these to outstanding degrees and was better than adequate in terms of the last, although it was not as good clinically as Vienna.

Yet this flawed educational system was to be a training ground for the faculties of the leading medical schools in America up to and for a time after World War I. To what extent the transplantation of German medical education to America is responsible for some of our own difficulties will be discussed later in this work. However, in considering the latter decades of the 19th century, it appears that the popularity of German scientific medicine among American teachers trained in Europe was largely due to the extensive facilities and enthusiastic teaching that the Americans received there. These far exceeded what was available elsewhere in Europe and certainly in our country. The product, German scientific medicine, was displayed to advantage, and perhaps the display made acceptance of the product easier, although it did receive some other help in America.

While French medicine was struggling to maintain its excellence, with varying results, and German laboratory-based medicine was astounding much of the world, especially America, the events in Great Britain, which continued its high standards of performance in clinical medicine, should not be ignored. Notable clinicians were numerous. Biochemistry, especially at Cambridge, showed marked development, but more as an independent science than as a part of medicine. The growth of physiology was less attention-getting but nevertheless was significant. Perhaps the quiet way in which physiology grew in Great Britain is exemplified by Sharpey.

A graduate of Edinburgh who studied for a time in Paris under Dupuytren and Lisfranc, and then in Germany during the *Naturphilosophie* period of retrogression, Sharpey returned to teach anatomy and physiology at Edinburgh and then at University College in London. He held the latter chair for 38 years and came to be regarded as influential a teacher as Muller in Germany, although much less prolific as an original investigator. Through his influence the number of physiological laboratories in Great Britain grew, and they were staffed by men of high competence (Taylor, 1971). The solid work of these physiologists was less in the direction of sensational originality than in bringing order into a field that had grown not only rapidly but incoherently. For example, after Brown-Sequard carried out his less-than-superb experiments on the adrenal glands and Schiff conducted his experiments on the thyroid gland (which Kocher's work subsequently clarified), English physiologists were bringing order into endocrinology, a field that showed tantalizing promise but lacked structure. Gull's clinical demonstration that dessicated cattle thyroid glands could cure human thyroid deficiency was an important stimulus to medical thinking. However, it was the work of the physiologists Schafer (at London's University College and later Edinburgh) and Starling (Schafer's successor at London) which turned the field into a science (Borell, 1978). One of Sharpey's assistants was Foster, who moved to Cambridge as Praelector of Physiology in 1870 and made that university the site of a major school of physiology, in which that science developed as an independent discipline. Its graduates included Martin (later of Johns Hopkins University), Langley, Gaskell, Bancroft, Adrian, and many other distinguished scientists. For a long time Great Britain lacked the great number of full-time medical scientists and extensive research and teaching facilities that the German universities possessed. Nor did the English medical school teachers exhibit as much evangelical enthusiasm for scientific medicine or propensity for theorizing and dogmatizing as did the Germans. Hence the number of Americans attracted to Great Britain for medical training was not large in the late 19th century, but it increased later.

Reference has been made to the part played by German philosophical systems in influencing ideas about medicine either directly or indirectly, by creating an intellectual climate in which certain ideas about medicine could become acceptable. Since this chapter is concerned with contrasting happenings in Germany and France, it is of interest to mention the status of relevant portions of

French philosophy. In fact, the decline of French scientific thinking, relative to the German, during and after the Second Empire and its subsequent renaissance by the end of the century have been linked causally to changes in French philosophy (Nye, 1979). If, indeed, this is the case, I believe it is only because they developed in parallel fashion. If anything, the change in French philosophy occurred later, in that it was a manifestation of a climate of thought already evident in French medical science. This is difficult to ascertain accurately because, unlike their German counterparts, French medical sciences were unwilling to make the all-encompassing generalizations. Accordingly, this view of the temporal relationship may be incorrect. However, the new French philosophy did describe prevailing French ideas of the period and, therefore, should be discussed.

The new philosophy had its formal beginning in a thesis by Boutroux entitled, *De la Contingence des Lois de la Nature* (1874). Boutroux was a Frenchman who went to Heidelberg in the late 1860s to study philosophy and its history. He greatly admired the German worship of learning and the manner in which the different learned disciplines criticized and influenced each other. He was impressed by the important role of philosophy there, and he wrote harsh criticisms of French learning, in which he said that each discipline maintained its own isolated status. He left Germany because of the war and in 1871 became a Professor of Philosophy at Caen, where he became friendly with men interested in philosophy, mathematics, symbolic logic, and related subjects. One of his friends, Tannery, had emphasized in the early 1870s that the seeming rigor of science was false, owing to its use of symbols. He made the remarkable statement that "mathematicians are so used to their symbols and have so much fun playing with them, that it is sometimes necessary to take their toys away from them in order to oblige them to think." In his 1874 thesis Boutroux asserted that fundamental scientific principles are, in fact, abstractions from reality; that is, not actual reality, but only a creation of the mind. Hence, he stated that the so-called "laws of nature" so important to German scientists were valid only in the mind's abstraction of reality, and not in reality itself. His

brother-in-law, Poincaré, was known also as a chief proponent of what came to be called the "conventionalist philosophy." Of course, that was the restatement of an ancient idea. There is no way of knowing to what extent
concepts such as those influenced physicians' thinking
about the role of laboratory science in the human problems
of medicine; but, that philosophy, which emphasized the
uncertainty of science, was quite different from the scientific materialism that was being promoted by German
physician-polemicists. When uncertainty in science finally
did reach Germany, it took a different route and had a
different and more limited form - Heisenberg's uncertainty
principle - which was so removed from the world as physicians knew it, as to be of no consequence to them.

At any rate, the viewpoints that were expressed
formally in the writings of Boutroux and later Poincaré
made it impossible to grant any validity to the scientific
reductionism popular in German medicine. That reductionism, while pretending to have been the ultimate in rationalism, had to distort the world and man in order to make
them coincide with the extant physicochemical dogmas.
Those doctrines, by claiming to be extensions of laboratory
science, actually had the effect of evoking skepticism toward the idea that science was the only way to study
man. Such skepticism by no means excluded laboratory
science from the study of man, sick or well, but that science was only one of the methods used, albeit one of the
more uncertain. French philosophy of the late 19th century emphasized the idea of uncertainties in human thinking; German philosophies assumed and preached the certainty of their concepts, and that was particularly true of
the Scientific Materialists who, for a time, occupied influential positions in German academic medicine.

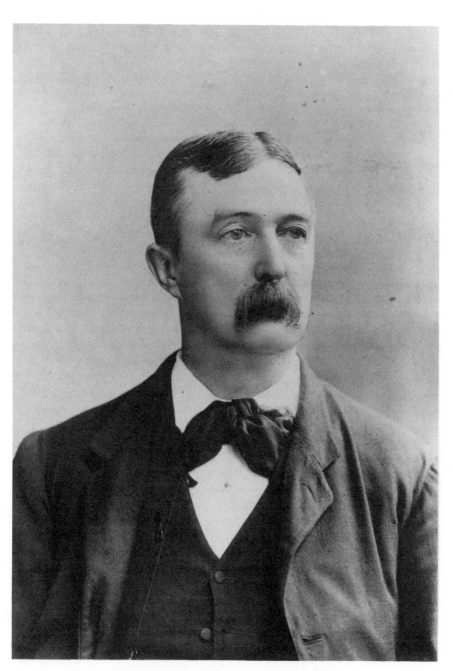

John Shaw Billings, 1838–1913

Chapter 18: The German Influence on American Medical Education: The Flexner Report

IN THE LATE 18TH CENTURY THE AMERICAN ENTHUSIASM for Edinburgh medicine was such that men trained at that school achieved high position in medical practice or education in American coastal cities (with the notable exception of Boston); a few Edinburgh men became prominent even west of the Alleghenies. Certain features of Edinburgh medical education consequently became established in America. Similarly, when Paris became the place for American physicians or students to enhance their training, many of these Paris-trained men achieved high position in American medicine prior to and just after the Civil War. This was most striking in Boston, where the highest-ranking faculty members at Harvard were Paris men, but it also occurred in Philadelphia, New York, and some other cities. In these cities the degree to which the ways of Paris medicine were adopted differed, being more marked in Boston than in the other cities. The same processes occurred when the German-speaking nations became the places to which American physicians went for training. The number of Americans who did so between the Civil War and World War I was very large. However, a majority of the Americans went to Vienna for clinical training, and when they returned to America many entered into practice or teaching as specialists in the newly defined clinical specialties. A minority, mostly academicians, studied at the German schools, where many were impressed by the following: (1) the belief of evangelizing German academic physicians that certain sciences were the essence of medicine, with clinical practice a relatively minor dependent; (2) the belief that clinical services were to be responsible for the laboratory research needed to secure progress in medicine; (3) the notion that the organization of hospitals to be used for teaching should make those hospitals appendages of a university, with the physicians becoming full-time employees of it (in contrast to the London system, where the medical school was an appendage of a hospital); (4) the conviction that increased time should be allotted to basic science in the medical school curriculum; and (5) the idea that premedical education should be extended and strengthened, a view already expressed by Eliot of Harvard and a little later by others.   In all of those areas the influence of German ideas about medicine and the education for it were to have a considerable influence on American medical education and later, in a blunted way, medical practice.   The most striking consequence of the German academic influence in America has been the maximizing of the role of laboratory sciences in medical practice.   That evangelizing movement succeeded because of two factors: (1) the activities of some American physicians; and (2) the fact that America had begun to produce a crop of millionaire industrialists, some of whom wanted to spend a portion of their money doing good, and a few of whom wanted to do it in the field of medicine. We should understand at once that however praiseworthy the motives underlying these enterprises, the intentions did not necessarily guarantee the quality of the results.   The business world has taught us that a man may have great skill in making money, which does not imply necessarily that he will have skill in spending it.

The German influence was very evident in the founding of a great new medical school in America in 1876.   It was a time when reductionism and the consequent overemphasis of the role of science in medicine was being touted strenuously in Germany.   The idea of founding the new school had its beginning when Peabody and Hopkins met in 1886.   Peabody, a native of Danvers, Massachusetts, had prospered in London and had become an outstanding philanthropist on both sides of the Atlantic. He persuaded Hopkins to follow the road of philanthropy, and in January of 1867 Hopkins incorporated the Johns Hopkins Hospital and the Johns Hopkins University (Parker, 1960).   In his thinking about the hospital he may have been influenced to some extent by the pamphlet written by his neighbor and business associate, Macaulay (French, 1953).   Macaulay followed the German line in advocating a close connection between hospital and university, as well as a greater emphasis on science in medical teaching.   In

Baltimore the importance of good hospital facilities was acknowledged widely. One physician wrote, "The rise and prosperity of all medical schools in Europe during the last century has been directly in proportion to the hospital advantages they could offer and to the importance attached to clinical teaching. The reputation of London for its medical teaching is in great part due to its hospitals. The Hotel Dieu has been the origin and center of the Paris school; the Allegemeine Krankenhaus has given a reputation to the Vienna school; and the Charité has brought to Berlin much of the fame that its university has gained in medicine." He added that placing the hospital under the control of a university, "with which its interests and successes are intimately connected" was a very decided advance (van Bibber, 1879). However, it is clear that it was Billings who actually carried out Hopkins' ideas about the union of school and hospital and who developed other ideas about the functions of the two institutions. Billings filled an important role as advisor to the trustees of the newly incorporated institution. In preparing his plans, he traveled extensively in Europe and corresponded with many there, including Florence Nightingale (Cope, 1957), but for the most part he developed his ideas in accordance with Hopkins' intention to create a teaching hospital tied to a university-controlled medical school. His views on the importance of science in premedical education were strongly similar to those that Gilman, the first president of Johns Hopkins University, had expressed in 1878, some years before the hospital and medical school opened (Chesney, 1936). Billings deserves some comment as one of America's most remarkable physicians. The fact that his career did not begin in Edinburgh, London, or an American coastal city may account for the little general recognition given him in the present century, although lately his reputation has been growing.

Billings was born in Indiana of Mayflower stock. As a boy he was a great reader, teaching himself Latin and Greek in the process of acquiring a wide literary background. He entered Miami University in Oxford, Ohio, where his poverty forced him to live very frugally. He graduated in 1857 and a year later entered the Medical College of Ohio in Cincinnati. As a student he served as intern at two of the hospitals in that city.   After receiving the M.D. degree, he became Demonstrator in Anatomy, a post he held for two years.   Offered an opportunity to become wealthy as assistant to Cincinnati's leading surgeon, he chose instead to join the Union Army, receiving his commission in April of 1862 at the age of 24.   He quickly attracted attention and was put in charge of a hospital, after which he was given the task of converting a barracks into another hospital.   He was given field duty beginning in March of 1863 and, after Chancellorsville, he was responsible for moving a hospital filled with wounded to the rear during the retreat.   He had charge of a divisional hospital that handled a large number of the wounded at Gettysburg, and he served in the headquarters of the Army of the Potomac during the bloody Wilderness campaign and the siege of St. Petersburg.   Shortly before the War's end, he was moved to the Surgeon-General's Office in Washington.   He was detached to make a survey of the Marine hospitals, and that material, together with his report on Army Barracks and Hospitals, was published in 1870.   At once he was recognized as an outstanding authority on hospital construction, organization, and management.   In 1876 he assumed his duties as planner and supervisor of the construction of the buildings of the hospital and medical school at Johns Hopkins.   Two of his important papers were published in 1878: One, in the American *Journal of Medical Sciences*, was a "Review on Higher Medical Education," an analysis of the European and American systems; the other, published by the Trustees of Johns Hopkins University, consisted of the talks he gave as Lecturer in the History of Medicine.   Those two documents were highly important statements on medical education. They discussed the requirement of studies leading to the arts degree previous to admission, the need for expertness in Latin and modern languages, the thorough study of logic and sciences related to medicine during the four-year medical course, the provision of a hospital building not only to house patients but to make available rooms for teaching, the insistence on extensive and close contact of the students with patients, the visiting of patients in their homes, the close association of university and hospital with control by the former, the adequate salaries for teaching by clinicians and scientists, and the need for research on clinical conditions. All of those items testify to the breadth and excellence of Billings' thinking. Although many are made uneasy by the idea of a university controlling a hospital, the propositions Billings put forward are eminently acceptable.

Billings went further (Chesney, 1938), writing the following,

> Even those Professors in the Medical Faculty whose duties are not purely clinical, must have more or less to do with the Hospital and Hospital Staff. The teacher of Pathological Anatomy or Pathological Chemistry must keep in view therapeutics and diagnosis as well as his own special branch and must be familiar with the latest advances in these subjects or the value and interest of his work will soon begin to diminish. Insofar as the teachers are students - and students they must be - the Hospital is their special field of study.

Abel, the pharmacologist at Hopkins, later concurred strongly with that idea (Macht, 1940). Billings also emphasized the importance of making observations as they occurred in nature, a process today scornfully called "birdwatching" by ultrascientific biologists. Billings wrote,

> In Physics, Chemistry, and to a certain extent in Natural History, the facts are either frequently repeated or can be reproduced at pleasure. In Medicine, as in Political or Social Science, the case is otherwise; we must depend upon observation of conditions which may occur very rarely. Chance may present to the most obscure practitioner an opportunity for observation which the greatest master may never meet, and whether he will avail himself of it or not will depend very much upon whether as a student his attention

has been called to the possibility of the occurrence of such a case....

Billings' ideas received much wider currency than
did the earlier reforms instituted at Harvard by Eliot, although the latter were presented in the Midwest by one of
the earlier writers on medical education reform, Wiley
(later the originator of the famous Food and Drug Act of
1906).   Wiley graduated from Hanover College, a small
Presbyterian institution in southern Indiana, his schooling
having been interrupted by service in the Union Infantry.
He then entered Harvard College, graduating *cum laude* in
chemistry, and receiving his diploma from the very hands
of President Eliot in 1873.   Returning to his home state
(which was also Billings' home state), he was appointed
Professor of Chemistry in the Indiana Medical College
(Fox, 1962).   There, in February of 1874, he wrote his paper on medical education, repeating some of Eliot's ideas
on the subject.   (The paper was read for him because he
was gravely ill on the appointed day.)   Eliot's reforms
mainly referred to length and content of the curriculum,
the requirements, and the running of the school, plus the
introduction of the new sciences as they developed.   He
did not mention research on patients, and Harvard always
has rejected the principle of full-time clinical teachers.
The excellence of Billings' conceptions and the
strength of the Hopkins' Trustees' support, albeit merely
nominal in some respects, make the circumstances of the
founding of the School an important landmark.   The acceptance of Billings' ideas did not result always in appropriate action.   For example, the organization of laboratories
as part of clinical services, after the German model, did
not occur until after Osler's resignation and the appointment of Barker as Professor of Medicine.   At that time
scientific laboratories established as part of clinical services were springing up in a number of places in this
country, but they combined research and diagnostic service
and pursued the teaching of clinical pathology to students.
This is what happened, for example, at the Peter Bent
Brigham Hospital in Boston.   It is probably a coincidence
that Barker, like Christian of the Brigham, was originally a
pathologist who rose to be Professor of Medicine at one of

the great American hospitals. Moreover, at Hopkins the full-time system for clinical teachers was not instituted for some decades after the Hospital opened. It is probably only a coincidence that the two features omitted by Eliot at Harvard were slow to be instituted at Johns Hopkins.

In considering the high quality of Billings' analysis of medical education, we must recognize its originality, as evidenced by the rejection of some of the more peculiar aspects of the German medicine, although, on the whole, he admired and respected it. Billings never mentioned the reductionism and the scientific materialism popular in Germany, the notion that all life phenomena can be explained by the simple laws of physics and chemistry (of the mid-19th century at that!). Similarly, he never mentioned Virchow's idea that medicine was only pathological physiology as studied in the laboratory, with the bedside and the autopsy room as peripheral and minor areas. After performing his services for Johns Hopkins, Billings went on to plan many other hospitals, including Boston's Peter Bent Brigham Hospital, but his most notable contribution was the creation of the Surgeon General's Index Catalogue of Medical Literature. The last of its 16 volumes was published in 1895, the year of his retirement from the Army. Garrison continued the work later. The next year Billings was appointed Director of the New York Public Library and changed its previous bewildering chaos to effective order.

Regrettably, some of the men Billings recruited for the Hopkins faculty were not as sensible as he, notably Mall and Welch. Mall, German-trained in microscopy, was made Professor of Anatomy at Johns Hopkins. He was an excellent microscopist, the "father of American embryology," but he scorned the teaching of anatomy, an attitude that evoked resentment among those students hoping to become surgeons (Bernheim, 1949). Since that was an internal affair at Hopkins, it is of no consequence to this work, except that it tells us something about the man. What is of interest is his fervently expressed admiration of almost everything German, which probably caused him to take a prominent part in promoting the Flexner Report, as will be discussed later. He was, without a doubt, one of the world's great embryologists, and Harvard wanted him to head the department that taught the subject separately. Mall claimed that the cost of living was so high in Boston as to make it necessary for him to have a larger salary than he was getting at Baltimore. Harvard offered it. He then played the two schools against each other in a kind of auction, finally remaining at Hopkins because their offer in the end was higher than Harvard's. When recruiting began for the basic scientists who were to teach their specialties at the University and its future Medical School, the high standing of German science was recognized and the new courses followed German approaches. Such was the case at the University as well as the Medical School. Thus in the latter decades of the 19th century it was Johns Hopkins, together with the Smithsonian Institution, which kept American physics abreast of the rest of the world.

All of the science positions, however, were not given to German-trained men. For example, the man President Gilman chose to be Professor of Physiology was trained as a physician and physiologist in London and had a fine career there; subsequently, he served purely as a physiologist under Foster at Cambridge. He had fine ideas, but he died too young to implement them. Henry Newell Martin was born in 1848 in County Down, his father coming from the South of Ireland and his mother from the North. His father was a Congregational minister who gave up that calling to become a schoolmaster, and Henry, the eldest of 12 children, was educated mostly at home. Just before his 16th birthday he entered the University of London to study at the medical school of University College. He also became apprentice to a local physician. He met Foster, then Sharpey's assistant and a lecturer in physiology, and the two became friends. In 1870 Martin received a scholarship to Cambridge, where Foster had become Head of Physiology. Martin worked as Foster's assistant in a course in elementary biology and later as assistant to Thomas H. Huxley in a similar course at the Royal College of Science. (In 1876 Huxley and Martin published a popular text called *Practical Biology*.) In 1873 he took his bachelor's degree in physiology with honors at Cambridge and at the same time took his medical degree at London. In 1876 he joined the faculty at Johns Hopkins after Foster and Huxley had recommended him to President Gilman. Martin married a much older woman, a beautiful and fascinating widow of a Confederate general, and entered actively into the social life of Baltimore and other cities. By the time the Medical School was almost ready to open in 1893, his health failed and, hence, he did not teach in the school.

With two pupils, Howell (ultimately his successor) and Donaldson, Martin developed the heart-lung preparation around 1882, although today he receives little credit for it. During the next 30 years the use of that preparation led Starling in England to formulate his Law of the Heart, a physiological generalization that has been used greatly in medicine (Breathnach, 1969). As a result of Martin's research on the heart, he, with Sedgewick (later of the Massachusetts Institute of Technology) proved wrong Brucke's contention that the aortic valve leaflets closed off the coronary arteries when the heart contracted. Martin also studied the vasomotor nerves of the heart and did work on respiration. It is interesting that in 1888 he railed against the information explosion, characterizing most of it as trash, and also criticized the view that advances in knowledge depend solely on money. He wrote, "Science cannot for any long period advance safely in chains, even if these chains be golden." These words can apply to the imposition of error and dogma in medicine through the agency of misguided financial support, a phenomenon that has adverse effects on medicine in our own time. He remarked that "theories are necessary to guide and systematize a scientist's work and lead to its prosecution in new directions, but they must be servants and not masters." We shall never know that he was no evangelical reformer of medicine in the German style of Ludwig or Virchow.

The story of Welch is more complicated. He was not an outstanding clinician - he scorned clinical medicine - and his work in the experimental laboratory was largely unimpressive. Although he did make a fine contribution with his work on the bacillus of gas gangrene, now appropriately named *Bacillus Welchii*, his studies on experimental lung edema, on the other hand, were trivial, and his other scientific publications were few. He was an excellent teacher, although he taught very little after the early 1900s, and was also an outstanding editorial critic of other men's works. His excellence in that regard was negated largely by his inability to meet deadlines except by inspired last-minute work; however, when the inspiration failed, the work was finished late or never. Except for one close friendship with Frederick Dennis, a New York physician who had helped him find a place in medicine, he had no close associates. The friendship dissolved in anger when Welch went to Baltimore instead of staying in New York. In Baltimore he had companions who joined him in banqueting and carrying out sophomoric practical jokes. He ate enormously - on occasion eating nothing but a succession of desserts - and he resented the moderation of others in this regard. A box of chocolates always was close at hand (Flexner and Flexner, 1941). He loved to give and attend large formal dinners, and also thoroughly enjoyed music, opera, theatre, and visual arts, but never as a participant. The word "sex" was never associated with him in any way, and gynecologic matters made him uncomfortable. Having women in the medical school embarrassed him. (Women were admitted after difficulties in the Baltimore and Ohio Railroad caused the stock, of which most was of the endowment of the Hopkins, to fall. The Medical School could not be opened until a group of wealthy women donated $500,000.) He was fond of a number of young girls and they of him, but, his biographers assure us, those relationships never deviated from the proper. Welch would go anywhere to make a speech or give a lecture, but his speeches appear pedestrian today and, remarkably, are rarely mentioned except by subject in contemporary accounts. Since, however, they usually were given after one of the gargantuan banquets of the period, they probably served their purpose. On the other hand, his lectures to students, physicians, or medical scientists on medical subjects usually were described as enthralling. They very well may have been, for he usually discussed matters about which his listeners had never heard.

Welch was born in 1850 into a Connecticut family that included several generations of medical practitioners. His earliest American ancestor was one who had been kidnapped as a boy by Cromwell's army in Ireland and ultimately had ended up in America as an indentured apprentice. His father was an extremely busy country doctor of whom he saw little, and his mother died when he was young. Welch seemingly had no close ties as a child, although his neighbors and schoolmates liked him. Revealed religion was much in his thoughts, but he never had the inspirational experience many young people had at the time. After preliminary schooling he went to Yale and had the ambition to teach Greek only there. He was unable to obtain such a post and taught elsewhere, and when that position was terminated, he became an apprentice to his father in medical practice, deciding on medicine as a career. He entered the College of Physicians and Surgeons in New York and apparently did well. The Professor of Practice, Clark, had been trained in Paris, as had several others of the faculty, and although there was no commitment to French methods such as Harvard maintained, the French approach did influence New York teaching. Professor Clark had a strong interest in post-mortem studies and this apparently attracted Welch more than did clinical work. Enrolled in a course in neurology with Seguin, one of Charcot's men, he won a microscope as a prize and became interested in microscopic anatomy. After graduation he did some work in pathology in New York with Delafield, during which time he became acquainted with Jacobi. Although he was a communist revolutionary who had served a prison term in Germany, Jacobi was full of the nationalist spirit that grew in Germany after 1848 (and worsened after 1870) and urged Welch to go nowhere but Germany for study (Temkin, 1950). In 1876 he went to Strasbourg where von Rechlinghausen was in charge of gross pathology. There were also several men from the College of Physicians and Surgeons there. Welch seemed to have made little impression on von Rechlinghausen and others of the faculty, including Hoppe-Seyler, with whom he studied physiological chemistry. He then went to Leipzig, but not to study with Ludwig; but, his other plans having proved unfeasible, he entered Ludwig's laboratory. He was entranced at once by Ludwig's strict quantitative methods - ignoring the fact that some of his methods were grossly inaccurate - and became convinced by the German stand that German laboratory science as applied to medicine was on the frontier of medical advance. He also became convinced that the reductionist view of medicine was not only the correct view, it was the only view. While working in Ludwig's laboratory in Leipzig in 1878 he wrote to his sister that the laboratory sciences were "about the only branch of medicine which yet deserve the name of science, the rest is a collection of unexplained facts, or supposed facts founded upon experience." He also wrote to her that the American lack of appreciation of this role of science in medicine made American medical education "horrible." He had heard of the planned program at Johns Hopkins and wrote to his sister, "I hope that Johns Hopkins will be able to teach German methods of teaching and study."

Welch developed a strong ambition to be head of pathology at Johns Hopkins once he had met Billings, who was on a recruiting trip for Johns Hopkins in Germany in 1877. Billings liked what he saw in Welch and reassured him by pointing out that the Hopkins would not open for some years and, hence, Welch could get more training in Germany. At the urging of Ludwig, Welch went to Breslau, which was far to the east, to study with Cohnheim. Cohnheim, although head of a pathological institute, did little pathology, leaving that job to his assistant, Weigert. Cohnheim held that "general pathology knows no other direction and no other classification than that which obtains in physiology." In that statement he referred to laboratory physiology as taught by Ludwig and others, and specifically minimized histology as being not truly physiological. Although Welch met Koch there, he was not impressed by the latter's work, for that period was one of derogation of the medical role of bacteriology by German pathologists and clinicians. While in Cohnheim's laboratory, Welch conducted a study on edema of the lungs which evoked great acclaim in Germany and elsewhere, but when read today, it appears conceived and carried out with astonishing naivete.

While in Germany, Welch and Mall saw a great deal of each other, fueling each other's enthusiasm for German scientific medicine. On his way home from Germany, Welch spent a few days in Paris, but did not bother to visit Pasteur (On more than one occasion Welch revised the history of his professional life and later claimed that he had visited Pasteur's laboratory.) On his return to New York he was given a pathology laboratory in Bellevue Hospital, at that time an independent medical school. (It later entered into a union with New York University.) He was highly regarded as a teacher and came to the attention of Flint, who asked him to write sections of his great text. Flint, one of the outstanding clinicians of his time, occasionally sent patients to Welch, who showed no interest in clinical practice. In 1884 he took a second trip to Europe, this time to study with Koch, whose work he had come to appreciate. He also visited other medical centers. Particularly revealing was his comment about Vienna, which he did not like because the men giving the courses while he was there were not famous and only talked about practical aspects of medicine. His concept of medicine was that of Germany in the years 1876 to 1878, scientific medicine taught by famous scientists (Temkin, 1950).

Returning to America, Welch became Professor of Pathology and Dean at Johns Hopkins, affronting his New York friends who had supported him with the idea, perhaps not justified, that he was going to bring his new ideas back to a school in that city. He had been recommended highly by Cohnheim, whose ideas he had espoused. As Professor of Pathology at Hopkins, he combined a modicum of traditional pathology with a large amount of pathological physiology and bacteriology, certainly an advance (Long, 1962). Welch made dozens of speeches, and three may be chosen as revealing his stand: those of 1888, 1893, and 1908. He believed that the medical school was to be a branch of a university with full-time salaried teachers. In this he echoed, in part, what Billings had proposed: "The aim of the School will be primarily to train practitioners of medicine and surgery, that is to qualify persons to take care of diseased and injured conditions of the body. We hold that the medical art should rest upon a thorough training in the medical sciences and that, other things being equal, he is the best practitioner who has this thorough training." Echoing Cohnheim and others, medicine was best studied, according to Welch, by reproducing its manifestations in animals or parts of them. (Those who were not willing to dissect dogs or cats could study rats or frogs which would reveal just as well, he thought, the secrets of disease in humans.)   Welch held that medicine was the application of what one might learn in that way. As Virchow had claimed, the laboratory of pathological physiology was the only important part of medicine; the findings at the bedside and in the autopsy room were secondary.   Fortunately one of the things that Welch had not learned in Germany was their rigidly authoritarian way of running a scientific organization.   Accordingly, although Welch was Dean, his views were circumvented easily. Abel, in his preclinical course, put what happened in the patient first, because it had to validate what his laboratory showed.   Osler, as Professor of Medicine, went even further, when he introduced greatly extended clinical experience for the students; however, Osler left, as did some others who did not like the situation.

Nevertheless, the permissive atmosphere that prevailed at the Hopkins, together with the fact that they had one of the finest faculties that money could buy, made Johns Hopkins one of the great medical schools of the country.   However, what was of concern was Welch's role in the development of the Flexner Report, some of whose markedly deleterious consequences will be discussed later. Before the subject of Welch is closed mention should be made of his career.

Welch's activities as a medical politician interfered with his academic and hospital duties, and he did less and less as time progressed.   Others assumed his duties, but finally, in 1917, he resigned as Professor of Pathology.   He was appointed Professor of the History of Medicine in 1926 and was instrumental in raising the money to found the Institute of the History of Medicine at Hopkins.   Johns Hopkins University had established the *Journal of Experimental Medicine* with Welch as editor.   Its first volume, published in 1896, contained his paper on gas bacillus, his only notable contribution to medical science.   In a letter describing its founding, he expressed his total lack of interest in practical medicine.   He was unable to run the *Journal*, and it collapsed in 1902 (Fishbein, 1962).   Subsequently, it was taken over by the Rockefeller Foundation, with Eugene Opie and Simon Flexner as editors.   Simon Flexner had been in Welch's department for some years, and when the decision was made to found the Rockefeller Institute, Flexner became its Director. Welch was outstanding as the first of the great medical politicians able not only to persuade wealthy donors of the value of the ideas he espoused (not necessarily his own), but also to obtain the huge sums needed to put them into effect.

While Mall and Welch continued their vigorous propaganda efforts in support of the German-inspired reductionist medicine, which they believed should be the American medicine of the future, the practical problem arose of finding a Professor of Medicine who adhered to the same beliefs. The problem apparently was solved in the person of Osler. By that time Osler was not only an outstanding clinical teacher and practitioner, but also someone who used clinical pathology and bacteriology more than was the common practice. At least equally important in the mind of Welch was Osler's statement in 1884 that medicine should be practiced and taught by fully salaried men in a university setting that included adequate laboratories as part of the clinical services. Osler then seemed to be the perfect choice for the position at Johns Hopkins. However, after a few years of experience he reversed his stand on laboratory medicine and the full-time physician, although that did not become known generally until many years later. At any rate, his greatness as a clinical teacher, together with his refusal to accept the Virchow-Welch concept of clinical medicine as a minor branch of pathophysiology, had the effect of creating a legend of Hopkins' greatness which was different from the one predicated and propagandized by Welch and his followers.

It was mentioned previously that most of the great clinicians of the 18th and early 19th centuries had histories with a common pattern: (1) Their interest in science was in natural science, that is, in observation more than experiment; and (2) Their interest in humanistic pursuits equaled or even exceeded their interests in the scientific. Osler's history fitted this pattern and perhaps should have predicted that he would become a clinician rather than a scientist working in the field of medicine.

Osler was born in 1849 in a small town in upper Canada, the son of an immigrant English clergyman. During his early schooling Osler came under the influence of several men who led him to develop what proved to be a strong lifelong interest in classical as well as English literature. He remained an omnivorous reader throughout his life and accumulated a notable library of medical classics. As a youth he was a good athlete, and his high spirits often involved him in mischief. His fondness for practical jokes persisted throughout most of his life. He showed an early interest in natural history. Although at first he planned to enter the clergy, he later decided on medicine, starting at the Toronto Medical School in 1868, but transferring in 1870 to McGill, where the clinical facilities were better. There he was influenced by Professor Howard, an excellent clinical observer himself, who introduced Osler to the writings of the great Scottish, Irish, and English clinicians of the early 19th century.

After graduation Osler spent the years 1872 to 1874 studying at clinics in Great Britain, Vienna, and Berlin, but occupied most of his time by working in physiology and histology (considered a branch of physiology) at the University College Hospital in London. Returning to Canada in 1874, he started in practice, but a year later became Lecturer in the Institutes of Medicine at McGill. (Today that subject would be called pathophysiology and pathological anatomy °including histology§.) He also had clinical duties and continued to read widely. He started a journal club, wrote articles for medical journals, attended medical meetings, donated specimens to museums and, in general, exhibited energetic interest in all branches of clinical medicine. In 1876 he became Pathologist to the Montreal General Hospital, where he gave a succession of outstanding conferences and wrote in his own hand the records of his many post-mortem examinations. Osler was also a Professor at the Veterinary Hospital and continued to show his interest in the broader aspects of disease. Initially inclined to accept German ideas about the overriding role of pathophysiology, he later rejected this view. He was made "Full Physician" to the Montreal General Hospital in 1874 and then spent a year studying with the great clinicians of London. His paper in the January of 1884 *Canadian Medical and Surgical Journal* came out strongly for a full-time paid medical school faculty and better laboratories associated with the clinical services. He was offered the post of Professor of Clinical Medicine at the University of Pennsylvania in 1884, and his decision to leave Montreal was determined by a flip of the coin. In Philadelphia he continued to demonstrate his outstanding qualities as a clinical observer and teacher, as well as his great interest in the use of gross pathology, histology, and bacteriology in teaching and in diagnosis.

Osler went to the Johns Hopkins Hospital as Physician in Chief in 1888, one year before the Hospital opened. His being chosen for the post was due to not only his extraordinary abilities as a clinical teacher accustomed to using laboratory data, but probably also to his previously expressed conviction that medicine was best carried on in a university setting by full-time physicians trained to use the laboratory as the basis of their teaching. Although Osler's disillusionment with full-time, science-oriented university medicine became evident during his tenure at Hopkins, his able and enthusiastic teaching made Hopkins famous among physicians. His remarkable *Principles and Practice of Medicine*, published first in 1891 and later in many other editions, carried his fame and that of Hopkins to even greater heights. That book became the bible to physicians all over the world, and there has been nothing in its class since. Osler, who never made a scientific discovery, soon came to differ sharply from Mall and Welch; for he believed that medicine could be learned only by experience at the bedside, supported by work in the autopsy room and, to a limited extent, the clinical laboratory. In fact, by January of 1893, as he said in his letter to Porter, the Harvard physiologist, he had "thrown away the manometer and tambour for the microscope and stethoscope." Hopkins' fame among physicians was due to Osler, the greatest clinician and clinical teacher of the century. The fame of Hopkins among laymen, including foundation directors, was ascribed to the activities of Welch, as preached by his prophet Abraham Flexner (Simon's brother). Osler had an opportunity to leave Hopkins in 1905, when he became Regius Professor at Oxford, and probably was more comfortable among the remarkable group of active English clinicians than he had been among the clincians at Hopkins.

Osler was followed at Hopkins by a succession of outstanding clinicians, and for nearly a century Hopkins was one of America's greatest clinical centers. It never fulfilled Welch's and Flexner's loudly proclaimed promise of a new laboratory-based medicine as delineated by Virchow; of course, some of the men and women of Hopkins' outstanding faculty, particularly the preclinical personnel, made important discoveries in the sciences related to medicine. However such discoveries may have changed, sometimes only temporarily, what clinicians did *to* and *with* their patients, they were not intended to change *how* they did it.

The "instrument" that gave German reductionist medicine of the 1870s its dominating position in American medical education was Abraham Flexner, an unusual man born in Louisville, Kentucky, in 1867 into a strict but not rigid Jewish family. After early schooling locally, he entered Johns Hopkins University at the age of 17, having chosen that institution because of its justifiably great reputation in advanced studies. Owing to a shortage of money, he accelerated his studies and took his A.B. degree in 1886, only two years later. (This was a year after Welch had become Professor of Pathology and Dean of the Medical School.) From 1886 until 1890 he taught in the Louisville High School and then opened his own academy with five students. He was highly successful in preparing difficult students for admission to Ivy League colleges. In 1905 Flexner closed his school and entered Harvard in order to prepare himself for what he himself called a career in "educational reform." Among his professors at Harvard was Munsterberg, whom he thought was not highly competent. Munsterberg welcomed his withdrawal from the course. In 1906 Flexner went to Europe and made his way "with throbbing heart to Berlin." (His emotion is reminiscent of that of the medieval Margery Kempe, who went on a pilgrimage to the Holy Land, riding a donkey the last few miles to Jerusalem. On catching sight of that city, she was so overcome with emotion that she "like to fall off her ass.")

Flexner believed that democracy might fail to appreciate excellence, something that could not occur in Germany at that time. He worked on his book, *The*

American College, which was really a critique of Harvard. When Pritchett, president of the Carnegie Foundation for the Advancement of Teaching, read it, he asked Flexner to make a survey of American medical schools, stating that "This is a layman's job, not a job for a medical man." Pritchett had been an astronomer at the United States Naval Observatory and later had become President of the Massachusetts Institute of Technology. His original suggestion to Carnegie was to set up a foundation to provide pensions for college professors, which was done, and afterward he organized the foundation for the study of teaching. Pritchett suggested that Flexner should have an advisory committee of physicians, but Flexner rejected the idea.

Flexner relied heavily on Billroth's account of German medical education, in which German and Austrian education were lumped together despite their obvious differences. Others found that book less than rewarding. Flexner believed that the proper person to study medical education was "a layman with a general educational experience, not a professor in a medical school." Some might differ with that view. Nevertheless, the product of this enterprise was the famous *Flexner Report, Bulletin Number Four of the Carnegie Foundation for the Advancement of Education*, published in 1910. The circumstances of its creation, formerly ambiguous, have begun to be clarified recently (Berliner, 1975, 1977). Those who read the *Report* will note that it is clearly two works.

The first part is a sound, if elementary and verbose, account of medical education, its history, and optimal format. It definitely was written by a person, or persons, who knew the field and, in fact, it strikingly resembled an earlier document written by Simon Flexner and Welch. The *Report* promoted the idea that good medicine was impossible without good training in physics, chemistry, and biology; however, it was lacking in important details - such as mention of the work of Billings, whose ideas created the Johns Hopkins Hospital and Medical School, and indication of an appreciation of the self-reform that medicine was undergoing by then - although it did mention, albeit inadequately, the events at Harvard.

The second portion of the *Report* is clearly by another hand. In 1910 it created a sensation in the lay
press and a good deal of resentment among medical educators and other physicians. In 1907 the American Medical
Association had reported the results of its inspection of
medical schools, which was followed by the closing of 40
of them, owing chiefly to the refusal of the State Boards
of Registration to accept the graduates of those schools
for examination. Less than a year later Bevan, Chairman
of the American Medical Association's Council on Medical
Education, approached the Carnegie Foundation with a suggestion for a cooperative study. After 1900 the chronology of the activities of the American Medical Association
in medical education, and the Association's interaction with
the Carnegie Foundation for the Advancement of Teaching
is as follows:

1904   Council established as permanent
standing committee of the AMA

1905   First national conference on medical
education

1906   First survey of US medical schools;
every school 1907 visited by a member of the
Council and/or the secretary

1907   First report on medical schools; their
classification as A, acceptable; B, borderline;
C, unacceptable

1908   Carnegie Foundation for the Advancement of Teaching asked to carry out independent study of U.S. medical schools

1909   Carnegie study made by Abraham
Flexner, 1910 accompanied on all of his medi-
cal school visits by Council Secretary Colwell;
Flexner Report published in 1910

1911   Council made third inspection of all
medical schools, and thereafter made regular

periodic reviews of schools with a formal approval or accreditation system

In 1909 Pritchett, President of the Foundation, persuaded its trustees to conduct studies of professional education, starting with the legal profession. He apparently was rebuffed, but the Foundation later published a limited account of law-school teaching. Actually, in December of 1908 Pritchett and Flexner already had attended a meeting of the AMA's Council on Medical Education. In November of 1909 Pritchett acknowledged that his Foundation was working "hand-in-glove" with the Council, but for reasons not stated he considered it best not to emphasize that fact. The *Report's* total lack of mention of the Council's work was not anticipated, however, and generated much ill will. In addition, any close relationship between the AMA's Council and the Foundation began to dissolve, owing to differences in the way each ranked medical schools. The Foundation's problems were not related solely to those growing differences with the American Medical Association; there were internal problems as well. Pritchett had had a hard time persuading the Foundation's trustees to designate Flexner as the man to make their survey. By that time Abraham Flexner's brother Simon had become Head of the Rockefeller Institute, and Welch at Hopkins had become President of the American Medical Association. (Until after World War I the AMA was a society of medical academicians.) Hence the choice of Abraham Flexner seemed to be sound if the criteria were purely political, however unsound it might be otherwise. After Abraham Flexner began his survey in 1909, Pritchett found it necessary to defend his choice of Flexner and minimize other people's concern about Flexner's uncertain judgment and "erratic tendencies." His unsatisfactory performance during his visit to Harvard was mentioned. At any rate, the second portion of what is called the *Flexner Report* is fragmentary, superficial and, at times, scurrilous. It has had little effect on medical education *per se* (Berliner, 1977), but it did ensure that those foundations sponsoring it, directly or indirectly, would offer the schools money. Such money was to be used to pursue alleged improvement along the lines recommended by Billings and others, and exemplified by the creation of the Johns Hopkins. The *Flexner Report, Bulletin Number Four* of *the Carnegie Foundation*, consistently used the Hopkins as a model (without stating that it was the Hopkins of Billings, not that of Welch and the Flexners). However, the *Report*, and the later report by one of the Rockefeller's General Education Board, supported the views expressed by the Hopkins' Dean, Welch, and some others, that family physicians not trained in the laboratory must disappear, that the only road to medical education was through laboratory science, and that the four-year premedical education was to consist of chemistry, physics, and biology. (What did the students do with the rest of their time?) It stated repeatedly, with no supporting evidence whatsoever, that medical practice could be pursued successfully only as a science. It did not go so far as to state, in so many words (as had Virchow, Cohnheim, and Welch), that medical practice was nothing but a minor offshoot of pathological physiology as developed in laboratories of animal experimentation, but it specifically did not exclude this peculiar dogma. Certainly the schools that accepted foundation money did not adhere to the dogma.

Flexner's autobiography (Flexner, 1960) is difficult to use as a source of data, since its content is highly selective and its approach is self-congratulatory, except when it celebrates German medicine and Johns Hopkins University. According to that work, many prominent men held Flexner in high esteem, including Flexner himself. Despite difficulties created in evaluating the data (owing to his exuberant self-congratulation), it is clear that he was a man of great brilliance and an inspiring teacher of the classics to Louisville adolescents (although his attempt to set up a similar school in New York City was not successful). He was clearly a man with other, perhaps greater, talents, for he quickly persuaded Rockefeller to donate $50,000,000 (before the days of tax benefits) and subsequently persuaded individuals, foundations, and state legislators to provide at least 12 times that amount in the furtherance of ideas that, he claimed, were entirely original. Consistency, except in self-praise, was not his forte. For example, in one section he derided an American visitor to a German laboratory who wanted to spend only a day

learning what was going on there and, in another, he gleefully boasted that in his survey of 155 medical schools,
each took him "several hours." He scolded some American
schools for admitting unqualified persons and boasted that
although he could not pass the entrance examinations, he
was admitted to Johns Hopkins University through the influence of a Baltimore rabbi.

Flexner hardly could qualify as an expert on medical
education. He, and evidently his sponsors also, did not
recognize that American medical education was changing
along lines defined by its earlier history. When American
began to grow beyond the Alleghenies, there was a great
shortage of doctors in the new lands, a problem that the
new states solved by abolishing the licensing of physicians.
A large number of schools were organized quickly to provide, at best, joint discussion of books by instructors and
students and, at worst, nothing but a device by which a
student could get a diploma - the only manifestation of
legitimacy in the absence of licensing - and from which
the teachers could earn extra money, both by collecting
fees for teaching and also by acting as consultants when
their ill-trained students needed help. Most of those substandard schools were beyond the Alleghenies. Twenty
percent of the schools Flexner wanted to abolish were in
the two cities of Chicago and Louisville. One of the substandard Louisville schools, which Flexner (gleefully)
claimed to have destroyed, graduated his elder brother Simon, who won a fellowship at Hopkins, rose to the rank of
Professor of Pathology under Welch, and ultimately became
Head of the Rockefeller Institute. A few substandard
schools also opened in the East, but some of the Eastern
schools that had closed produced competent physicians.

By the latter decades of the 19th century, some of
the substandard schools and others began to unite with
universities in an attempt to achieve improved administrative standards and stability. For example, Bellevue Hospital Medical School, a hospital-organized school after the
London fashion, had an outstanding faculty and teaching
staff (for a time including Welch, who, therefore, actually
worked at a non-university medical school); it later joined
New York University. Tufts College Medical School grew
out of an inferior Boston proprietary school. A few

schools, such as Maryland, actually created universities, which Flexner dismissed with contempt. Today Jefferson Medical College, one of the great medical schools of the post-Civil War period and later, is in the process of creating a university around itself. Flexner also chose to ignore or underplay the reform of medical education then occurring at Harvard and at Vanderbilt. In addition, he ignored the efforts of the American Medical Association by the turn of the century to improve the quality of the schools. Flexner thought that Dr. Colwell, who was responsible for the data of the AMA reports, was unnecessarily tactful while making inspections and describing the results. How much of the AMA data Flexner used without attribution is not known. It is known, however, that in 1907 Welch and Simon Flexner put together a report for the Rockefeller Foundation which seems to have been incorporated later in Abraham Flexner's 1910 report (Berliner, 1977).

The General Education Board had been established by John D. Rockefeller in 1902, with Buttrick as Secretary and Gates as a member, the latter becoming Chairman in 1907. It was Gates who initiated the founding of the Rockefeller Institute in 1905, with Abraham Flexner's brother Simon as Head. Carnegie became a member in 1908. The General Education Board praised the Hopkins and supported its endowment. In 1913 Flexner became Assistant Secretary of the General Education Board and, in 1914, a member. The interlocking interests and activities, with respect to medical education, of the Carnegie Foundation for the Advancement of Education and the General Education Board were revealed in many ways, including the language of the latter's report in 1925.

Flexner's arrogance was well known, and it was especially prominent in his attempted relations with Harvard. (If anybody was going to be arrogant, it was going to be Harvard.) The trouble between Harvard and Flexner was more due to the man's boorish behavior than to differences over principle at the time. Christian, at Harvard, and Flexner were in the midst of discussions, not about the nature of medicine, but about the possibility of having Harvard's clinical teaching done only by fully salaried instructors. Christian, supported by another professor, Cushing, held that only junior instructors should be salaried fully to encourage them to elect an academic career in preference to practice. Flexner insisted that all clinical teachers, starting with the professors, be totally full-time. While these informal discussions were in progress, Flexner presented Christian's idea to the Rockefeller Foundation as an official proposal from Harvard, despite the fact that it had not been voted on by the Medical School Faculty or approved by the Dean of the School or the President of the University. The Foundation rejected that supposed formal proposal, which was the first time that Harvard University's President, Lowell, heard about a proposal, and the Medical School's Dean, Bradford, knew little more. Their reactions, although not recorded in any accessible documents, can be imagined.

Whatever Flexner's qualities, good or bad, the main criticism evoked by his *Report* was that it had no basis. He had no way of establishing what good medical practice was (he ignored it), and he made no effort to prove its dependence on what he had come to believe was the only good medical education. His only criterion with respect to the latter was whether or not it was German. In one place he unwittingly revealed his true bias by declaring that German medical education resembled that which was obtained at Johns Hopkins. Anything that was like German or Hopkins' medical education was good; anything else was bad. He stated that most American medical schools should be abolished and the survivors rebuilt along German-Hopkins lines, including a German authoritarian organization of the laboratories. When in Germany inspecting its medical schools, he had, he thought, a stroke of good luck: Mall came along to discuss matters with him. When asked by Gates, Rockefeller's advisor on medical affairs, what he would do if he had $1,000,000. with which to begin reforming medical education, he replied that he would give it to Welch. The fact that Abraham Flexner knew little about medical education in America, was biased against all types of such education except German, and made no attempt to prove that German education produced doctors better able to practice medicine then, for example, the French, the English, or even the best of the American, might be taken for the harmless foolishness of an overenthusiastic mind. However it was not harmless, for it carried money with it - hundreds of millions of dollars. Although that undoubtedly led to progress in the sciences related to medicine, there was no evidence that it improved medical practice, in fact, quite the contrary. Here is an example of how Flexner's supporters - men who were skillful in making money - could be foolish in spending it: The *Report*, its attendant and subsequent publicity, and the schools' need to obtain foundation money created a state mind in which laboratory science came first, and clinical pursuits, if mentioned at all, were represented as totally dependent on those sciences.

Later, when Osler came to reject completely the Virchow-Welch concept of medicine as a laboratory science with minor clinical components, he criticized the *Flexner Report*. He had had experience with some of the aspects of this mode at Hopkins and had indicated his skepticism of it. After the *Flexner Report* was published in 1910, Osler wrote a letter to President Remsen of Hopkins in which he discussed the *Report* and related matters in remarkably vigorous language. The letter was sent to Remsen in 1911, yet was published in the *Canadian Medical Association Journal* on October 6, 1962. In it he warned against the appointment of medical faculties on the basis of their laboratory and research reputations instead of on their interest in students and patients. Osler prophesied that laboratory professors would not have the necessary background, would be out of touch with the conditions under which their students would live and practice, would be forgetful of the wider claims of a clinical teacher, and would be pure laboratory men. He also warned that "the school would narrow as teacher and student chase each other down the fascinating road of research." Osler believed that a man did not have to be a research person in order to teach; in fact, he strongly stated, "A research man often was not fit to teach medical students." In his conclusion he expressed his belief, chiefly (and one that has been on the minds of many physicians since), that it was necessary to divert the ardent souls who wanted to be full-time professors away from the medical school, in which they were not at home, to the research institutes to which they properly belonged and in which they could do their best work. (Osler's advice never was followed in this country, and his gloomy view of the future of American medicine has become a reality.)

The French and English varieties of medical education were based on the view that laboratory science, like anything else that might prove useful (as sociology and anthropology later came to be), should be pursued with, but ultimately subsidiary to, bedside medicine. The sciences so used were called "accessory sciences" in France and "collateral sciences" in England. In 19th-century Germany and in the writings of the Welch-Flexner school (misrepresented as Johns Hopkins), the laboratory sciences were called "basic sciences" and were to be considered the substance of whatever might happen at the bedside. The concept of laboratory sciences as "contributory" to bedside medicine was different only in one word from the concept of laboratory sciences as "basic" to bedside medicine. Nevertheless, there was an enormous difference between the two concepts. What happened for a time in some German-speaking countries - acceptance of the ideas espoused by Ludwig and the other mid-century reductionists as well as by Virchow, Cohnheim, and Welch - was never accepted in Austria. In Germany, after creating a furor over a period of a few decades, it began to lose its appeal after the turn of the century. It would be foolish to imply that a specific way of looking at things is typical of a whole country.

Reductionism in medicine was not practiced universally or even admired in 19th-century Germany. At first it was prominent, mainly in cities of northeastern Germany, chiefly Berlin and Leipzig. Nevertheless, for convenience, modern reductionism (as distinguished from the reductionism of the iatrochemists and iatromathematicians) in this work is called "German." When it spread in Germany, it was given a distinctive name so as to indicate its difference from the ordinary practice of medicine. From around 1880 until after World War I it was called *innere medizin*, erroneously translated in America as "internal medicine." The German word *innere* has many meanings, and the meaning applied to reductionist medicine in Germany implied that it was the true essence of medicine. Many of the American medical academicians who studied in Germany after 1880 brought back that German notion. In effect, adopting such a concept of medicine rejected patient-oriented medicine in favor of disease-oriented or, worse still, theory-oriented medicine.

Those notions about the role of medical sciences held in Germany in the years around 1875 to 1880 ultimately were given lasting acceptance only in America. That acceptance was induced in this country mainly by money, first from foundations and subsequently in much larger amounts from federal agencies. It created the setting for a major change in medical practice which has downgraded clinical skills and the medical care that depends on them. But then, America is the land of Noble Experiments.

The other main portion of Flexner's master plan for American medical education involved its control by universities, with all the faculty as salaried members of them. University control has come to prevail in America and, in fact, the trend started long before Flexner's day. It was mentioned that on the Continent formal medical education from the Renaissance onward was mainly a university function. There were some exceptions, notably the teaching at Jewish medical schools that flourished in the south of France after the expulsion of the Jews from Spain.

The medical school at Leyden was a main force in medical education in the 17th and 18th centuries, and that school was part of a university as well. Leyden's heir, the medical school at Edinburgh, was also university-controlled, although medical teaching had begun in Edinburgh earlier under other auspices. In England the story was quite different. The medical schools attached to the two old universities, Oxford and Cambridge, were notably backward. The best formal medical teaching was carried on in independent teaching hospitals and at private medical schools. Not until the middle decades of the 19th century did London have a university and a connected medical school. The English pattern, in which progress was seemingly at a standstill in the universities and was restored only by non-university schools, should not be taken as the rule for the entire world. Certainly the university medical teaching at Padua, Leyden, and Edinburgh in the 16th through 18th centuries was progressive with respect to clinical matters, although it was regressive at the two latter institutions due to their acceptance of iatrochemical superstitions.

In America the earliest medical education was by apprenticeship, although many leading physicians crossed the Atlantic Ocean to obtain some or most of their training at established schools in Great Britain or, less often, on the Continent. The first American medical schools, established in the 18th century, were university-connected, although a number of private medical schools were established early in the next century. Both types of schools went through ups and downs, and some private schools closed. In the State of Vermont, for example, the university medical school barely survived while private medical schools throve for a time, until the reverse occurred. In Boston, although the medical school at Harvard was established securely, its educational approach in the early 19th century was not progressive, and members of its faculty, notably Bigelow and Holmes, established a private medical school to teach clinical medicine after the methods then used in London and Paris.

In the 19th century the American medical schools not connected with universities did poorly as a rule. Many closed, mainly because of their own problems or because of the reform activities of the American Medical Association. Others joined universities, and some actually created universities. Today all new schools are university-connected. There is no doubt that a university connection is an advantage to a medical school. It promises, although it does not guarantee, academic stability and financial security. The propensity of some universities to support old dogmas or to adopt (or invent) new ones is common but not universal. This need not affect medical education adversely, so long as the university connection does not impair the functional independence of a medical school's clinicians.

Epilogue

The Reverend John Trusler (1736-1820), eccentric divine, superintendent for a time of the Library Society whose purpose was to abolish publishers, founder of an academy for teaching oratory, wholesale purveyor of ghost-written sermons for clergymen, and sometime student of medicine at Leyden, is best known today for his commentary on Hogarth's works. Those works first were collected in 1768 and published again in 1821, 1831, 1838, and 1861-1862. In his commentary on Hogarth's satirical engraving, "The Consultation of Physicians," Trusler wrote,

> It has been said of the ancients that they began by attempting to make physic a science and failed; of the moderns, that they began by attempting to make it a trade, and succeeded.

His first proposition to some extent was inaccurate, since not only the ancients but Trusler's contemporaries had tried to make medicine a science, and others have tried since then, all without success.

When shamanism ceased to be a main characteristic of medicine, the explaining of diseases as effects of possession by demons or other exogenous intelligences became unacceptable. Similarly, astrology had its day and then vanished, except of course in some of today's popular magazines. The subsidence of medical interest in astrology by no means ended the occurrence of superstition in medicine - it has not ended yet, nor probably ever will it. With the Renaissance, physics and chemistry began to grow, not only in content but in attractiveness to physicians. Clinical manifestations of disease were explained by the then fragmentary and erroneous data of those sciences, and the superstitions of iatrochemistry and iatromathematics became main preoccupations of some of the great 17th-century European clinicians.

In combination with vestiges of ancient Galenic humoral concepts, the physical and chemical superstitions of the 17th century persisted well into the 19th. Such collective superstitions disintegrated when their inadequacies were revealed by bedside observations, and their disappearance was hastened by newer chemical and physiological observations in diseased and healthy animals. The assimilation of the latter data into medicine went on during the 19th century in England and France, and only slightly less actively in Austria.

The events in Germany were startlingly different, for a revolution, today called "scientific medicine" developed there. That nation in the early 19th century was far behind Great Britain, Ireland, France, and Austria. It lacked their tradition of the continuous growth of medical knowledge and the prompt application of the new information to bedside medicine. There were, of course, some fine clinicians in the German states, but they were few in number, and some of them were replaced by medical scientists after 1848. The idea enunciated by leading German medical scientists such as Virchow and Cohnheim - that the practice of medicine was to be derived only from laboratory studies - manifestly was absurd, but it maintained an anomalous existence as part of Welch's plan for the reform of American medical education. Welch's specific legacy to American education, propagated by certain foundations and by journalists who agreed with Abraham Flexner that Welch was the savior of medicine in this country, was the late 19th-century German superstition of scientific medicine. The persistence of this notion in America - it was never more than a notion - led to certain developments that adversely have affected clinical medicine.

One factor that exaggerated the importance of the role of laboratory science in modern medicine was the use of the word "basic" to describe it, and that led inevitably to the expansion of the scientific segment of the medical school curriculum. The reasoning was that if laboratory science were basic to medicine (as Virchow, Cohnheim, Welch, and some laymen connected with certain foundations held), then the more science in the curriculum the better the subsequent medical practice.   That reasoning ignored several important facts: (1) Physicians trained only in laboratory sciences, even when those sciences were medicine-related, were unable to practice medicine unless also trained as clinicians.   There was nothing to indicate that men whose main interest was science before they became physicians fared any better in medical practice than those whose main interests were (and very likely continued to be) history, the arts, or philosophy.   If anything, the data point in a somewhat opposite direction. (2) Almost all material published in scientific journals today has no evident relationship to clinical medicine, even if one accepts its scientific validity by itself, which does not make it applicable to living organisms.   The fact that almost all such data are too artifactual to be applied to intact living organisms should not be forgotten.   Also to be remembered is that the greater part of this data, even when considered in its intrinsic scientific state (*i.e.*, not yet applied to clinical medicine) is too tentative, too controversial, or too closely dependent on some unnatural method to be acceptable in any broad sense, either in or outside clinical medicine.

These facts raise questions about what the role of the medicine-allied sciences is in medical education, for they certainly have an important role.   For one thing, certain portions of this scientific material explain the manifestations of disease, albeit not necessarily accurately, and hence make some disease phenomena intelligible when they otherwise might be confusing.   It is regrettable that for some teachers a phenomenon does not exist unless an explanation for it is known or can be expected to be made knowable soon.   This role is a limited one, for the greatest usefulness of science is to be found in physiologic or biochemical studies of intact animals or whole organs, studies that are relatively few in number.   The usefulness of data obtained in subcellular systems is dubious except in some genetic diseases, most of which are uncommon. Moreover all of these data, even when usable, merely illuminate the disease process, possibly explaining some of the physical findings, and they are of limited usefulness in explaining the nature and occurrence of symptoms.   Symptoms are manifestations experienced by a person and cannot be appreciated - sometimes not even recognized - without knowing a good deal about the person. However, having students use medicine-related sciences merely as stepping stones to clinical medicine - a role considered important by most medical educators and primary by some like Welch - is not valid. It does not accurately describe the place of laboratory science in medical education, for, in the words of Bacon, it causes the former to be "degraded most unworthily to the situation of a handmaid and made to wait upon medicine...and to wash the immature minds of youth and imbue them with a first dye, that they may afterwards be more ready to receive and retain another." Many students clearly have an interest in the medicine-related sciences which is not merely utilitarian, having developed such an interest in one or another of the sciences in their premedical years; some want to maintain the interest in the changing science as a hobby.

The main role of science in medicine is more general. Celsus observed that medicine was the earliest of the sciences to use experiment, and most physicians since then have realized that while it may be possible to practice medicine satisfactorily without a knowledge of laboratory science, it is not possible to do any thinking about medicine without such knowledge. However, many good practitioners do not need to do much thinking about medicine. Some clinicians of extensive experience will have acquired so many responses to cues of which they are not conscious that they perform better when reacting than when thinking. Of course, a clinical teacher must then figure out what he was reacting to and for what reason. The preclinical sciences have their greatest utility in the development of diagnostic or therapeutic approaches, but they do not teach doctors how to use them. It must be remembered that these developments primarily were made by non-physicians. Another point that should be emphasized is that medicine created most of the sciences (Raven, 1960) and that fertilizing effect is of the utmost importance. The development of sciences along lines determined by medical needs has always led to enrichment of these sciences in other directions. Accordingly, the fact that the medical discovery of the vitamins was a main factor in the development of a large segment of enzymology should not make that part of enzymology a part of medicine or medical education, as a result.

The "Introduction" to this work lists the comments of recent great physicians who decried attempts to make clinical medicine a form of applied science. But such warning began long ago.

Overemphasis of the importance of laboratory sciences was recognized early in modern times. Billings, whose tour of German schools in 1877 led to the creation of the Johns Hopkins Medical School wrote, "The student is led to think that his highest aim should be to do some experiment which no one has done before, and for this purpose he may work for a year in a laboratory and yet acquire but a tithe of the knowledge which he goes there to obtain." Osler likewise censured the neglect of teaching in the German university for "the more seductive pursuit of the 'bauble reputation.'" However, the idea of replacing American - basically French - methods by Virchow's could be instituted only with money, as at Johns Hopkins. Few schools other than Harvard had enough money. At Harvard President Eliot, an enthusiastic admirer of Virchow, attempted to use general university funds to shape the medical school curriculum. (Beecher and Altschule, 1977). The clinical faculty was prosperous and powerful through their control of the city's medical practice and was not forced to accept Eliot's bribes. They kept Harvard a medical school and not a research institute.

However greatly German medicine may have been respected and admired 100 years ago, at the time when Welch was dreaming his dreams about transplanting German medical science to America, other American physicians were expressing much sounder views about the limited role of the laboratory sciences in medical teaching and practice. The state of some of the medical thinking in America is well exemplified by what happened at the Harvard Medical School. There, the first full-time chairs in America in physiology (1869) and in physiological chemistry (1908) were established, clearly in the German pattern. However, the clinical specialties were established earlier in the 19th century, after the fashion of Vienna

(Beecher and Altschule, 1977).   Science was recognized as having something to contribute.   The first chief of psychiatry at the Boston Psychopathic Hospital was a pathologist, appointed in 1914, just as Meynert had been appointed at Vienna.   Several Professors of Medicine had been pathologists - Fritz and, as late as 1912, Christian - clearly a reflection of the Parisian mode.   Cabot, whose first fame came from his book on the examination of the blood in 1896 was an outstanding clinician and went on to found the first hospital social service department in any American hospital at the Massachusetts General Hospital in 1906 (William, 1950).   Nevertheless, the German emphasis on laboratory work was widely adopted in America. Rollerston in England commented tactfully on that fact in 1907, writing that "The thoroughness of the work in the clinical laboratory is no doubt in part due to the influence of German clinics, to which recently qualified American men resort very freely.   It is impossible to exaggerate the value of clinical laboratory work, and this is so confidently relied upon in everyday practice that there is, perhaps, some danger that the routine physical examination of patients may be less thorough than in the past."

Mark Twain's comment is pertinent here: "There is something fascinating about science.   One gets such wholesale returns of conjecture out of such a trifling investment of fact."

In much the same vein, Pickering (1978) emphasized that science was infinitely replicable and impersonal whereas an art was not necessarily replicable, but was personal.   The latter statement accounts for the vast differences in the competence of medical practitioners.   What is called the art of medicine consists of an understanding of every aspect of the patient's problem as influenced by his personality as well as his physical state.   That understanding only can come from listening to the patient and appreciating what he is saying.   Hearing the patient's message is the basic quality in good medical practice.   The physician cannot, however, evoke that message unless he shows by word, facial expression, and manner that he is interested in what the patient is trying to convey, that he understands it or will continue his questioning until he does, and that he has sympathy to appreciate it and knowledge to begin to help it.   He certainly cannot evoke such a message by his absence.

Perhaps the clearest expression of concern over the place of the laboratory in medicine was given by Peabody in his 1922 paper in the *Boston Medical and Surgical Journal* (now know as *The New England Journal of Medicine*) and elucidated in Minot's discussion, which followed it.   Peabody deserves a word of comment, for he was instrumental in creating the atmosphere of the Thorndike Memorial Laboratory at the Boston City Hospital, which early exemplified the proper role of the laboratory in medical practice, teaching, and research.   He was born in Cambridge in 1881, the son of a Unitarian minister who was also a Harvard professor.   William James was a neighbor, and the Peabody family saw much of the Jameses.   The Peabody family traveled to Europe twice, and young Peabody learned German there.   He almost died of typhoid fever in Venice in 1899, at which time his brother died of the disease.   Peabody graduate *cum laude* from Harvard College and then entered the Medical School.   In April 1906, as Vice-President of the Boylston Medical Society (then the highest student position), he presented a paper on diabetes mellitus, in which he said, as a *third-year student*, "We must not forget in treating diabetes that we are treating a man and not a disease."   Fitz advised him to enter a career of academic medicine.   At that time Pratt had just returned to Harvard from his training at Johns Hopkins under Osler and Welch, and later in Germany.   He offered an elective course in medical research for fourth-year students, and Peabody was his first pupil.   Laboratory space was provided in the newly opened Medical School buildings, and Peabody worked there on typhoid fever.   As an intern he developed a method for growing the organism out of the bloodstream and reported it before the American Medical Association in 1908.   The audience may have been surprised to hear the young intern conclude that the early diagnosis of typhoid fever led not only to better treatment and better nursing, but also perhaps to more adequate domestic arrangements, an unusual conclusion for a scientific paper.

After his internship Peabody had two years at the Hopkins, one in clinical medicine and the other in pathology, followed by a year in Germany studying chemistry under Fischer.   Then he was Resident Physician at the new research hospital of the Rockefeller Institute, and during this time he helped prepare a classic *clinical* description of poliomyelitis.   His next position was as Chief Resident of the newly opened Peter Bent Brigham Hospital in Boston from 1913 to 1915, and during that period he again spent time in Europe, much of it with Krogh in Copenhagen. From 1915 to 1921 he was engaged in making clinical applications of the methods of physiology to heart and lung disease.   He visited China and Rumania for the Rockefeller Foundation and became recognized worldwide as a leader in American medicine, albeit a young one.   He was offered the position of Professor of Medicine at Johns Hopkins, as well as Columbia, Yale, and Stanford, not to mention that of Dean at the new University of Chicago Medical School. He chose to remain in Boston, planning and directing the new Thorndike Memorial Laboratory at the Boston City Hospital.   Several hundred of the men who were trained there became professors elsewhere.   These details of Peabody's life are given to demonstrate his fitness to discuss the role of the laboratory in clinical medicine.   His statement (Peabody, 1922) and Minot's discussion immediately after it still are worth reading:

> The important part which the laboratory has come to play in medical science is generally accepted and appreciated, but the relation which it should bear to clinical practice remains to be satisfactorily defined.   It is obvious to all clinicians of experience that the laboratory never can become and never should become the predominating factor in the practice of medicine, but it is equally evident that sound medicine cannot be carried on without the support of the laboratory and that in the future the dependence of the clinic on the laboratory will probably increase rather than decrease....

> The leading exponents of clinical laboratory work are the large hospitals - espe-

cially the hospitals associated with teaching institutions - and these exert a profound effect on private medical practice....

Many of the laboratory data that fill the pages of carefully compiled hospital records do not have a direct diagnostic or therapeutic bearing on the individual case, but they contribute information which throws light on the pathological physiology and clarifies the disease process. Insofar as the accumulation of such accessory laboratory observations is instructive to those who are studying the patients, the work is more than justified, but if, as sometimes happens, particularly with the younger members of the staff, it leads to the idea that all these observations are necessary for the proper diagnosis and treatment of any given case, the result may be most unfortunate. Properly used, such laboratory observations are enlightening and broadening; improperly used, they are blinding and narrowing....

From this point of view, much hospital laboratory work may be regarded as of indirect significance for the individual patient, but aimed at the training of better clinicians. When, as sometimes happens, it results in the production of poor clinicians, unable to interpret disease except through the eyes of the laboratory, its purpose has failed and failed seriously.....

Even so-called thoroughness should be tempered by reason, and the reason that must dictate the part which laboratory tests shall play in any given case must be the result of a combination of clinical experience with an understanding of the physiological significance of the available tests....

It is frequently alleged that many of our medical schools and teaching hospitals are producing "laboratory men" instead of clinicians.   If it is true that the graduates of these institutions enter the practice of medicine handicapped by their dependence on the laboratory, then the system of training is wrong or - what seems more probable - it is imperfectly carried out.   When schools and hospitals do their full duty, their graduates will have had an opportunity to study disease intensively, checking and controlling their bedside observations by a variety of exact laboratory investigations.   Such an experience will enable them to correlate the clinical manifestations of disease with the underlying physiological processes so that they can subsequently understand and interpret disease without recourse to all the laboratory procedures which were necessary in their student days....

Minot's subsequent discussion also was notable:

I think that Dr. Peabody has concisely pointed out the relation of the physician to the laboratory.   As he has said the future development is for better clinicians rather than better technicians.   Good technicians are, of course, indispensable.   Laboratory findings must be considered simply as additional clinical symptoms.   They should be used to assist in, rather than to determine, the diagnosis, prognosis, or treatment.   We must not forget that the patient is the center of our professional life, and not some isolated data directly or indirectly referable to the individual.

It is not uncommon to see patients who think they have been thoroughly studied and have obtained an undoubtedly correct opinion because they have had an endless number of tests made and have been furnished with extensive reports, often meaningless. In turn, the physician at times seems to feel that "if all the tests are done" then he has overlooked nothing; such a man often gives little attention to the accuracy of the tests and loses sight of the fact that proper interpretation of the results is fundamental. In other words, in utilizing the laboratory, one must use his mind and not make acceptance of dogma. In obscure cases for study, all forms of tests may be justifiable and desirable, but to undertake these blindly is wasteful and useless. Such a procedure without medication tends to lead one to not making use of our best methods of diagnosis, namely, what we see upon looking at the patient and what he tells us by his own words, together with well-directed questions on our part....

Figures tend to lead one to a sense of false security. Clinical information is seldom appraised in figures. Laboratory data, on the other hand, is often expressed in figures which are apt to lead one to the conclusion that such data are final and judgment is not required. This is incorrect, for judgment is often the sole method of arriving at the figure. Likewise, figures presented by a technician must be judged as to correctness and evaluated by the clinician. One is apt to be satisfied with figures and to believe they express exactness, forgetting that when used for certain laboratory data they may vary widely with technic and that they often express only approximate values....

One must bear in mind that positive results usually should have clinical evidence to support them and that negative examinations

are to be cautiously interpreted and repeated
if other clinical symptoms do not agree....

Both of those men emphasized that the focus of
laboratory studies in clinical medicine had to be fixed on a
patient with a disease and not on some physiologic theory.
That is noteworthy, for both men had extensive training in
laboratory sciences.   How did their eminently sound conception of laboratory medicine become submerged?   In his
Care of the Patient, Peabody (1923) days:

> When   one   considers   the   amazing
> progress of science in its relation to medicine
> during the last thirty years, and the enormous
> mass of scientific material which must be
> made available to the modern physician, it is
> not surprising that the schools have tended to
> concern themselves more and more with this
> phase of the educational problem.   And while
> they have been absorbed in the difficult task
> of digesting and correlating new knowledge, it
> has been easy to overlook the fact that the
> application of the principle of science to the
> diagnosis and treatment of disease is only one
> limited aspect of medical practice.   The prac-
> tice of medicine in its broadest sense includes
> the whole relationship of the physician with
> his patient.

Accordingly, a large part of the physiological and
chemical research in medicine is of greater value and interest to beginning students in clinical medicine and their
teachers than to any other groups.   This phenomenon is
interesting in itself, for it has no exact counterpart in the
other professions, such as law and the clergy.   It may
suggest an explanation for the fact that many of the best
teachers in medicine also do research; indeed, in many
instances their work in the laboratory is an expression of
their   fundamental   inclination   toward   teaching.   This is
entirely laudable, provided that it does not interfere with
or, worse, replace clinical teaching.   The fact that many
good teachers of medicine do research regrettably has led

to the error that the mark of the good teacher is his list of published research papers. It is not rare today, as was the case in Germany a century ago, for a man to be put in charge of a clinical unit because of his laboratory research, not because he is competent in patient care or in bedside teaching. In such cases, the unit may produce some good clinicians not due to the teaching and example of the professor, but in spite of it. That deplorable state of affairs has been compounded by government policies that make available vast sums of money to support those in university-hospital clinical posts doing research - research often related to medicine only tangentially, if at all. In such circumstances those who might be excellent physicians and clinical teachers must find their own rewards, for they receive none from granting agencies.

Medical students trained by laboratory scientists to think superficially like medical scientists nevertheless may refuse to take that road. Peabody did, through his own thinking and efforts, and many others have and will. However, the number grows smaller yearly, for such students receive little encouragement from their teachers. Moreover, recent years have seen the extraordinary development of laboratory tests and devices that purport to describe (they merely measure) one or another aspect of the clinical state. The sheer mass of data - produced by machines believed to be free from not only any possibility of error but also any misconception in design - is likely to push to one side other data unable to be expressed in numbers. The belief in the absolute accuracy and validity of such data is an error in itself, for the interpretation of laboratory data is no sure and simple task. In the past there were many practitioners who were inexpert in history-taking and physical examination; today, with the progress made by science and technology, many physicians, in addition, are unable to interpret laboratory reports adequately.

The pitfalls in the interpretation of clinical laboratory data are ignored almost universally by those taking them seriously and using them for other than cynical reasons. (Cynical reasons include wanting to be considered up-to-date by patients, hoping to avoid a possibility of malpractice suits instigated by unscrupulous or ignorant patients and their similarly motivated attorneys, and desiring the additional income the tests may bring to physicians.) To those who perform the tests for cynical reasons, the interpretations do not matter. What matters is that the tests were done and the results - any results - appear in the record. The physicians who genuinely believe the tests to be helpful, as they often are, and who want to use them effectively in their work are the ones who have problems with the data. Most physicians had little or no instruction as medical students with respect to the sources of error and the limits of valid interpretation of those tests used in practice. Few physicians have at their command the available critical information, such as Kozinn's excellent paper (1978), or knowledge of its use. Since every test may give false answers at times (leaving to one side errors introduced by poor laboratory technique), a normal or abnormal result is not absolute. If a physician has taken into account the probability of false answers, which varies with each test and each method used to carry out a particular test, he now is faced with having to distinguish between, on the one hand, statistically significant data (defined mathematically) and, on the other hand, that which is clinically significant (determined by the degree to which the abnormality affects some bodily function). The assumption that small deviations from the normal - undetectable by inspection, but detectable only by statistical evaluation - *must* signify physiological effects is one of the major superstitions responsible for poor medical practice today. We may describe such a powerful superstition as one that believes disease to be defined by two standard deviations from the mean; although nearly 5% of all normal findings are outside that range, any such findings indicate sickness and must, at all costs, be made to fall within the range. That superstition is based on bad statistics and certainly is bad medicine. Attempting to return to normal the measurement of drastic medications or procedures may create a disease that never existed before that time, because *all* medications and procedures have untoward effects in some patients. The converse superstition, that any measurement within two standard deviations of the normal mean cannot be abnormal, has prevented or slowed the use of effective treatment in more than one case.

We thus see laboratory medicine increasing, not decreasing, fallibility of inadequate physicians, while it helps the good ones only to a small degree in their practice. Seeking the help of laboratory medicine when needed is admirable, but allowing it to displace thinking and minimize interaction with the patient destroys the doctor-patient relationship and thereby destroys medicine. It has led to the habit of judging a sick man's restoration to health by a number on the laboratory data report, ignoring his clinical state. Many physicians now judge the effect of a medication by its level in the blood rather than by those changes it produces in the clinical manifestations. It encourages the treatment of minor or questionable deviations from so-called "normal ranges" by medications or procedures with a high frequency of untoward side-effects, side-effects that not only may not change the measurement significantly or at all, but also may create a new illness. Worst of all, the reliance on numbers on a chart permits or, even worse, encourages physicians to neglect the personal care of patients. As one critic, not known for the temperateness of his comments, has stated, physicians are more preoccupied with the laying on of tools than with the laying on of hands (Lown, 1978). I believe he has underestimated the evils of laboratory-oriented medicine, which have spread beyond the confines of clinical practice. That kind of medicine encourages the belief that all patients with a given set of measurements are alike, whereas any good physician knows that no two people are ever alike. The error leads to the conclusion that a medication ineffective in at least 95% of patients with (what seems to be) the same illness should not be used, despite evidence that some such drugs are the only ones able to help some of the remaining 5%.

It has been pointed out that the strongest critics of modern laboratory-oriented medical practice are those who have distinguished themselves in medicine-related laboratory sciences as used in research.

To quote Peabody's *The Care of the Patient* again, "It is probably fortunate that most systems of education are constantly under the fire of general criticism, for if education were left solely in the hands of teachers, the chances are good that it would soon deteriorate." It is interesting to hear that voice from more than a half-century ago express distrust of academic medicine, for such an idea is to be found repeatedly in recent medical writings.

It is of great importance to realize that the sciences themselves are not under attack here; rather it is their current application to American medical education which is suspect. The sciences have their own inherent validity. The history of medicine records repeatedly the inclusion of content or concept from one science or another, but always with its subsequent modification or elimination of some or all incorporated material. History also records medicine's absorption of content or concept from the humanities, but that has usually escaped emphasis, the notable exception being the contributions of the pictorial arts to anatomical illustration. The contributions of the other humanities arouse far less than those of the physical sciences, and hence are less suitable for use in journalism. If this book has done anything, it has pointed out how important the pursuit of humanistic activities has been in the lives of nearly all great clinicians. This suggests that such pursuits, important in shaping the personality of a good physician, result in the evolution of an outstanding clinician.

The reliance today upon scientific data and concepts as explanations of medical phenomena is nothing new. In earlier eras, such explanations drew from the scientific theory of the times - Galenism, iatrochemistry, or iatro-mathematics. Today's scientific data are much less likely to be erroneous than were the data of earlier days, but they are still too few, too fragmentary, and too uncertain to permit the formulation of satisfactory systems of ideas. The main problem of medical practice based on scientific data is the shortage of reliable and relevant data. Since the academic physician largely justifies his profession by correlating, as best he can, the manifestations of disease with what currently is accepted in science, he must credit scientific data with a volume and a degree of reliability that is not deserved. This phenomenon was evident in an extreme form in 18th-century medicine. Today, science that might (by stretching inference) be applicable to clinical medicine is emphasized to a degree that exaggerates its significance. Under such circumstances, scientific theory ceases to be the servant; it becomes the master. The failure of laboratory science to justify its dominant role in medicine today, curiously, is made evident by the fact that many academic physicians devote their research efforts to what they call "Basic" research, which turns out to be laboratory research that is related to medicine only tangentially, if at all.

Perhaps medicine again will be simply the relationship between doctor and patient, as stated by Peabody:

> The treatment of a disease may be entirely impersonal; the care of a patient must be completely personal. The significance of the intimate personal relationship between physician and patient cannot be too strongly emphasized, for in an extraordinarily large number of cases both diagnosis and treatment are directly dependent on it, and the failure of the young physician to establish this relationship accounts for much of his ineffectiveness in the care of patients.

As is perhaps inevitable, things have come full circle. The conception of clinical medicine as whatever transpires between a doctor and a patient emphasizes that clinical medicine exists only in the doctor-patient relationship. That idea, expounded a half-century ago by Henderson, with his accustomed clarity and precision, was accepted automatically by good physicians of the past. Similar considerations apply to those machines and other devices whose use has become so large a part of medicine. Here we need only repeat the comment of Richards - who won a Nobel Prize for *physiological* studies - that no medical instrument can work without a human at each end, on being the patient, the other, a doctor. Today's physicians, often discouraged, dissuaded, or actually prevented from maintaining a good doctor-patient relationship by the ascendancy of laboratory-based medicine, find themselves unable to be first-rate physicians, unfortunately a fact soon discovered by their patients.

We also find ourselves able to agree with Garrison's comment about the patients' belief in earlier eras that they were being treated successfully by physicians who, by modern scientific standards, knew little that was correct scientifically.   This is not a plea for ignorance, since comparisons of mortality statistics of the past with those of the present immediately invalidate that notion; rather, it is merely recognition of the fact that clinical experience affords the doctor a degree of competence that predominant reliance on laboratory data does not.   Such an idea has been expressed widely by those both within and outside clinical medicine; yet, it has had only slight effects with respect to changing medical education and, subsequently, medical practice.   Whatever the future may hold for medical teaching, we can assert that any medical practice derogating or interfering with the doctor-patient interrelationship is medicine deformed.

A main thesis of this work is that the excessive and uncritical use of the laboratory in medicine has impaired clinical practice by attenuating the doctor-patient relationship.   There is another factor that will cause further deterioration of the situation: changes in the results of scientific research on which laboratory medicine now depends. As many writers have noted (*e.g.*, Henry Adams in his *Education of Henry Adams*), the productivity of scientific pursuits follows an S-shaped curve.   Today we are clearly on the rapidly rising part of the curve, but in time the rate of increase will lessen and the curve ultimately will become nearly horizontal as growth slows.   Although the total production of technology-based science may not decrease noticeably for some time, the production of first-rate material slackens first.   The rate of production of first-rate work, and even that of inferior work, decreases rapidly, while the rate of growth of marginal research may remain high for some time.   Under these circumstances the ratio between the trivial and the highly important grows *exponentially* larger (Rescher, 1978; Glass, 1979).   Hence those physicians who are committed to a practice of medicine based on laboratory data will find themselves relying more and more on material of either decreasing validity or diminishing significance, or both.   Some scientists believe that this never can happen, but others see the future deterioration of science as inevitable.   I believe, as do some others (Glass, 1979), the we already are experiencing such deterioration in the biological sciences. When it occurs finally to a marked and unmistakable degree, the custom of giving the products of the laboratory preference over the products of direct intellectual activity will cease to be acceptable.   Then will there be physicians trained in a practice of medicine based on doctor-patient interactions?

REFERENCES

- A -

Abel-Smith B: The Hospitals, 1800-1948. Cambridge, Harvard University Press, 1964

Abrahams HJ: A summary of Lavoisier's proposals for training in science and medicine. Bull Hist Med 32:389-407, 1958

Ackerknecht EH: Paul Bert's triumph. Bull Hist Med (Suppl) 3:16-31, 1944

Ackerknecht EH: Elisha Bartlett and the philosophy of the Paris clinical school. Bull Hist Med 24:43-60, 1950

Ackerknecht EH: Broussais, or a forgotten medical revolution. Bull Hist Med 27:320-343, 1953

Ackerknecht EH: Rudolf Virchow: Doctor, Statesman, Anthropologist. Madison WI, University of Wisconsin Press, 1953

Ackerknecht EH: Historical notes on cancer. Med Hist 2:114-119, 1958

Ackerknecht EH: Medicine at the Paris Hospital, 1794 - 1848. Baltimore, Johns Hopkins University Press, 1967

Ackerknecht EH: Cellular theory and therapeutics. Clio Med 5:1-5, 1970

Ackerknecht EH: The history of the discovery of the vegetative (autonomic) nervous system. Med. Hist. 18:1-8, 1974

Adelmann HB: Marcello Malpighi and the Evolution of Embryology. Ithaca, Cornell University Press, 1966

Adelmann HB (ed): The Correspondence of Marcello Malpighi, 5 vols. Ithaca, Cornell University Press, 1975

Agnew RAL: The achievement of Dominic John Corrigan. Med Hist 9:230-240, 1965

Albury WR: Physiological explanation in Magendie's manifesto of 1809. Bull Hist Med 48:90-99, 1974

Allen P: Medical education in 17th-century England. J Hist Med 1:115-143, 1946

Allen P: Early American animalcular hypotheses. Bull Hist Med 21:734-743, 1947

Altschule MD: Roots of Modern Psychiatry, 2nd ed. New York, Grune and Stratton, 1965

Altschule MD: Origins of Concepts in Human Behavior. Washington, Hemisphere Publishing Company, 1977

Amacher MP: Thomas Laycock, I.M. Sechenov, and the reflex arc concept. Bull Hist Med 38:168-183, 1964

Anning ST: The General Infirmary at Leeds, 2 vols. Edinburgh, E & S Livingstone, 1963

Appleby JH: John Grieve's correspondence with Joseph Black and some contemporaneous Russo-Scottish medical intercommunication. Med Hist 29:401-413, 1985

Ayala FJ, Dobzhansky T (eds):   Studies in the Philosophy of Biology. Reduction and Related Problems. London, Macmillan Publishing Company, 1974

- B -

Baker AB: Artificial respiration, the history of an idea. Med Hist 15:336-351, 1971

Baker F: The Two Sylviuses. An Historical Study. Bull Johns Hopkins Hosp 20:329-339, 1909

Baker, JR: Abraham Trembley of Geneva, Scientist and Philosopher, 1710-1784. London Edward Arnold & Co, 1952

Baker KM: Condorcet: From Natural Philosophy to Social Mathematics. Chicago, Univ of Chicago Press, 1975

Bariety M: Louis et la méthode numérique. Clio Med 7:177-183, 1972.

Barkam L: Nature's Work of Art. The Human Body as Image of the World. New Haven, Yale University Press, 1975

Barrett NR: A Tribute to John Snow, M.D., London 1813-1858. Bull Hist Med 19:517-535, 1946.

Bates DG: The background of John Young's thesis on digestion. Bull Hist Med 36:341-361, 1962

Bates DG: Sydenham and the medical meaning of "method." Bull Hist Hed 51:324-338, 1977

Bauer D de F: Elisha Bartlett, a distinguished physician with complete transposition of the viscera. Bull Hist Med 17:85-92, 1945

Bean WB: Origin of the term "internal medicine." New Engl J Med 306:182-183, 1982

Bedford DE: An early account of aortic incompetence by Thomas Cuming (1798-1887). MedHis 11:398-401, 1967

Bedford DE, Hartston W, Drew R: An early account of rheumatic heart diseas by Joseph Brown (1784-1868). Med Hist 20:76-79, 1976

Beecher HK Altschue M.D: Medicine at Harvard. Hanover NH: University Press of New England, 1977

Beekman F: William Hunter's education at Glasgow, 1731-1736. Bull Hist Med 15:284-297, 1944

Beekman F: Teacher and pupil: the brothers William and John Hunter from 1748 to 1760. Bull Hist Med 28:501-514, 1954

Beer RR: Der Grosse Haller. Sackingen, Hermann Stratz Verlag, 1947

Behrman S: John Farre (1775-1862) and other nineteenth century physicians at Moorfields. Med Hist 6:73-76, 1962

Behrman S: Thomas Young, the physician. Clio Med 10:277-284, 1975

Belloni L (ed): Opere Scelte di Marcello Malpighi. Turin, Unione Tipografico-Editrice Torinese, 1967

Belloni L: De la théorie atomistico-mécaniste à l'anatomie subtile (de Borelli à Malpighi) et de l'anatomie subtile à l'anatomie pathologique (de Malpighi a Morgagni). Clio Med 6:99-107, 1971

Bennett, JA: A note on theories of respiration and muscular action in England c. 1660. (Christopher Wren) Med His 20:59-60, 1976

Berlin I: Nationalism: Past neglect and present power. Part Rev 46:337, 1979

Berliner HS: A larger perspective on the Flexner Report. Int J Health Serv 5:573-592, 1975

Berliner HS: New light on the Flexner Report: Notes on the AMA-Carnegie Foundation background. Bull Hist Med 51:603-609, 1977

Bernard C: Lectures on the Phenomena of Life Common to Animals and Plants. (Hoff, HE, Guillemin R, Guillemin L[trans]). Springfield, IL CC Thomas, 1974

Bernheim BM: The Story of the Johns Hopkins. New York, Whittlesey House, 1949

Best AE: Reflections on Joseph Lister's Edinburgh experiments on vaso-motor control. Med Hist 14:10-30, 1970

Bigelow HJ: Medical Education in America. Cambridge, Welch, Bigelow and Company, 1871

Billroth T: The Medical Sciences in the German Universities. New York, The Macmillan Company, 1924

Bishop PJ: A list of papers etc., on Leopold Auenbrugger (1722-1809) and the history of percussion. Med Hist 5:192-196, 1961

Black DAK: Johnson on Boerhaave. Med His 3:325-329, 1959

Blick EM French influences on early American medicine. Mt Sinai Hospital J 24:499-509, 1957

Blumenthal H: American and French Culture, 1800-1900. Interchange in Art, Science Literature and Society. Baton Rouge, Louisiana State Univ, 1976

Bluth EI: James Hope and the acceptance of auscultation. J Hist Med 25:202-210, 1970

Boas EP: A refugee doctor of 1850. J Hist Med 3:65-94, 1948

Boksay G: Dr. Richard Bright and Lake Balaton. Med Hist 14:106-107, 1970

Bonner TN: American Doctors and German Universities. Lincoln, NE University of Nebraska Press, 1963

Borrell M: Setting the standards for a new science: Edward Schafer and endocrinology. Med Hist 22:282-290, 1978

Breathnach CS: Sir David Barry's experiments on venous return. Med Hist 9:133-141, 1965

Breathnach CS: Henry Newell Martin (1848-1893). A pioneer physiologist. Med Hist 13:271-279, 1969

Breathnach CS: The development of blood gas analysis. Med Hist 16:51-62, 1972

Brechka FT: Gerard van Swieten and his World 1700-1772. The Hague, Martin Nijhoff, 1970

Brednow W: Dietrich Georg Kieser, Sein Leben und Werk. Weisbaden, Franz Steiner, 1970

Bridenbaugh C: Dr. Thomas Bond's essay on the utility of clinical lectures. J Hist Med 2:10-19, 1947

Brieger GH: American surgery and the germ theory of disease. Bull Hist Med 40:135-145, 1966

Brieger GH: Review of Coulter HL, Divided Legacy: A History of the Schism in Medical Thought. Isis 69:103-105, 1978

Brock WH: The life and work of William Prout. Med Hist 9:101-126, 1965

Brockbank W: Portrait of a Hospital, 1752-1948. London, William Heineman, 1952

Brockbank W: The Honorary Medical Staff of the Manchester Royal Infirmary, 1830-1848. Manchaster, Manchester University Press, 1965

Brown, TM: The College of Physicians and the acceptance of iatromechanism in England, 1665-1695. Bull Hist Med 44:12-30, 1970

Brown TM: Physiology and the mechanical philosophy in mid-seventeenth century England. Bull Hist Med 15:25-54, 1977

Brown Sequard CE: Advice to Students. Cambridge, John Wilson & Son, 1867

Bruce-Chwatt LJ, Bruce-Chwatt J: Nicolas Copernicus, MD. Bull NY Acad Med 49:895-905, 1973

Bruce-Chwatt LJ: John Macculloch, MD, FRS (1775-1835) The precursor of the discipline of malariology. Med Hist 21:156-165, 1959

Buess H: Albrecht von Haller and his "Elementa physiologiae" as the beginning of pathological physiology. Med Hist 3:123-131, 1959

Bullough VL: The development of the medical university at Montpellier to the end of the fourtheenth century. Bull Hist Med 30:508-523, 1956

Bulloch W: The History of Bacteriology. London, Oxford University Press, 1938

- C -

Campbell WC: History of trichinosis. Paget, Owen and the discovery of Trichinella Spiralis. Bull Hist Med 53:520-442, 1969

Cannon SF: Science in Culture. The Early Victorian Period. New York, Neale Watson, 1978

Cantu JQ, Cantu RC: The psychiatric efforts of William Heberden, Jr. Bull Hist Med 41:132-139, 1967

Carter KC: The germ theory, beriberi, and the deficiency theory of disease. Med Hist 21:119-136, 1977

Cassedy JH: The flamboyant Colonel Waring. An anti-contagionist holds the American stage in the age of Pasteur and Koch. Bull Hist Med 36:163-176, 1962

Castiglioni A: A History of Medicine. (Krumbhaar EB [trans; ed]), pp 601-608. A A Knopf, 1941

Chance B: Richard Bright, traveller and artist (illus). Bull Hist Med 8:909-933, 1940

Cheever DW: The professional horizon. Harvard Med Assoc Bull 4:11-18, 1893

Chesney AM Two documents relating to medical education at the Johns Hopkins University. A report by Daniel C. Gilman, first President of the Johns Hopkins University, and a letter by Henry W Acland, F.R.S., Regius Professor of Medicine in the University of Oxford. Bull Inst Hist Med 4:477-504, 1936

Chesney AM: Two papers by John Shaw Billings on medical education. Bull Inst His Med 6:285-359, 1938

Chitnis AC: Medical Education in Edinburgh, 1790-1826, and some Victorian social consequences. Med Hist 17:173-185, 1973

Choulant JL: History and Bibliography of Anatomic Illustration (Frank M [trans; ed]). Chicago, University of Chicago Press, 1920

Churchill FB: Rudolf Virchow and the pathologist's criteria for the inheritance of acquired characteristics. J Hist Med 31:117-148, 1976

Clark G: Bernard Mandeville, MD and eighteenth century ethics. Bull Hist Med 45:430-443, 1971

Clark-Kennedy AE: The London: A Study in the Voluntary Hospital System. London, Pitman Publishing Company, 1962

Cohen of Birkenhead, Lord: James Carson, MD, FRS, of Liverpool. MedHist 7:1-12, 1963

Cohen of Birkenhead, Lord: The Liverpool Medical School and physicians (1642-1934). Med Hist 16:310-320, 1972

Coley NG: Alexander Marcet (1770-1822), physician and animal chemist. Med Hist 12:394-402, 1968

Collin V: Des Diverses Méthodes d'Exploration de la Poitrine. Paris, J B Ballière, 1824

Cooter RJ: Phrenology and British alienists, c. 1825-1845. Med Hist 20:1-21,135-151, 1976

Cope Z: John Shaw Billings, Florence Nightingale and the Johns Hopkins Hospital. Med Hist 1:367-368, 1957

Cope Z: Extracts from the diary of Thomas Laycock, chiefly written when he was a medical student, 1833-1935. Med Hist 9:169-176, 1965

Cope Z: The influence of the free dispensaries upon medical education in Britain. Med Hist 13:29-36, 1969

Copeman WSC: Doctors and Disease in Tudor Times. London, Dawson, 1960.

Corvisart des Marets JN: An Essay on the Organic Diseases and Lesions of the Heart and Great Vessels (J Gates [trans]) facsimile of 1812 edition with introduction by DW Richards. New York, Hafner, 1962

Coulter HL: Divided Legacy. A History of the Schism in Medical Thought, 3 vols. Washington, DC, Wehawken Book Company, 1975, 1977

Coury C: L'école médical de l'hôtel-Dieu de Paris au XIXe siècle. Clio Med 2:307-326, 1967

Cowen DL: A note on John Locke. J Hist Med 12:516, 1957

Cowen DL: Comments on Dr. Romanell's article on Locke and Sydenham. Bull Hist Med 33:173-180, 1959

Cragg RH: Thomas Charles Hope (1766-1844). Med Hist 11:186-189, 1967

Cranefield PF: The organic physics of 1847 and the biophysics of today. J Hist Med 12:407-423, 1957a

Cranefield PF: Charles E. Morgan's Electrophysiology and Therapeutics: An unkown English version of du Bois-Reymond's Thierische Elekitricitat. Bull Hist Med 31:172-181, 1957b

Cranefield PF: The philosophical and cultural interests of the biophysics movement of 1847. J Hist Med 21:1-7, 1966

Cranefield PF: The Way In and the Way Out: Francois Magendie, Charles Bell, and the Roots of the Spinal Nerves. Mt. Kisco NY: Futura Press, 1973

Crillin JK: William Cullen: His calibre as a teacher, and an unpublished inroduction to his A Treatise of the Materia Medica (London, 1773). Med Hist 15:79-87, 1971

Crellin JK: Chemistry and 18th-century British medical education. Clio Med 9:9-21, 1974

Croslan MP: Historical Studies in the Language of Chemistry. Cambridge, Harvard University Press, 1962

Cummins NM: Some Chapters of Cork Medical History. Cork, Cork University Press, 1957

- D -

Dainton C: The Story of England's Hospitals. Springfield CC Thomas, 1962

Daston LJ: British responses to psycho-physiology, 1860-1890. Isis 69:192-208, 1978

Davis AB: Circulation Physiology and Medical Chemistry in England 1650-1680. Lawrence, KA, Coronado Press, 1973

Debus AG: The English Paracelsans. London, Oldbourne, 1965

Debus AG: The Chemical Dream of the Renaissance. Cambridge, Heffer, 1968

Debus AG: The Paracelsans and the chemists: The chemical dilemma in Renaissance medicine. Clio Med 7:185-199, 1972

Debus AG (ed): Science, Medicine and Society in the Renaissance. New York, Science History Publications, 1972

Debus AG (ed): Medicine in Seventeenth-Century England. Berkeley, University of California Press, 1974

DeGuistino D: Conquest of Mind. Phrenology and Victorian Social Thought. London, Croom Helm, 1975

de Saussure D: Haller and la Mettrie. J Hist Med 4:431-449, 1949

Dewhurst K: Sydenham on "A dysentary." Bull Hist Med 29:393-400, 1955

Dewhurst K: A Symposium on trigeminal neuralgia. With contributions by Locke, Sydenham, and other eminent seventeenth century physicians. J Hist Med 12:21-36, 1957

Dewhurst K: Sydenham's original treatise on smallpox with a preface, and dedication to the Early of Shaftesbury, by John Locke. Med Hist 3:278-302, 1959

Dewhurst K: An essay on coughs by Locke and Sydenham. Bull Hist Med 33:366-374, 1959

Dewhurst K: Locke's essay on respiration. Bull Hist Med 34:257-273, 1960

Dewhurst K: Thomas Sydenham (1624-1689), reformer of clinical medicine. Med Hist 6:101-118, 1962

Dewhurst K: A review of John Locke's research in social and preventive medicine. Bull Hist Med 36:317-340, 1962

Dewhurst K: John Locke 1632-1704: Physician and Philosopher. London, Wellcome Historical Medical Library, 1963

Dewhurst K: Some letters of Dr. Charles Goodall (1642-1712) to Locke, Sloane, and Sir Thomas Millington. J Hist Med 17:487-508, 1962

Dewhurst K (ed): Oxford Medicine. Oxford, Sandford Publications, 1970

Dewhurst K: Dr. Thomas Sydenham (1624-1689), His Life and Original Writings. Berkeley, University of California, 1966

Dewhurst K, Reeves N: Friedrich Schiller. Medicine, Psychology and Literature. Berkely, University of California Press, 1978

Dible JH: DJ Larrey, a surgeon of the Revolution, Consulate, and Empire. Med Hist 3:100-107, 1959

Dols MW: The Black Death in the Middle East. Princeton, Princeton Univeristy Press, 1976

Doolin W: Dublin's contribution to medicine. J Hist Med 2:321-336, 1947

Dubos RJ: Louis Pasteur. Free Lance of Science. Boston, Little Brown & Company, 1950

Duclaux EP: Pasteur: The History of a Mind (Smith EF and Hedges F [trans]). Philadelphia, Saunders, 1920

Duveen DI, Klickstein HS: Antoine Laurent Lavoisier's contributions to medicine and public health. Bull Hist Med 29:164-179, 1955

Dvoichenko-Markov E: American doctors in the Crimean War. J Hist Med 9:362-367, 1954

- E -

East CFT: The Story of Heart Diseases. London, William Dawson & Sons, 1957

Eckman J: Anglo-American Hostility in American medical literature of the nineteenth century. Bull Hist Med 9:31-71, 1941

Edelstein L: Sydenham and Cervantes. Bull Hist Med (Suppl) 3:55-61, 1944

Edgar II: Modern Surgery and Lord Lister. J Hist Med 16:145-160, 1961

Edwards G: John Snow and the Institute of France. Med Hist 3:249-251, 1959

Entralgo PL: Sensualism and vitalism in Bichat's "Anatomie Générale." J Hist Med 3:47-64, 1948

- F -

Farley J, Geison GI: Science, politics and spontaneous generation in nineteenth century France: The Pasteur-Pouchet debate. Bull Hist Med 48:161-198, 1974

Finch JS: Sir Thomas Browne. A Doctor's Life of Science and Faith. New York, Schuman, 1950

Finlayson R: The vicissitudes of sputum cytology. Med Hist 2:24-35, 1958

Finney JMT: The Physician. New York, Charles Scribner & Sons, 1923

Fishbein M: Some great medical editors. Bull Hist Med 36:70-82, 1962

Flamm ES: The neurology of Jean Cruvilhier. Med Hist 21:343-355, 1977

Flaxman N: A history of heart-block. Bull Inst Hist Med 5:115-130, 1937

Flaxman N: The Hope of cardiology. James Hope (1801-1841). Bull Inst Hist Med 6:1-21, 1938

Fleetwood J: History of medicine in Ireland. Dublin, Browne and Nolan, 1951

Flexner A: Medical Education in the United States and Canada (with introduction by Pritchett HS). New York, Carnegie Foundation for the Advancement of Teaching, 1910

Flexner A: Abraham Flexner: An Autobiography (rev). New York, Simon & Schuster, 1960

Flexner S, Flexner JT: William Henry Welch and the Heroic Age of American Medicine. New York, Viking Press, 1941

Follis RH Jr: A note on the centenary of John Goodsir's "Anatomical and Pathological Observations." Bull Hist Med 18:438-444, 1945

Foster WD: Lionel Smith Beale (1828-1906) and the beginnings of clinical pathology. Med Hist 2:269-273, 1958

Foster WD: The early history of clinical pathology in Great Britain. Med Hist 3:173-187, 1959

Foster WD, Pinniger JL: History of pathology at St. Thomas's Hospital, London. Med Hist 7:330-347, 1963

Foucalt M: The Birth of the Clinic. An Archeology of Medical Perception. London, Tavistock Publications, 1973

Fox WL: "What is wanting":Dr. Harvey W Wiley's view of American medical education (1874). Bull Hist Med 36:268-274, 1962

Foxe AN: Plague; Laennec (1781-1826): The Invention of the Stethoscope and Father of Modern Medicine, 2nd ed. New York, Hobson Book Press, 1947

Frank MH, Weiss JJ (trans): "Introduction," Ludwig C: Textbook of Human Physiology. Med Hist 10:76-86, 1966

French JC: Mr. Johns Hopkins and Dr. Macaulay's "Medical Improvement." Bull Hist Med 27:562-566, 1953

French RK: Robert Whytt, The Soul, and Medicine. London, Wellcome Institute, 1969

French RK: Sauvages, Whytt and the motion of the heart: Aspects of eighteenth-century animism. Clio Med 7:35-54, 1977

Frenk E: Johann Rudolph Burkhard's Syllogae Phainomenon Anatomikon. Aarau, Verlag HR Sauerlander, 1958

Friedenwald H: Notes on Moritz Schiff (1823-1896). Bull Inst Hist Med 5:589-602, 1937

- G -

Galaty DH: The philosophical basis of mid-nineteenth century German reductionism. J Hist Med 29:295-316, 1974

Galdston I: Some notes on the early history of chemotherapy. Bull Hist Med 8:806-818, 1940

Gale BG: The dissolution and the revolution in London hospital facilities. Med Hist 11:91-96, 1967

Garrison FH: An Introduction to the History of Medicine 4th ed. Philadelphia and London, WB Saunders Company, 1929

Gaskell E: Early American English Translations of European medical works. Med Hist 14:300-307, 1970

Geddes LA, Hoff HE: The capillary electrometer. The first graphic recorder of bioelectric signals. Arch Int Hist Sci 14:275-290, 1961

General Education Board, The: An Account of its Activities 1902-1914. New York, General Education Board, 1915

Gibbon JH: London Surgery in the early part of the nineteenth century. Ann Med Hist 4:80-85, 1922

Gibson WC: The biomedical pursuits of Christopher Wren. Med Hist 14:331-341, 1970

Glass B: Milestones and rates of growth in the development of biology. Quart Rev Biol 54:31-53, 1979

Gloyne SR: John Hunter. Baltimore, Williams and Wilkins, 1950

Goldschmid E: The influence of the social environment on the style of pathological illustration. J Hist Med 7:258-270, 1952

Goodman DC: The application of chemical criteria to biological classification in the eighteenth century. Med Hist 15:23-44, 1971

Goodman DC: Chemistry and the two organic kingdoms of nature in the nineteenth century. Med Hist 16:113-130, 1972

Gordon-Taylor G, Walls EW: Sir Charles Bell, His Life and Times. Edinburgh, E & S Livingstone, 1958

Grange KM: Pinel or Chiarugi? Med Hist 7:371-380, 1963

Gray TC: History of anaesthesia in Liverpool. Med Hist 16:375-382, 1972

Gray J: History of the Royal Medical Society, 1737-1937 (Guthrie D [edl]). Edinburgh, Edinburgh University Press, 1952

Green JHS: Marshall Hall (1790-1857): A Biographical Study. Med Hist 2:120-133, 1958

Gregory F: Scientific Materialism in Nineteenth-century Germany. Boston, D Reidel, 1977a

Gregory F: Scentific versus dialectical materialism: A clash of ideologies in nineteenth-century German radicalism. Isis 68:206-223, 1977b

Gruber H, Gruber V: Hermann von Helmholtz: Nineteenth-century polymorph. Scientific Monthly 83:92-99, 1956

Gruman GJ: The rise and fall of prolongevity hygiene 1558-1873. Bull Hist Med 35:221-229, 1961

Gubser A: The Positiones variae medicae of Franciscus Sylvius. Bull Hist Med 40:72-80, 1966

Guillain, G: JM Charcot, 1825-1893: His Life - His Work (Bailey P [trans; ed]). New York, Paul B Hoeber, 1959

Guthrie D: Lord Lister: His Life and Doctrine. Baltimore, Williams and Wilkins, 1949

Guthrie D: The influence of the Leyden school upon Scottish medicine. Med Hist 3:108-122, 1959

Guthrie D: Extramural Medical Education in Edinburgh. Edinburgh, E & S Livingstone, 1965

- H -

Haigh E: The roots of the vitalism of Xavier Bichat. Bull Hist Med 49:72-86, 1975

Haigh EL: Vitalism, the soul and sensibility: The physiology of Theophile Bordun. J Hist Med 31:30-41, 1976

Haigh EL: The vital principle of Paul Joseph Barthez: The clash between monism and dualism. Med Hist 21:1-14, 1977

Hall M: Principles of the Theory and Practice of Medicine (Bigelow J, Holmes OW [eds]), 1st American ed. Boston, Little & Brown, 1839

Hamey WB (ed): The case reports and Autopsy records of Ambrose Pare. Springfield, IL, Charles C Thomas, 1960

Handler CE (ed): Guy's Hospital - 250 Years. London, Guy's Hospital Gazette, 1976

von Harnack A: History of Dogma, 3rd German ed, p 140 (Buchanan N [trans]). New York, Dover, 1961

Harvey AM: Adventures in Medical Research. A Century of Discovery at Johns Hopkins. Baltimore, Johns Hopkins University Press, 1976

Harvey AM: John Shaw Billings: Forgotten hero of American medicine. Perspect Biol Med 27:35-51, 1977

Heaton CE: Medicine in New Amsterdam. Bull Hist Med 9:125-143, 1941

Heaton CE: Medicine in New York, during the English Colonial Period, 1664-1675. Bull Hist Med 17:9-37, 1945

Heller R: Officers de sante: The second-class doctors of nineteenth-century France. Med Hist 22:25-43, 1978

Henderson LJ: Introduction in Claude Bernard, An Introduction to the Study of Experimental Medicine. New York, Macmillan Company, 1927.

Henderson LM: The practice of medicine as applied sociology. Trans Assoc Am Physicians 51:8-22, 1936

Herrick JB: Certain textbooks on heart disease of the early nineteenth century. Bull Hist Med 10:136-147, 1941

Hoeldtke R: The history of associationism and British medical psychology. Med Hist 11:46-65, 1967

Hoff EC, Hoff PM: The life and times of Richard Lower, physiologist and physician (1631-1691). Bull Inst Hist Med 4:517-535, 1936

Hoff HE: The history of vagal inhibition. Bull Hist Med 8:461-496, 1940

Hoff HE: Claude Bernard's Introduction. A review. Bull Hist Med 36:177-181, 1962

Hoff HE, Geddes LA: The rheotome and its prehistory: A study in the historical interrelation of electrophysiology and electromechanics. Bull Hist Med 31:212-234, 1957

Hoff HE, Geddes LA: Graphic registration before Ludwig; the antecedents of the kymograph. Isis 50:5-21, 1959

Hoff HE, Geddes LA: A historical perspective on physiological monitoring: Chauveau's projecting kymograph and the projecting physiograph. Cardiovas Res Center Bull (Baylor) 14:3-35, 1975

Holmes FL: The milieu interieur and the cell theory. Bull Hist Med 37:315-335, 1963

Holmes FL: Claude Bernard and Animal Chemistry: The Emergence of a Scientist. Cambridge, MA, Harvard University Press, 1974

Howard-Jones N: Fracastonio and Henle: A re-appraisal of their contribution to the concept of communicable diseases. Med Hist 21:61-68, 1977

Howell TH: Geriatrics one hundred years ago. Med Hist 17:199-203, 1973

Huard P: Les échanges médicaux Franco-Anglais au XVIIIe siècle. Clio Med 3:41-58, 1968

Huard P: Sciences, Médicine, Pharmacie, de la Révolution à l'Empire (1789-1815). Paris, Roger Dacosta, 1970

Huard P: Quelques idées sur la structure de la matière vivante au XIXème siècle; leur incidence sur la pratique médicale. Clio Med 9:57-64, 1974

Huard P, Imbault-Huard MJ: La clinique Parisiènne avant et apres 1802. Clio Med 10:173-182, 1975

Hughes RE: George Budd (1808-1882) and nutritional deficiency diseases. Med Hist 17:127-135, 1973

Hughes RE: James Lind and the cure of scurvy: An experimental approach. Med Hist 19:342-351, 1975

Hume EE: Francis Home, MD (1719-1813), the Scottish military surgeon who first described diptheria as a clinical entity. Bull Hist Med 11:48-68, 1942

Hume EE: Surgeon John Jones, US Army, father of American surgery and author of America's first medical book. Bull Hist Med 13:10-32, 1943

Hunter P: Fernand Widal. Med Hist 7:56-61, 1963

Huntley FL: Sir Thomas Browne, MD, William Harvey, and the metaphor of the circle. Bull Hist Med 25:236-247, 1951

Hurzeller H: Robert Whytt (1714-1766) und seine physiologesehin Schriffen. Zurich, Juris Druck, 1973

- I -

Illingworth CFW: The Story of William Hunter. Edinburgh and London, E & S Livingstone, 1967

Irons EE: Theophile Bonet 1620-1689. His influence on the science and practice of medicine. Bull Hist Med 12:623-665, 1942

Isler H: Thomas Willis (1621-1675), Doctor and Scientist (trans). New York, Hafner, 1968

Itokawa Y: Kanehiro Takaki (1849-1920). A biographical sketch. J Nutr 106:583-588, 1976

- J -

Jackson J: Preface in Louis P: Researches on the Effects of Bloodletting in Some Inflammatory Diseases. Boston, Hilliard, Gray & Company, 1836

Jacobs MS: Paul Ehrlich and his relation to modern chemotherapy. Bull Hist Med 8:956-964, 1940

Jarcho S: Giovanni Battista Morgagni: His interests, ideas, and achievements. Bull Hist Med 22:503-527, 1948

Jarcho S: A review of Auenbrugger's Inventum Novum, attributed to Oliver Goldsmith. Bull Hist Med 33:470-474, 1959

Jarcho S: Morgagni and Auenbrugger in the retrospect of two hundred years. Bull Hist Med 35:489-496, 1961

Jarcho S (trans; ed): Practical Observations on Dropsy of the Chest. Breslan Leopoldine Academy of Scientists 1706, Philadelphia, 1971

Jevons FR: Boerhaave's biochemistry. Med Hist 6:343-362, 1962

Johnstone RW: William Cullen. Med Hist 3:33-46, 1959

Jolley N: Leibniz on Locke and Socinianism. J Hist Ideas 39:233-250, 1978

Joens EWP: The life and works of Guilhelmus Fabricius Hildanus (1560-1634). Med Hist 4:196-209, 1960

Jones RM: American doctors in Paris, 1820-1861: A statistical profile. J His Med 25:143-157, 1970

Jones RM: American doctors and the Parisian medical world, 1830-1840. Bull Hist Med 47:40-65, 177-204, 1973

Jones RM: The Parisian education of an American surgeon: Letters of Jonathan Mason Warren (1832-1835). Philadelphia, American Philosophical Society, 1978

Jones MJA, Gemmill CL: The notebook of Robley Dunglison, student of clinical medicine in Edinburgh, 1815-1816. J Hist Med 22:261-273, 1967

Jones VA: John Hall: Seventeenth-century physician of Stratford upon Avon. Proc Roy Soc Med 70:709-714, 1977

Joseph H: Shakespeare's Son-In-Law: John Hall, Man and Physician. Hamden, CT, Archon Books, 1964

- K -

Kargon R: John Graunt, Francis Bacon, and the Royal Society: The reception of statistics. J Hist Med 18:337-348, 1963

Kass IH, Bartlett AH: Thomas Hodgkin, MD (1798-1866): An annotated bibliography. Bull Hist Med 43:138-175, 1969

Keele KD: William Harvey: The Man, the Physician, and the Scientist. London, Nelson, 1965

Keele KD: Thomas Willis on the brain: An essay review. Med Hist 11:194-200, 1967

Keele KD: Addison on the "supra-renal capsules": An essay review. Med Hist 13:195-202, 1969

Keele KD: The application of the physics of sound to 19th century cardiology: With particular reference to the part played by CJB Williams and James Hope. Clio Med 8:191-221, 1973

Keele KD: The Sydenham-Boyle theory of morbific particles. Med Hist 18:240-248, 1974

Keers RY: Two forgotten pioneers. James Carson and George Bodington. Thorax 35:483-489, 1980

Keil H: Dr. William Charles Wells and his contribution to the study of rheumatic fever. Bull Hist Med 4:789-816,1936

Kelly T: George Birkbeck, Pioneer of Adult Education. Liverpool, Liverpool University Press, 1959

Kennedy E: "Idealogy" from Destutt de Tracy to Marx. J Hist Ideas 40:353-368, 1979

Kerran R: Laennec: His Life and Times (Abrahams-Curiel DC [trans]). Oxford, Pergamon Press, 1960

Keynes GL: Sir Thomas Browne, MD. St Bart Hosp J 19:158-161, 1912

Keynes GL: The Life of William Harvey. Oxford, Clarendon Press, 1966

Kieffer JE: Philadelphia controversy, 1775-1780. Bull Hist Med 11:148-160, 1942

King LS: Auscultation in England 1821-1837. Bull Hist Med 33:446-453, 1959

King LS: Empiricism and rationalism in the works of Thomas Sydenham. Bull Hist Med 44:1-11, 1970

Kisch B: Jacob Helm's observations and experiments on human digestion. J Med Hist 9:311-328, 1954

Kisch B: An early American report on Jacob Helm's work on human digestion. J Hist Med 10:230-232, 1955

Klemperer P: The pathology of Morgagni and Virchow. Bull Hist Med 32:24-38, 1958

Klemperer P: Notes on Carl von Rokitasky's autobiography and inaugural address. Bull Hist Med 35:374-380, 1961

Klickstein HD: A short history of the professorship of chemistry of the University of Pennsylvania School of Medicine 1765-1847. Bull Hist Med 27:43-68, 1953

Klickstein HS: David Hosack on the qualifications of a professor of chemistry in the medical department. Bull Hist Med 28:212-236, 1954a

Klickstein HS: Paris on chemistry in medicine. J Hist Med 9:460-464, 1954b

Kocher PH: Paracelsan medicine in England: The first thirty years (c. 1570-1600). J Hist Med 2:451-480, 1947

Kohler RE: Walter Fletcher, FG Hopkins, and the Dunn Institute of Biochemistry: A case study in the patronage of science. Isis 69:331-355, 1978

Kohler RE: Medical Reform and Biomedical Science - A Case Study, In Two Hundred Years in American Medicine. Philadelphia, University of Pennsylvania Press, 1979

Koller G: Des Leben des Biologen Johannes Muller, 1801-1858. Stuttgart, Wissenschaftliche Verlagsgessellschaft, 1958

Kozinn PJ: Critical evaluation and utilization of clinical laboratory reports. Infect Dis 8(7):4, 1978

Kramer HD: The germ theory and the early public health program in the United States. Bull Hist Med 22:233-247, 1948

Kraus M: American and European medicine in the eighteenth century. Bull Hist Med 8:679-685, 1940

Kruta V: JE Purkyne's contribution to the cell theory. Clio Med 6:109-120, 1971

- L -

Landing BH: Rollin R Gregg of Buffalo. A 19th century opponent of Pasteur and the germ theory of disease. Bull Hist Med 36:524-528, 1962

Langdon-Brown W: Some Chapters in Cambridge Medical History. New York, The Macmillan Company, 1946

Lawrence C: Physiological apparatus in the Wellcome Museum. 1. The Marey sphygmograph. Med Hist 22:196-200, 1978

Lawson G: Surgeon in the Crimea. London, Constable, 1968

Lehmberg SE: Sir Thomas Elyot, Tudor Humanist. Austin, University of Texas Press, 1960

Leibowitz JO: Thrombo-embolic disease and heart-block in Vesalius. Med Hist 7:258-264, 1963

Leibowitz JO: Thomas Hodgkin (1798-1866). Clio Med 2:97-101, 1967

Leibowitz JO: The History of Coronary Heart Disease. London, Wellcome Institute of the History of Medicine, 1970

Leigh D: John Haslam, MD (1764-1844): Apothecary to Bethlem. J Hist Med 10:17-44, 1955

Lesky E: Ignaz Philipp Semmelweis und die Wiener Medizinische Schule. Vienna, H Bohlaus, 1964

Lesky E: Purkyn's Weg: Wissenschaft, Bildung und Nation. Vienna, H Bohlaus, 1970

Lesky E: Structure and function in Gall. Bull Hist Med 44:297-314, 1970

Lesky E Wandruszka A (eds): Gerard Van Swieten und seine Zeit. Vienna, H Bohlaus, 1973

Lesky E: The Vienna Medical School of the 19th Century (Williams L, Leviz IS [trans]). Baltimore, Johns Hopkins University Press, 1976

Lilienfeld DE: "The greening of epidemiology": Sanitary Physicians and the London Epidemiological Society (1830-1870). Bull Hist Med 52:503-538, 1979

Lind HR (trans): Berengario da Carpi Jacopo: A Short Introduction to Anatomy (Isagogae breves). Chicago, University of Chicago Press, 1959

Lindeboom GA (ed): Boerhaave's Correspondence, Part I, 2 vols. Leiden, EJ Brill, 1962-1964

Lindeboom GA: Herman Boerhaave: The Man and His Work. London, Methuen, 1968

Lindeboom GA: Boerhaave and His Time. Leiden, EJ Brill, 1970

Lindeboom GA: Boerhaave's concept of the basic structure of the body. Clio Med 5:203-208, 1970

Lindeboom GA: Boerhaave's impact on the relation between chemistry and medicine. Clio Med 7:271-278, 1972

Lipman TO: The response to Liebig's vitalism. Bull Hist Med 40:511-524, 1966

Lipman TO: Vitalism and reductionism in Liebig's physiological thought. Isis 58:167-185, 1967

Livesley B: The resolution of lemon juice as a cure for scurvy. Bull Hist Med 35:123-132, 1961

Long ER: A History of American Pathology (enlarged, revised ed). New York, Dover Publications, 1965

Lough J: Locke's Travels in France, 1675-1679. Cambridge, Cambridge University Press, 1953

Louis PCA: Researches on Phthisis, 2nd ed (Walshe WH [trans]). London, Sydenham Society, 1844

Lown B: Post-Mi care: How to manage your patient's arrhythmas. Mod Med 46(16):60-77, 1978

Luckhardt AT: Introduction. In von Helmholtz H: On Thought in Medicine. Bull Inst Hist Med 6:117-119, 1968

Luisada AA: A short chronology of important events in cardiology. Bull Hist Med 3(Suppl):152-160, 1944

Lunsingh-Scheurleer THL: Posthumus-Meyjes GHM (eds): Leiden University in the Seventeenth Century: An Exchange of Learning. Leiden, EJ Brill, 1975

- M -

Macht DI: Personal reminiscences of Professor John J. Abel. Bull Hist Med 8:721-730, 1940

MacKinney LC: Early Medieval Medicine. Baltimore, The Johns Hopkins University Press, 1937

MacKinney LC: The beginnings of Western Scientific anatomy: New evidence and a revision in interpretation of Mondeville's role. Med Hist 6:233-239, 1962

MacNalty AS: The prevention of smallpox: From Edward Jenner to Monckton Copeman. Med Hist 12:1-18, 1968

Maddison F, Pelling, Webster C (eds): Essays on the Life and Work of Thomas Linacre c. 1460-1524. Oxford, Clarendon Press, 1977

Magnus-Levy A: The heroic age of German medicine. Bull Hist Med 16:331-342, 1944

Magnus-Levy A: Energy metabolism in health and disease. J Hist Med 2:307-320, 1947

Major RH: Antonio di Pagolo Benivieni. Bull Inst Hist Med 3:739-749, 1935

Major RH: Agostini Bassi and the parasitic theory of disease. Bull Hist Med 16:97-107, 1944

Maluf NSR: How a physiologist anticipated a physical chemist. Bull Hist Med 14:352-365, 1943

Marcus JR: Communal Sick-Care in the German Ghetto. Cincinnati, Hebrew Union College Press, 1947

Marshall ML: Dr. Holmes and American medical literature. Bull Hist Med 22:277-287, 1948

Marx OM: A re-evaluation of the Mentalists in early 19-century Germany psychiatry. Am J Psychiat 121:752-760, 1965

Marx OM: Nineteenth-century medical psychology. Theoretical problems in the work of Griesinger, Meynert, and Wernicke. Isis 61:355-370, 1970

Marx OM: Psychiatry on a neuropathological basis. Th. Meynert's application for the extension of his venia legendi. Clio Med 6:139-158, 1971.

Marx OM: Wilhelm Griesinger and the history of psychiatry: A reassessment. Bull Hist Med 46:519-544, 1972

Maulitz RC: Schwann's way: Cells and crystals. J Hist Med 26:422-437, 1971

Mayer CF: Metaphysical trends in modern pathology. Bull Hist Med 26:71-81, 1952

McConaghy RMS: Sir George Baker and the Devonshire colic. Med Hist 11:345-360, 1967

McConaghy RMS: Sir William Blizard and his poems. Med Hist 2:292-297, 1958

McGrew RE: The first cholera epidemic and social history. Bull Hist Med 34:-61-73, 1960

McHenry LC Jr.: Samuel Johnson's "The Life of Dr. Sydenham." Med Hist 8:181-187, 1964

McHenry LC Jr.: Dr. Johnson and Dr. Herberden (sic). Clio Med 11:117-123, 1976

McInness EM: St. Thomas's Hospital. London, George Allen & Unwin, 1963

McKusick VA: Rouanet of Paris and New Orleans. Experiments on the valvular origin of the heart sounds 125 years ago. Bull Hist Med 32:137-151, 1958

McKusick VA, Wiskind HK: Osborne Reynolds of Manchester. Contributions of an engineer to the understanding of cardiovascular sound. Bull Hist Med 33:116-136, 1959

McKusick VA, Wiskind HD: Felix Savart (1791-1841), physician physicist. Early studies pertinent to the understanding of murmurs. J Hist Med 14:411-423, 1959

Medvie VC, Thompson JL (eds): The Royal Hospital of St. Bartholomew. London, The Royal Hospital of St. Bartholomew, 1974

Meikeljohn A: The Life, Work and Times of Charles Turner Thachrah, Surgeon and Apothecary of Leeds (1795-1833). Edinburgh and London, E & S Livingstone, 1957

Meyer A, Hierons R: Observations on the history of the "Circle of Wills." Med Hist 6:119-130, 1962

Meyer A, Hierons R: On Thomas Willis's concepts of neurophysiology. Med Hist 9:1-15, 142-155, 1965

Michaelis AR: EJ Morey - physiologist and first cinematographer. Med Hist 10:201-203, 1966

Middleton WS: Turner's Lane Hospital. Bull Hist Med 40:14-42, 1966

Miller JGF: The background of Laennec. Bull Med 40:411-414, 1967

Moorman LJ: William Withering: His work, his health, his friends. Bull Hist Med 12:355-366, 1942

Mora GA: Heinroth's Contributions to Psychiatry. In Heinroth JCA: Textbook of Disturbances of Mental Life. Baltimore, Johns Hopkins University Press, 1975

Moravia S: From homme machine to homme sensible: Changing eighteenth-century models of man's image. J Hist Ideas 39:45-60, 1978

Morgan AD: Some forms of undiagnosed coronary disease in nineteenth-century England. Med Hist 12:344-358, 1968

Morris WIC: Brotherly love. An essay on the personal relations between William Hunter and his brother John. Med Hist 3:20-32, 1959

Morton RS: Dr. William Wallace (1791-1837) of Dublin. Med Hist 10:38-43, 1966

Moschcowitz E: Louis Pasteur's credo of science. Bull Hist Med 22:451-466, 1948

Muller HJ: The Uses of the Past. New York, Oxford University Press, 1952

Multhauf R: Medical chemistry and "the Paracelsans." Bull Hist Med 28:101-126, 1954

Musser R, Kantz JC, Jr: The friendship of William Withering and Erasmus Darwin. Bull Hist Med 8:844-847, 1940

- N -

Nash P, Kasamias AM, Perkinson HJ: The Educated Man. Studies in the History of Educational Though. New York, John Wiley and Sons, 1965

Navarro V: Medicine under Capitalism. New York, Prodist, 1976

Neale AV: Some thoughts and experiments on respiration and on asthma, with special reference to Henry Hyde Salter. Med Hist 7:247-257, 1963

Neuburger M: British medicine and the old Vienna Medical School. Bull Hist Med 12:486-528, 1942

Neuburger M: British medicine and the Gottingen Medical School in the eighteenth century. Bull Hist Med 14:449-466, 1943

Neuburger M: Some relations between British and German medicine in the seventeenth century. Bull Hist Med 3(Suppl):223-236, 1944

Neuburger M: Some relations between British and German medicine in the first half of the eighteenth century. Bull Hist Med 17:217-228, 1945

Meuburger M: John Floyer's pioneer work. Bull Hist Med 22:208-212, 1948

Meuburger M: Francis Clifton and William Black, eighteenth century critical historians of medicine. J Hist Med 5:44-49, 1950

Newman C: The Evolution of Medical Education in the Nineteenth Century. London, Oxford University Press, 1957

Newman C: Physical signs in the London hospitals. Med Hist 2:195-201, 1958

Niebyl PH: Science and metaphor in the medicine of Restoration England. Bull Hist Med 47:356-374, 1973 Norford DP: Microcosm and macrocosm in seventeenth-century literature. J Hist Ideas 38:409-428, 1977

Numbers RL, Orr WJ, Jr: William Beaumont's reception at home and abroad. Isis 72:590-612, 1981

Nye MJ: The Boutroux circle and Poincare's conventionalism. J Hist Ideas 40:107-120, 1979

- O -

Oberndorf, CP: The Psychiatric Novels of Oliver Wendell Holmes. New York: Columbia University Press, 1943

Ober WB (ed): Great Men of Guy's. New York, Scarecrow Reprint Company, 1973

Olby R: Cell chemistry in Miescher's day. Med Hist 13:377-382, 1969

Olmsted JMD: The contemplative works of Claude Bernard. Bull Inst Hist Med 3:335-354, 1935

Olmsted JMD: Francois Magendie, Pioneer in Experimental Physiology and Scientific Medicine in XIX Century France. New York, Schumann, 1944

Olmsted JMD: Charles Edouard Brown-Sequard. Baltimore, Johns Hopkins University Press, 1946

O'Malley CD: English Medical Humanists: Thomas Linacre and John Caius. Lawrence, KA, Univeristy of Kansas Press, 1965

O'Malley CD: The lure of Padua. Med Hist 14:1-9, 1970

O'Malley CD, Russel KF: Daniel Edward's Introduction to Anatomy 1532. A facsimile reproduction with English translation and an Introductory Essay on Anatomical Studies in Tudor England. London, Oxford University Press, 1961

O'Malley CD, Saunders JB de CM: Vesalius as a clinician. Bull Hist Med 14:594-608, 1943

Onuigbo, WIB: Lung cancer in the nineteenth century. Med Hist 3:69-77, 1959

Onuigbo, WIB: Historical trends in cancer surgery. Med Hist 6:154-161, 1962

Onuigbo WIB: The paradox of Virchow's views on cancer meastasis. Bull Hist Med 36:444-449, 1962

Onuigbo WIB: Thomas Hodgkin (1798-1866) on cancer cell carriage. Med HIst 11:406-411, 1967

Oppenheimer JM: New Aspects of John and William Hunter. New York, Henry Schuman, 1946a

Oppenheimer JM: A note on William Blake and John Hunter. J Hist Med 1:41-45, 1946b

Oppenheimer JM: John Hunter, Sir Thomas Browne and the experimental method. Bull Hist Med 21:17-32, 1947

Oppenheimer JM: John and William Hunter and some contemporaries in literature and art. Bull Hist Med 23:21-47, 1949

- P -

Pace A: Notes on Dr. John Morgan and his relations with Italian men and women of science. Bull Hist Med 18:445-453, 1945

Pachter HM: Paracelsus, Magic into Science. New York, H. Schuman, 1951

Pagel W: The Religious and Philosophical Aspects of van Helmont's Science and Medicine. Baltimore, Johns Hopkins University Press, 1944

Pagel W: The speculative basis of modern pathology. Jahn, Virchow and their philosophy of pathology. Bull Hist Med 18:1-43, 1945

Pagel W: Paracelsus. An Introduction to Philosophical Medicine in the Era of the Renaissance. Basel, S. Karger, 1958

Pagel W: Harvey's role in the history of medicine. Bull Hist Med 24:70-73, 1950a

Pagel W: The circular motion of the blood and Giordano Bruno's philosophy of the circle. Bull Hist Med 24:398-399, 1950b

Pagel W: William Harvey's Biological Ideas. Selected Aspects and Historical Background. Basel, S. Karger, 1967

Pagel W: New Light on William Harvey. Basel, S. Karger, 1976

Parker F: Influences on the founder of the Johns Hopkins University and the Johns Hopkins Hospital. Bull Hist Med 34:148-153, 1960

Peabody FW: The physician and the laboratory. Bost Med Surg J 187:324-327, 1922

Penman WR: The introduction of the Edinburgh quizzing system into American medical education. Bull Hist Med 52:89-95, 1978

Peterson MJ: The Medical Profession in Mid-Victorian London. Berkeley, University of California Press, 1978

Philip R: Robert Koch's discovery of the tubercle bacillus. Am Rev Tuberc 26:637-652, 1932

Pickstone JV: Globules and coagula: Concepts of tissue formation in the early nineteenth century. J Hist Med 28:336-356, 1973

Pickstone JV: Vital actions and organic physics: Henri Dutrochet and French physiology during the 1820's. Bull Hist Med 50:191-212, 1976

Pinero JML: The relation between the "alte Wiener Schule" and the Spanish medicine of the enlightenment. Clio Med 9:109-123, 1974

Plaut A: Rudolph Virchow and today's physicians and surgeons. Bull Hist Med 27:236-251, 1953

Porter IA: Alexander Gordon, M.D., of Aberdeen, 1752-1799. Edinburgh and London, Oliver & Boyd, 1958

Porter IA: Thomas Trotter, M.D., naval physician. Med Hist 7:155-164, 1963

Porter IH: The nineteenth-century physician and cardiologist Thomas Bevill Peacock (1812-1882). Med Hist 6:240-254, 1962

Porter IH: Thomas Bartholin (1616-1680) and Niels Steensen (1636-1686) master and pupil. Med Hist 7:99-123, 1963

Power DA: The evolution of the surgeon in London. St Bartholomew's Hosp J 19:83-93, 1912

Poynter FNL: A unique copy of George Armstrong's printed proposals for establishing the Dispensary for Sick Children, London, 1769. Med Hist 1:65-73, 1957

Poynter FNL: Chemistry in the Service of Medicine. London, Pitman Medical Publishing Company, 1963

Poynter FNL: The Evolution of Hospitals in Britain. London, Pitman Medical Publishing Company, 1964

Poynter FNL: Medicine and Man. London, Penguin Books, 1973

Poynter FNL: Sydenham's influence abroad. Med Hist 17:225-234, 1973

Poynter FNL, Bishop WJ: A Seventeenth-Century Doctor and his Patients; John Symcotts, 1592-1662. Streatly, Bedfordshire, Bedfordshire Historical Record Society, 1951

Pridon D: Rudolph Virchow and social medicine in historical perspective. Med Hist 8:274-278, 1964

Proskauer C: A civil ordinance of the year 1846 to combat phosphorus necrosis. Bull Hist Med 11:561-569, 1942

- Q -

Quen JM: Isaac Ray and his "Remarks on Pathological Anatomy." Bull Hist Med 38:113-126, 1964

- R -

Rae I: Knox, The Anatomist. Springfield IL, Thomas, 1965

Rath G: Neural pathology. A pathogenic concept of the 18th and 19th centuries. Bull Hist Med 33:526-541, 1959

Rather LJ (trans): Disease, Life, and Man. Selected Essays by Rudolph Virchow. Stanford, CA, Stanford University Press, 1958

Rather LJ: Rudolph Virchow's views on pathology, pathological anatomy, and cellular pathology. Arch Pathol 82:197-204, 1966

Rather LJ: Virchow's review of Rokitansky's Handbuch in the Preussische medizinal - Beitung, Dec. 1846. Clio Med 4:127-140, 1969a

Rather LJ: Some relations between eighteenth-century fiber theory and nineteenth-century cell theory. Clio Med 4:191-202, 1969b

Rather LJ: Langenbeck on the mechanics of tumor metastasis and the transmission of cancer from man to animal. Clio Med 10:213-225, 1975

Rather LJ, Rohl ER: An English trnaslation of the hitherto untranslated part of Rokitansky's Einleitung to volume I of the Handbuch der Allgemeinen Pathologie (1846) with a bibliography of Rokitansky's published works. Clio Med 7:215-225, 1972

Rather LJ: The Genesis of Cancer. A Study in the History of Ideas. Baltimore, The Johns Hopkins University Press, 1978

Raven CE: Medicine - the mother of the sciences. Med Hist 4:85-90, 1960

Reill PH: The German Enlightenment and the Rise of Historicism. Berkeley, University of California Press, 1975

Rendle-Short J: William Cadogan, eighteenth-century physician. Med Hist 4:288-309, 1960

Rendle-Short M, Rendle-Short J: The Father of Child Care. Life of William Cadogan (1711-1797). Bristol, John Wright, 1966

Rescher N: Scientific Progress. University of Pittsburgh Press, 1978

Richmond PA: Some variant theories in opposition to the germ theory of disease. J Hist Med 9:290-303, 1954a

Richmond PA: American attitudes toward the germ theory of disease (1860-1880). J Hist Med 9:428-454, 1954b

Riese W: Claude Bernard in the light of modern science. Bull Hist Med 14:281-294, 1943

Riese W: The Legacy of Phillipe Pinel: An Inquiry into Thought on Mental Alienation. New York, Springer Publishing Company, 1969

Riesman D: The Dublin Medical School and its influence upon medicine in America. Ann Med Hist 4:86-96, 1922

Risse GB: The quest for certainty in medicine: John Brown's system of medicine in France. Bull Hist Med 45:1-12, 1971

Risse GB: The Brownian system of medicine: Its theoretical and practical implications. Clio Med 5:45-51, 1970

Risse GB: Kant, Schelling, and the early search for a philosophical 'science' of medicine in Germany. J Hist Med 27:145-158, 1972

Risse GB: Doctor William Cullen, Physician, Edinburgh. A consultation practice in the eighteenth century. Bull Hist Med 48:338-351, 1974

Risse GB: Schelling "Naturphilosophie" and John Brown's system of medicine. Bull Hist Med 50:321-334, 1976

Roddis LH: James Lind, Founder of Nautical Medicine. New York, Henry Schuman, 1950

Rodin AE: The Influence of Matthew Baillie's Morbid Anatomy: Biography, Evaluation and Reprint. Springfield IL, CC Thomas, 1973

Rolleston HD: Medicine and medical schools in America. Brit Med J 2:1845-1846, 1907

Rommanell P: Locke and Sydenham: A fragment on smallpox (1670). Bull Hist Med 32:293-321, 1958

Rook A: Medicine at Cambridge (1660-1760). Med Hist 13:107-122, 1969a

Rook A: Robert Glynn (1719-1800), physician at Cambridge. Med Hist 13:251-259, 1969b

Rosen G: John Eliotson, physician and hypnotist. Bull Inst Hist Med 4:600-603, 1936a

Rosen G: Carl Ludwig and his American students. Bull Inst Hist Med 4:609-650, 1936b

Rosen G: The medical aspects of the controversy over factory conditions in New England, 1840-1850. Bull Hist Med 15:483-497, 1944

Rosen G: The philosophy of ideology and the emergence of modern medicine in France. Bull Hist Med 20:328-339, 1946

Rosen G: Some recent European publications dealing with Paracelsus. J Hist Med 2:537-548, 1947

Rosen G: Romantic medicine: A problems in historical periodization. Bull Hist Med 25:149-158, 1951

Rosen G: Problems in the application of statistical analysis to questions of health. Bull Hist Med 29:27-45, 1955

Rosen G: A History of Public Health. New York, MD Publications, 1958

Rosen G: Mercantilism and health policy in eighteenth-century French thought. Med Hist 3:259-277, 1959

Rosen G: Patterns of health research in the United States, 1900-1960. Bull Hist Med 39:201-221, 1965

Rosen G: Christian Fenger, medical immigrant. Bull Hist Med 48:129-145, 1974

Rosenberg JC: Friendships between Viennese physicans and musicians. Bull Hist Med 32:366-369, 1958

Rosenblatt MB: Emphysema in the nineteenth century. Bull Hist Med 43:533-552, 1969

Rothschuh KE: Was ist Krankheit? Erscheinung, Erklarung, Singebung. Darmstadt, Wissenschaftliche Buchgessellschaft, 1975

Rousseau A: Une révolution dans la sémiologie médicale, le concept de spécificité lesionelle. Clio Med 5:123-131, 1970

Rousseau A: Gaspard-Laurent Bayle (1774-1816). Le Théoricien de l'Ecole de Paris. Clio Med 6:205-211, 1971

Roux PJ: Relations d'un Voyage Fait a Londres en 1814. Paris, Chez l'Auteur, 1815

- S -

Saunders JB de CM, O'Malley CD: The Illustrations from the Works of Andreas Vesalius of Brussels. Cleveland, World Publishing Company, 1950

Schiller F: Concepts of stroke before and after Virchow. Med Hist 14:115-131, 1970

Schiller J: Claude Bernard and Brown Séquard. The chair of general physiology and the experimental method. J Hist Med 21:260-270, 1966

Schiller J: Claude Bernard et les Problèmes Scientifiques de son Temps. Paris, Editions du Cedre, 1967

Schipperges H: Utopien der Medizin. Gesichte and Kritik der ärtzlichen Ideologie des 19 Jahrunderts. Salzburg, Otto Muller Verlag, 1968

Schöer H: Carl Ludwig, Begrunder der messenden Experimentalphysiologie. Stuttgart, Wessenschaftliche Verlags Gessellschaft, 1967

Schofield RE: Mechanism and Materialism: British Natural Philosophy in an Age of Reason. Princeton, Princeton University Press, 1970

Schott A: An early account of blood pressure measurement by Joseph Struthius (1510-1568). Med Hist 21:205-309, 1977

Schullian DM: On the origin of the phrase *Nihil est in intellect quod non prius fuerit in sensu.* J Hist Med 25:77-80, 1970

Schwab RN: The history of medicine in Diderot's Encyclopédie. Bull Hist Med 32:216-223, 1958

Scudamore C: Observations on M. Laennec's Method of Forming a Diagnosis of Diseases of the Chest by Means of the Stethoscope, and of Percussion. London, (for the author), 1826

Selwyn S: Sir James Simpson and hospital cross-infection. Med Hist 9:241-248, 1965

Selwyn S: Sir John Pringle: Hospital reformer, moral philosopher and pioneer of antiseptics. Med Hist 10:266 -274, 1966

Shapiro RW: James Currie - The physican and the quest. Med Hist 7:212-231, 1963

Shipley NR: Thomas Sutton, Tudor-Stuart Moneylender and Philanthropist. PhD dissertation. Boston, Harvard University, 1967

Shryock H: Nineteenth-century medicine: Scientific aspects. Cahiers d'Histoire Mondiale 3:881-908, 1957

Shryock RN: Germ theories in medicine prior to 1870: Further comments on continuity in science. Clio Med 7:81-109, 1972

Sigerist HE: The People's Misery: Mother of Diseases, an address delivered in 1790 by Johann Peter Frank. Bull Hist Med 9:81-100, 1941

Sigerist HE, Longcope WT: Maurice Arthus' philosophy of scientific investigation. Preface to De l'Anaphylaxie à l'Immunité, Paris 1921. Bull Hist Med 14:366-390, 1943

Singer C, Holloway SWF: Early medical education in England in relation to the pre-history of London University. Med Hist 4:1-17, 1960

Smeaton WA: Fourcroy, Chemist and Revolutionary, 1755-1809. Cambridge, England (for the author), 1962

Smith DC: The Emergence of Organized Clinical Instruction in the Nineteenth Century Cities of Boston, New York and Philadelphia. University of Minnesota Thesis, 1979

Snapper I: Meditations on Medicine and Medical Education, Past and Present. New York, Grune Stratton, 1956

Snell WE: Captain Cook's surgeons. Med Hist 7:43-55, 1963

Spriggs EA: John Hutchinson, the inventor of the spirometer - his North Country background, life in London, and scientific achievements. Med Hist 21:357-364, 1971

Stannard J: Materia medica in the Lock-Clarke correspondence. Bull Hist Med 37:201-225, 1963

Stern ES: Dr. Hodgin's relationship with his distinguished friend and patient, Sir Moses Montefiore, Bt, FRS. Med Hist 11:182-185, 1967

Stevenson LG: William Harvey and the facts of the case. J Hist Med 31:90-97, 1976

Stillé A: Medical Education in the United States. Philadelphia, Isaac Ashmead, 1846

Stillé A: Introductory Lecture of the One Hundred and Ninth Session of the Medical Department of the University of Pennsylvania. Philadelphia (by the class), 1874

Stokes W: Introduction to the Use of the Stethoscope. Edinburgh, Maclachlan & Stewart, 1825

Stolinski C: John Hunter: Pioneer of freeze-fracture. Med Hist 19:303-306, 1975

Stookey B: Samuel Clossy, AB, MD, FRCP of Ireland. First Professor of Anatomy, King's College (Columbia), New York. Bull Hist Med 38:153-167, 1964

- T -

Taylor DW: The life and teaching of William Sharpey (1802-1880) "Father of modern physiology in Britain." Med Hist 15:126-153, 241-259, 1971

Temkin O: The philosophical background of Magendie's physiology. Bull Hist Med 20:10-35, 1946a

Temkin O: Materialism in French and German physiology of the early nineteenth century. Bull Hist Med 20:322-327, 1946b

Temkin O: Medicine in 1847 - Continental Europe. Bull Hist Med 21:469-486, 1947

Temkin O: The European background of the young Dr. Welch. Bull Hist Med 24:308-318, 1950

Temkin O: Basic science, medicine, and the romantic era. Bull Hist Med 37:97-129, 1963

Temkin O: Galenism: Rise and Decline of a Medical Philosophy. Ithaca Cornell University Press, 1973

Thomas HQ: The old Poor Law and Medicine. Med Hist 24:1-19, 1980

Thomas KB: John Hunter and an amputation under analgesia in 1784. Med Hist 2:53-56, 1958

Thorwald J: The Dismissal. The Last Days of Ferdinand Sauerbruch (Winston R, Winston C [trans]). New York, Pantheon Books, 1961

Tickner FJ, Medvei VC: Scurvy and the health of European crews in the Indian Ocean in the seventeenth century. Med Hist 2:36-46, 1958

Trail RR: Sydenham's impact on English medicine. Med Hist 9:356-364, 1965

Triolo VA: The Institution for Investigating the Nature and Cure of Cancer. A Study of Four Excerpts. Med Hist 13:11-28, 1969

Trolle D: The development of our knowledge of foetal heart activity: With special reference to Denmark. Clio Med 10:111-128, 1975

- U -

Underwood EA: Boerhaave's Men at Leyden and After. Edinburgh, Edinburgh University Press, 1977

- V -

Valadez FM, O'Malley CD: James Keil of Northampton, physician anatomist, and physiologist. Med Hist 15:317-335, 1971

Van Bibber JR: The Future Influence of the Johns Hopkins Hospital on the Medical Profession of Baltimore. Baltimore, Innes & Company, 1879

Verso ML: Some notes on a contemporary review of early French hematology. Med Hist 5:239-252, 1961

Verso ML: The evolution of blood-counting techniques. Med Hist 8:149-158, 1964

Verso ML: Some nineteenth-century pioneers of haematology. Med Hist 15:55-67, 1971

Vess DM: Medical Revolution in France 1789-1796. Gainesville, FL, University of Florida Press, 1975

von Behring EA: Gesammelte Abhandlungen zur Atiologischen Therapie von Ansteckenden Krankheiten. Leipzig, Thieme, 1893

von Brunn WAL: Medizinische Zeitschriften im neunzehnten Jahrhundert. Stuttgart, George Thieme Verlag, 1963

von Engehardt D: Hegel und die Chemie. Weisbaden, Guido Dressler Verlag, 1976

von Harnack A: History of Dogma, 3rd German ed, p 140 (Buchanan N [trans]). New York, Dover, 1961

- W -

Waldron HA: James Hardy and the Devonshire colic. Med Hist 13"74-81, 1969

Walls EW: John Bell, 1763-1820. Med Hist 8:63-69, 1964

Watermann R: Theodor Schwann. Leben und Werk. Dusseldorf L: Schwann Verlag, 1960

Webster C: The Great Instauration: Science, Medicine and Reform, 1626-1660. London, Duckworth, 1976

Weiner DB: Le droite de l'homme à la santé - une belle idée devant l'Assemblée Constituante: 1790-1791. Clio Med 5:209-223, 1970

Weiss S: Clinical medicine as a university discipline. Harvard Med Alum Bull 10:37-42, 1946

Welch WH: Some of the advantages of the union of medical school and university. N Engl Yale Rev 13:145-163, 1888

Welch WH: The interdependence of medicine and other sciences of nature. Science 27:49-64, 1908

Welch WH: Address by William H Welch on the history of pathology. Bull Inst Hist Med 3:1-18, 1935

Westerbrink HGK: Biochemistry in Holland. Clio Med 1:153-158, 1966

Wetherill JH: The York Medical School. Med Hist 5:253-269, 1961

Wiggers CJ: Some significant advances in cardiac physiology during the nineteenth century. Bull Hist Med 34:1-15, 1960

Wightman WPD: The Emergence of Scientific Medicine. Edinburgh, Oliver & Wood, 1971

William TF: Cabot, Peabody and the care of the patient. Bull Hist Med 24:462-481, 1950

Willis T: The Anatomy of the Brain and Nerves (Feindel W [ed]). Montreal, McGill University Press, 1965

Wilson JW: Cellular tissue and the dawn of the cell theory. Isis 35:168-173, 1944

Wilson JW: Virchow's contribution to the cell theory. J Hist Med 2:163-178, 1947

Winslow CEA: A physician of two centuries ago: Richard Mead and his contributions to epidemiology. Bull Inst Hist Med 3:509-544, 1935

Wolfe DE: Sydenham and Locke on the limits of anatomy. Bull Hist Med 35:193-220, 1961

Woods EA, Carlson ET: The psychiatry of Philippe Pinel. Bull Hist Med 35:14-25, 1961

Wright-St. Clair RE: Doctors Monro: A Medical Saga. London, Wellcome Historical Monographs, 1964

Wyatt HV: James Lind and the prevention of scurvy. Med Hist 20:433-438, 1976

- Y -

Yandell DN: Address Before the American Medical Association. Louisville, JP Morton & Company, 1872

Young FG: Rise of Biochemistry Between 1800 and 1900. In Poynter FNL (ed): Chemistry in the Service of Medicine. London, Pitman Medical Publishing Company, 1963

Young JH: James Hamilton (1767-1839), obstetrician and controversialist. Med Hist 7:62-73, 1963

- Z -

Zakon SJ, Benedek T: David Gruby and the centenary of medical mycology. 1841-1941. Bull Hist Med 16:155-168, 1944

Zimmerman LM: Surgeons and the rise of clinical teaching in England. Bull Hist Med 37:167-178, 1963

Zuppinger H: Albert Kölliker (1817-1905) und die mikroskopische Anatomie. Zurich, Juris-Druck, 1974